THE NETTER COLLECTION
of Medical Illustrations
2nd Edition

Reproductive System
Endocrine System
Respiratory System
Urinary System
Integumentary System
Musculoskeletal System
Digestive System
Nervous System
Circulatory System

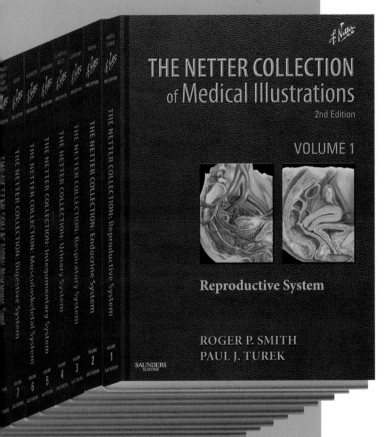

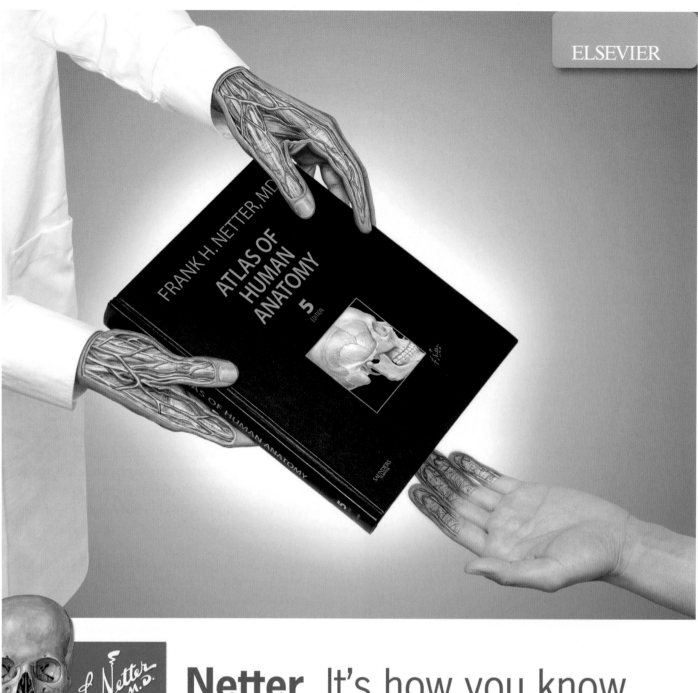

VOLUME 2

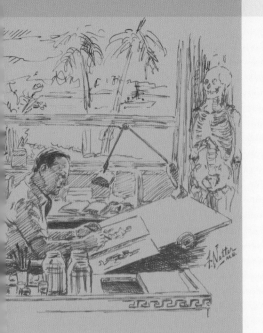

The Netter Collection
OF MEDICAL ILLUSTRATIONS:
Endocrine System

Second Edition

William F. Young, Jr., MD, MSc
Professor of Medicine, Mayo Clinic College of Medicine
Division of Endocrinology, Diabetes, Metabolism, and Nutrition
Mayo Clinic
Rochester, Minnesota

Illustrations by
Frank H. Netter, MD, and Carlos A. G. Machado, MD

CONTRIBUTING ILLUSTRATORS
James A. Perkins, MS, MFA
John A. Craig, MD
Kristen Wienandt Marzejon, MS, MFA

ELSEVIER
SAUNDERS

1600 John F. Kennedy Blvd.
Ste 1800
Philadelphia, PA 19103-2899

THE NETTER COLLECTION OF MEDICAL ILLUSTRATIONS: ISBN: 978-1-4160-6388-9
ENDOCRINE SYSTEM, Volume 2, Second Edition

ISBN: **978-1-4160-6388-9**

Acquisitions Editor: Elyse O'Grady
Developmental Editor: Marybeth Thiel
Editorial Assistant: Chris Hazle-Cary
Publishing Services Manager: Patricia Tannian
Senior Project Manager: John Casey
Designer: Lou Forgione

Printed in China
Last digit is the print number: 9 8 7 6 5 4 3 2 1

Dr. Frank H. Netter exemplified the distinct vocations of doctor, artist, and teacher. Even more important, he unified them. Netter's illustrations always began with meticulous research into the forms of the body, a philosophy that steered his broad and deep medical understanding. He often said, "Clarification is the goal. No matter how beautifully it is painted, a medical illustration has little value if it does not make clear a medical point." His greatest challenge—and greatest success—was chartering a middle course between artistic clarity and instructional complexity. That success is captured in this series, beginning in 1948, when the first comprehensive collection of Netter's work, a single volume, was published by CIBA Pharmaceuticals. It met with such success that over the following 40 years the collection was expanded into an eight-volume series—each devoted to a single body system.

In this second edition of the legendary series, we are delighted to offer Netter's timeless work, now arranged and informed by modern text and radiologic imaging contributed by field-leading doctors and teachers from world-renowned medical institutions and supplemented with new illustrations created by artists working in the Netter tradition. Inside the classic green covers, students and practitioners will find hundreds of original works of art—the human body in pictures—paired with the latest in expert medical knowledge and innovation, and anchored in the sublime style of Frank Netter.

Dr. Carlos Machado was chosen by Novartis to be Dr. Netter's successor. He continues to be the primary artist contributing to the Netter family of products. Dr. Machado says, "For 16 years, in my updating of the illustrations in the *Netter Atlas of Human Anatomy*, as well as many other Netter publications, I have faced the challenging mission of continuing Dr. Netter's legacy, of following and understanding his concepts, and of reproducing his style by using his favorite techniques."

Although the science and teaching of medicine endures changes in terminology, practice, and discovery, some things remain the same. A patient is a patient. A teacher is a teacher. And the pictures of Dr. Netter—he called them pictures, never paintings—remain the same blend of beautiful and instructional resources that have guided physicians' hands and nurtured their imaginations for over half a century.

The original series could not exist without the dedication of all those who edited, authored, or in other ways contributed, nor, of course, without the excellence of Dr. Netter, who is fondly remembered by all who knew him. For this exciting second edition, we also owe our gratitude to the authors, editors, advisors, and artists whose relentless efforts were instrumental in adapting these timeless works into reliable references for today's clinicians in training and in practice. From all of us at Elsevier, we thank you.

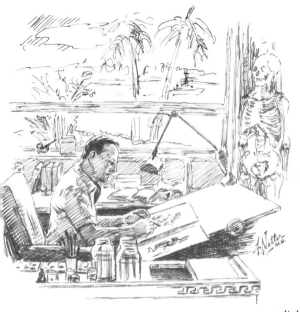

Dr. Frank Netter at work

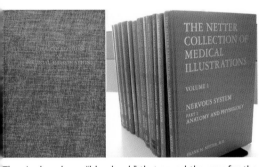

The single-volume "blue book" that paved the way for the multivolume *Netter Collection of Medical Illustrations* series, affectionately known as the "green books."

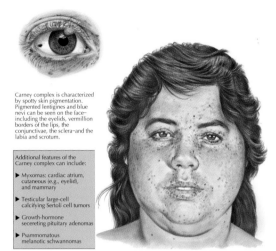

CUSHING'S SYNDROME IN A PATIENT WITH THE CARNEY COMPLEX

Carney complex is characterized by spotty skin pigmentation. Pigmented lentigines and blue nevi can be seen on the face–including the eyelids, vermillion borders of the lips, the conjunctivae, the sclera–and the labia and scrotum.

Additional features of the Carney complex can include:

▶ Myxomas; cardiac atrium, cutaneous (e.g., eyelid), and mammary

▶ Testicular large-cell calcifying Sertoli cell tumors

▶ Growth-hormone secreting pituitary adenomas

▶ Psammomatous melanotic schwannomas

PPNAD adrenal glands are usually of normal size and most are studded with black, brown, or red nodules. Most of the pigmented nodules are less than 4 mm in diameter and interspersed in the adjacent atrophic cortex.

A brand new illustrated plate painted by Carlos Machado, MD, for *The Endocrine System*, Volume 2, ed. 2

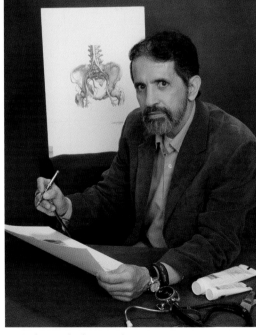

Dr. Carlos Machado at work

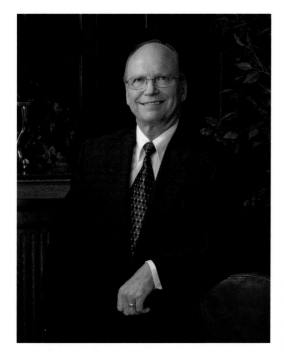

William F. Young, Jr, MD, MSc, is Professor of Medicine at Mayo Clinic College of Medicine, Mayo Clinic, Rochester, Minnesota, USA. He holds the Tyson Family Endocrinology Clinical Professorship in Honor of Vahab Fatourechi, MD. He received his bachelor degree and his medical degree from Michigan State University and his master of science degree from the University of Minnesota. Dr. Young trained in internal medicine at William Beaumont Hospital in Royal Oak, Michigan, and completed a fellowship in endocrinology and metabolism at Mayo Clinic in Rochester, Minnesota. He has been a member of the staff at Mayo Clinic since 1984. Dr. Young is the recipient of multiple education awards including the Mayo Fellows Association Teacher of the Year Award in Internal Medicine, the Mayo Clinic Endocrinology Teacher of the Year Award, the Mayo School of Continuing Medical Education Outstanding Faculty Member Award, and the H. Jack Baskin, MD, Endocrine Teaching Award from the American Association of Clinical Endocrinologists in recognition of his profound impact in teaching fellows in training. Professional honors include being a recipient of the Distinguished Mayo Clinician Award, the Distinction in Clinical Endocrinology Award from the American College of Endocrinology, and the Distinguished Physician Award from the Endocrine Society. Dr. Young's clinical research focuses on primary aldosteronism and pheochromocytoma. He has published more than 200 articles on endocrine hypertension and adrenal and pituitary disorders. Dr. Young has presented at more than 300 national and international meetings and has been an invited visiting professor at more than 100 medical institutions.

The second edition of the Endocrine System volume of the Netter Collection is designed to provide physicians at all stages of training and practice with a visual guide to the anatomy, physiology, and pathophysiology of the endocrine glands. The first edition was published in 1965. In the intervening 5 decades, there have been remarkable developments in our understanding of endocrine disorders. The text has been entirely rewritten, but most of the anatomic and clinical artwork of Frank H. Netter, MD, has stood the test of time. Since new endocrine disorders and treatment approaches have been recognized over the past 50 years, new artwork has been added in every section, including the following: current surgical approaches to remove pituitary tumors, tests used in the diagnosis of Cushing syndrome, adrenal venous sampling for primary aldosteronism, Cushing syndrome caused by primary pigmented nodular adrenocortical disease, treatment of type 1 and type 2 diabetes mellitus, multiple endocrine neoplasia types 1 and 2, and von Hippel–Lindau syndrome. Carlos Machado, MD, James A. Perkins, MS, MFA, Kristen Wienandt Marzejon, MS, MFA, and John Craig, MD, have contributed outstanding new plates to this edition, as well as adapted and updated existing artwork. The accompanying text serves to illuminate and expand on the concepts demonstrated in the images.

The book is organized in 8 sections, which correspond to the glands and components of the endocrine system: pituitary and hypothalamus, thyroid, adrenal, reproduction, pancreas, bone and calcium, lipids and nutrition, and genetics and endocrine neoplasia. In some cases, the Netter drawings are supplemented with modern diagnostic images (e.g., computed tomography and magnetic resonance imaging). The original Netter edition and the new illustrations focus on embryology, gross anatomy, histology, physiology, pathology, clinical manifestations of disease, diagnostic modalities, and surgical and therapeutic techniques.

Writing an "update" that spans 5 decades has been a daunting challenge. However, this new edition will serve to preserve and provide context for the original Netter illustrations well into the twenty-first century. This work is not a complete textbook of endocrinology, but rather it is a visual tour of the highlights of this medical discipline. I hope readers find the artwork and accompanying text useful guides as they navigate the world of endocrinology.

I gratefully acknowledge my colleagues and patients at Mayo Clinic who have provided me with the clinical experience, perspective, and insights to address the broad field of endocrinology. The editorial and production staffs at Elsevier have been very supportive at every step from initial general concepts to final publication. I am indebted to the incredible second generation of Netter artists. I also want to thank my daughter, Abbie L. Abboud, MS, CGC, ELS, for her invaluable help in medical editing and providing guidance on clarity of thought and concept. Finally, I dedicate this book to my family—their encouragement and support have been inspirational during the 2 years it took to produce the second edition of the *Endocrine System* volume of the Netter Collection.

William F. Young, Jr., MD, MSc
Rochester, Minnesota
November 2010

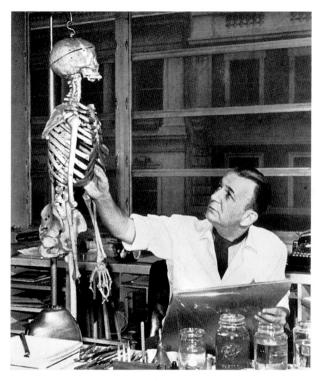

$\mathbf{M}$any readers of the CIBA COLLECTION have expressed a desire to know more about Dr. Netter. In response to these requests this summary of Dr. Netter's career has been prepared.

Frank Henry Netter, born in 1906 in Brooklyn, New York, received his M.D. degree from New York University in 1931. To help pay his way through medical school and internship at Bellevue, he worked as a commercial artist and as an illustrator of medical books and articles for his professors and other physicians, perfecting his natural talent by studying at the National Academy of Design and attending courses at the Art Students' League.

In 1933 Dr. Netter entered the private practice of surgery in New York City. But it was the depth of the Depression, and the recently married physician continued to accept art assignments to supplement his income. Soon he was spending more and more time at the drawing board and finally, realizing that his career lay in medical illustration, he decided to give up practicing and become a full-time artist.

Soon, Dr. Netter was receiving requests to develop many unusual projects. One of the most arduous of these was building the "transparent woman" for the San Francisco Golden Gate Exposition. This 7-foot-high transparent figure depicted the menstrual process, the development and birth of a baby, and the physical and sexual development of a woman, while a synchronized voice told the story of the female endocrine system. Dr. Netter labored on this project night and day for 7 months. Another interesting assignment involved a series of paintings of incidents in the life of a physician.

Among others, the pictures showed a medical student sitting up the night before the osteology examination, studying away to the point of exhaustion; an emergency ward; an ambulance call; a class reunion; and a night call made by a country doctor.

During World War II, Dr. Netter was an officer in the Army, stationed first at the Army Institute of Pathology, later at the Surgeon General's Office, in charge of graphic training aids for the Medical Department. Numerous manuals were produced under his direction, among them first aid for combat troops, roentgenology for technicians, sanitation in the field, and survival in the tropics.

After the war, Dr. Netter began work on several major projects for CIBA Pharmaceutical Company, culminating in THE CIBA COLLECTION OF MEDICAL ILLUSTRATIONS. To date, five volumes have been published and work is in progress on the sixth, dealing with the urinary tract.

Dr. Netter goes about planning and executing his illustrations in a very exacting way. First comes the study, unquestionably the most important and most difficult part of the entire undertaking. No drawing is ever started until Dr. Netter has acquired a complete understanding of the subject matter, either through reading or by consultation with leading authorities in the field. Often he visits hospitals to observe clinical cases, pathologic or surgical specimens, or operative procedures. Sometimes an original dissection is necessary.

When all his questions have been answered and the problem is thoroughly understood, Dr. Netter makes a pencil sketch on a tissue or tracing pad. Always, the subject must be visualized from the standpoint of the physician; is it to be viewed from above or below, from the side, the rear, or the front? What area is to be covered, the entire body or just certain segments? What plane provides the clearest understanding? In some pictures two, three, or four planes of dissection may be necessary.

When the sketch is at last satisfactory, Dr. Netter transfers it to a piece of illustration board for the finished drawing. This is done by blocking the back of the picture with a soft pencil, taping the tissue down on the board with Scotch tape, then going over the lines with a hard pencil. Over the years, our physician-artist has used many media to finish his illustrations, but now he works almost exclusively in transparent water colors mixed with white paint.

In spite of the tremendously productive life Dr. Netter has led, he has been able to enjoy his family, first in a handsome country home in East Norwich, Long Island, and, after the five children had grown up, in a penthouse overlooking the East River in Manhattan.

ALFRED W. CUSTER

In the early days the endocrine glands were looked upon as an isolated group of structures, secreting substances which, in some strange way, influenced the human organism. The thyroid gland was known to be an organ of considerable significance. The clinical syndromes of hyper- and hypothyroidism and the therapeutic effects of thyroid administration and thyroidectomy were recognized. Insulin had become available, and its use in controlling diabetes was being explored. It was known generally that the pituitary gland exerted some influence over the growth and sex life of mankind. Nonetheless, the endocrine glands were still considered as a system apart, secreting mysterious and potent substances. In the light of modern knowledge, however, this is not an isolated system at all but, rather, an essential and controlling mechanism of all the other systems; indeed, together with the nervous system, the integrator of biochemistry and physiology in the living organism.

Thus, although this volume was originally planned as an atlas on the endocrine glands, it was impossible to execute it intelligently without becoming involved in such basic and related subjects as carbohydrate, protein, and fat metabolism; the major vitamins; enzyme chemistry; genetics; and inborn metabolic errors. As a matter of fact, as I now survey the entire subject, it seems to me that the growth of our understanding of the function of the endocrine glands has come about as much or more from the study of the basic physiology of the glandular secretions as from study of the morphological effects of the endocrine system itself. I have also been tremendously impressed and awed by the painstaking,

patient, and unrelenting work of the men and women who have, bit by bit, unraveled and correlated the mysteries of these various fields. It has been my great pleasure, in creating this volume, to have worked with some of these pioneers or with their disciples. No words of appreciation for the help and encouragement I received from all my collaborators can completely convey the satisfaction I obtained from getting to know each of them and becoming their friend.

In finding my way through the uncharted space of the endocrine universe, I sorely needed a guide—one who could plot a course among the biochemical constellations, yet at all times would know his way back to earthly clinical considerations. Such a one I found in Dr. Peter H. Forsham, who took over the editorship of this volume upon the death of Dr. Ernst Oppenheimer, about whom I have written in the preceding pages. I shall always cherish the stimulating hours Dr. Forsham and I spent together in work and, occasionally, in play.

A creative effort such as that which this volume has demanded absorbs a great deal of one's time, effort, and dreams. In short, it tends to detach the artist from his surroundings and personal relationships and to make him difficult to live with! For these reasons I must express special appreciation to my wife, Vera, for patiently bearing with me through these tribulations. She always managed to return me to reality when I became too detached, bring a smile to my face when I was distressed, and help me in so many other ways during this challenging but rather awesome assignment.

FRANK H. NETTER, M.D.

ADVISORY BOARD

Plate 1-1   Pituitary and Hypothalamus

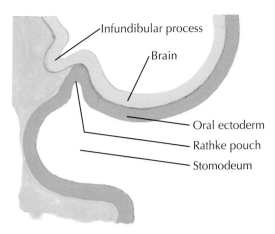

1. Beginning formation of Rathke pouch and infundibular process

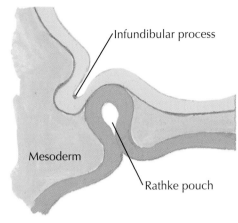

2. Neck of Rathke pouch constricted by growth of mesoderm

DEVELOPMENT OF THE PITUITARY GLAND

The pituitary gland, also termed the *hypophysis*, consists of two major components, the adenohypophysis and the neurohypophysis. The adenohypophysis (anterior lobe) is derived from the oral ectoderm, and the neurohypophysis (posterior lobe) is derived from the neural ectoderm of the floor of the forebrain.

A pouchlike recess—Rathke pouch—in the ectodermal lining of the roof of the stomodeum is formed by the fourth to fifth week of gestation and gives rise to the anterior pituitary gland. Rathke pouch extends upward to contact the undersurface of the forebrain and is then constricted by the surrounding mesoderm to form a closed cavity. The original connection between Rathke pouch and the stomodeum—known as the craniopharyngeal canal—runs from the anterior part of the pituitary fossa to the undersurface of the skull. Although it is usually obliterated, a remnant may persist in adult life as a "pharyngeal pituitary" embedded in the mucosa on the dorsal wall of the pharynx. The pharyngeal pituitary may give rise to ectopic hormone-secreting pituitary adenomas later in life.

Behind Rathke pouch, a hollow neural outgrowth extends toward the mouth from the floor of the third ventricle. This neural process forms a funnel-shaped sac—the infundibular process—that becomes a solid structure, except at the upper end where the cavity persists as the infundibular recess of the third ventricle. As Rathke pouch extends toward the third ventricle, it fuses on each side of the infundibular process and subsequently obliterates its lumen, which sometimes persists as Rathke cleft. The anterior lobe of the pituitary is formed from Rathke pouch, and the infundibular process gives rise to the adjacent posterior lobe (neurohypophysis). The neurohypophysis consists of the axons and nerve endings of neurons whose cell bodies reside in the supraoptic and paraventricular nuclei of the hypothalamus, forming a hypothalamic–neurohypophysial nerve tract that contains approximately 100,000 nerve fibers. Remnants of Rathke pouch may persist at the boundary of the neurohypophysis, resulting in small colloid cysts.

The anterior lobe also gives off two processes from its ventral wall that extend along the infundibulum as the pars tuberalis, which fuses to surround the upper end of the pituitary stalk. The cleft is the remains of the original cavity of the stomodeal diverticulum. The dorsal (posterior) wall of the cleft remains thin and fuses with the adjoining posterior lobe to form the pars intermedia. The pars intermedia remains intact in some species, but in humans, its cells become interspersed

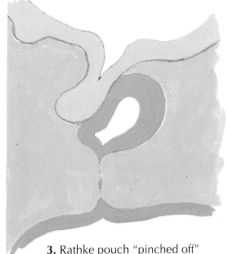

3. Rathke pouch "pinched off"

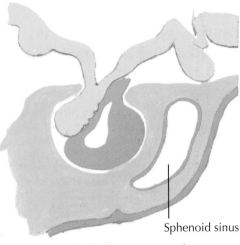

4. "Pinched off" segment conforms to neural process, forming pars distalis, pars intermedia, and pars tuberalis

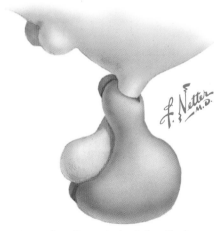

5. Pars tuberalis encircles infundibular stalk (lateral surface view)

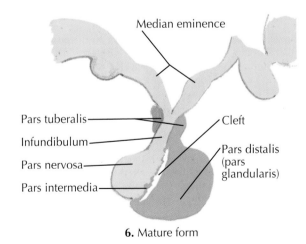

6. Mature form

with those of the anterior lobe, and it develops the capacity to synthesize and secrete pro-opiomelanocortin (POMC) and corticotropin (adrenocorticotropic hormone [ACTH]). The part of the tuber cinereum that lies immediately above the pars tuberalis is termed the *median eminence*.

Both the adenohypophysis and the neurohypophysis are subdivided into three parts. The adenohypophysis consists of the pars tuberalis, a thin strip of tissue that

surrounds the median eminence and the upper part of the neural stalk; the pars intermedia, the portion posterior to the cleft and in contact with the neurohypophysis; and the pars distalis (pars glandularis), the major secretory part of the gland. The neurohypophysis is composed of an expanded distal portion termed the *infundibular process*; the infundibular stem (neural stalk); and the expanded upper end of the stalk, the median eminence of the tuber cinereum.

Plate 1-2

Endocrine System

DIVISIONS OF THE PITUITARY GLAND AND RELATIONSHIP TO THE HYPOTHALAMUS

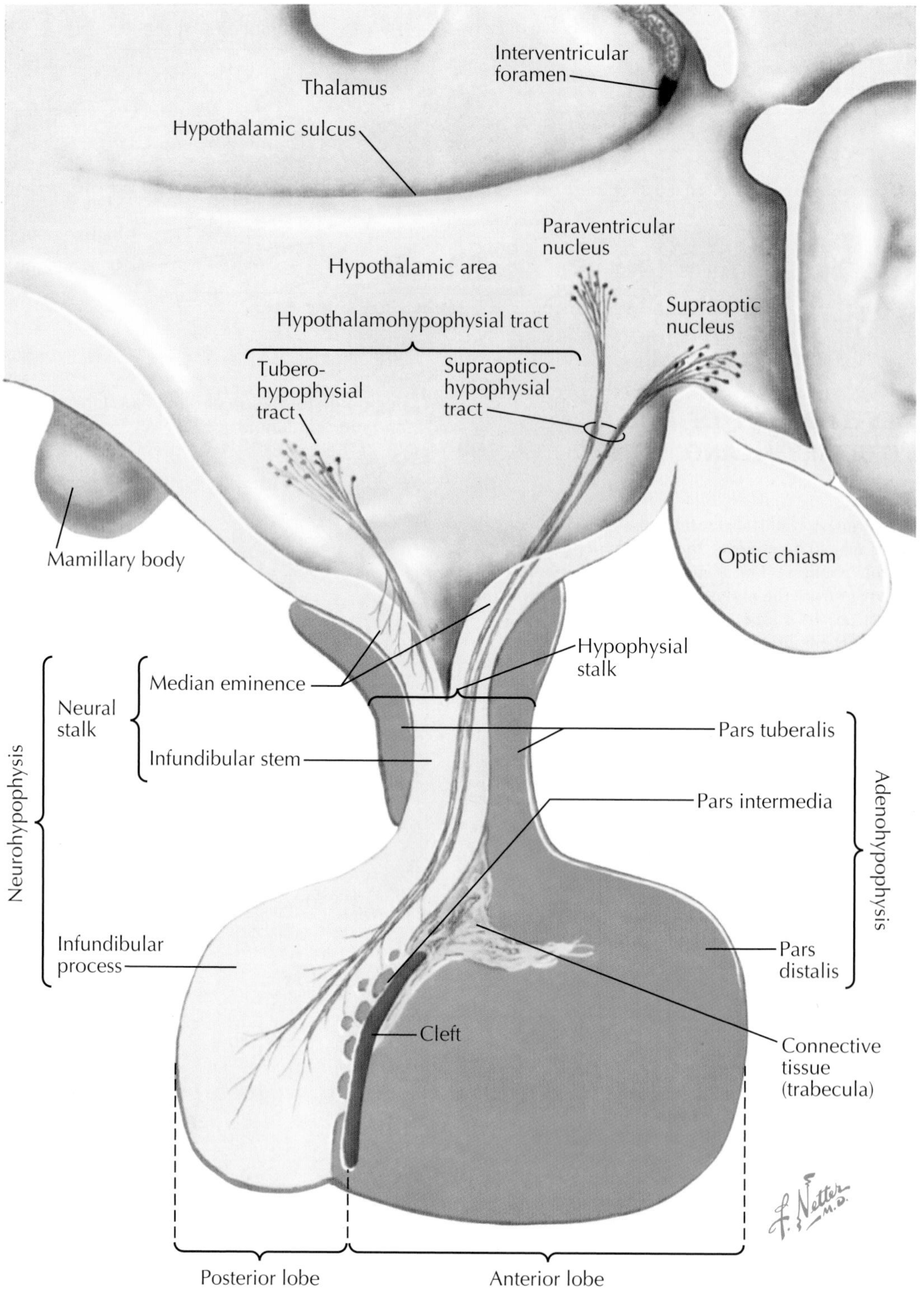

The pituitary gland (hypophysis) is composed of the neurohypophysis (posterior pituitary lobe) and adenohypophysis (anterior pituitary lobe). The neurohypophysis consists of three parts: the median eminence of the tuber cinereum, infundibular stem, and infundibular process (neural lobe). The adenohypophysis is likewise divided into three parts: the pars tuberalis, pars intermedia, and pars distalis (glandularis). The infundibular stem, together with portions of the adenohypophysis that form a sheath around it, is designated as the hypophysial (pituitary) stalk. The extension of neurohypophysial tissue up the stalk and into the median eminence of the tuber cinereum constitutes approximately 15% of the neurohypophysis. A low stalk section may leave enough of the gland still in contact with its higher connections in the paraventricular and supraoptic nuclei to prevent the onset of diabetes insipidus. Atrophy and disappearance of cell bodies in the supraoptic and paraventricular nuclei follow damage to their axons in the supraopticohypophysial tract. If the tract is cut at the level of the diaphragma sellae, only 70% of these cells are affected; if the tract is severed above the median eminence, about 85% of the cells will atrophy. Thus, approximately 15% of the axons terminate between these levels.

The main nerve supply, both functionally and anatomically, of the neurohypophysis is the hypothalamohypophysial tract in the pituitary stalk. It consists of two main parts: the supraopticohypophysial tract, running in the anterior or ventral wall of the stalk, and the tuberohypophysial tract in the posterior, or dorsal, wall of the stalk. The tuberohypophysial tract originates in the central and posterior parts of the hypothalamus from the paraventricular nucleus and from scattered cells and nuclei in the tuberal region and mamillary bodies. The supraopticohypophysial tract arises from the supraoptic and paraventricular nuclei. On entering the median eminence, it occupies a very superficial position, where it is liable to be affected by basal infections of the brain and granulomatous inflammatory processes. The tuberohypophysial tract in the dorsal region of the median eminence is smaller and consists of finer fibers. In the neural stalk, all the fibers congregate into a dense bundle lying in a central position,

leaving a peripheral zone in contact with the pars tuberalis, which is relatively free of nerve elements. The hypothalamohypophysial tract terminates mainly in the neurohypophysis.

The hypothalamus has ill-defined boundaries. Anteroinferiorly, it is limited by the optic chiasm and optic tracts; passing posteriorly, it is bounded by the posterior perforated substance and the cerebral peduncles. On sagittal section, it can be seen to be separated from the thalamus by the hypothalamic sulcus on the wall of the third ventricle. Anteriorly, it merges with the preoptic septal region, and posteriorly, it merges with the tegmental area of the midbrain. Its lateral relations are the subthalamus and the internal capsule.

A connective tissue trabecula separates the posterior and anterior lobes of the pituitary; it also extends out into the anterior pituitary lobe for a variable distance as a vascular bed for the large-lumened artery of the trabecula. The embryonic cleft, which marks the site of the Rathke pouch within the gland, may be contained, in part, in this trabecula. It is easier to see in newborns and tends to disappear in later life. Colloid-filled follicles in the adult gland mark the site of the pars intermedia at the junction between the pars distalis and the neurohypophysis. This boundary may be quite irregular because fingerlike projections of adenohypophysial tissue are frequently found in the substance of the neurohypophysis.

Plate 1-3

Pituitary and Hypothalamus

BLOOD SUPPLY OF THE PITUITARY GLAND

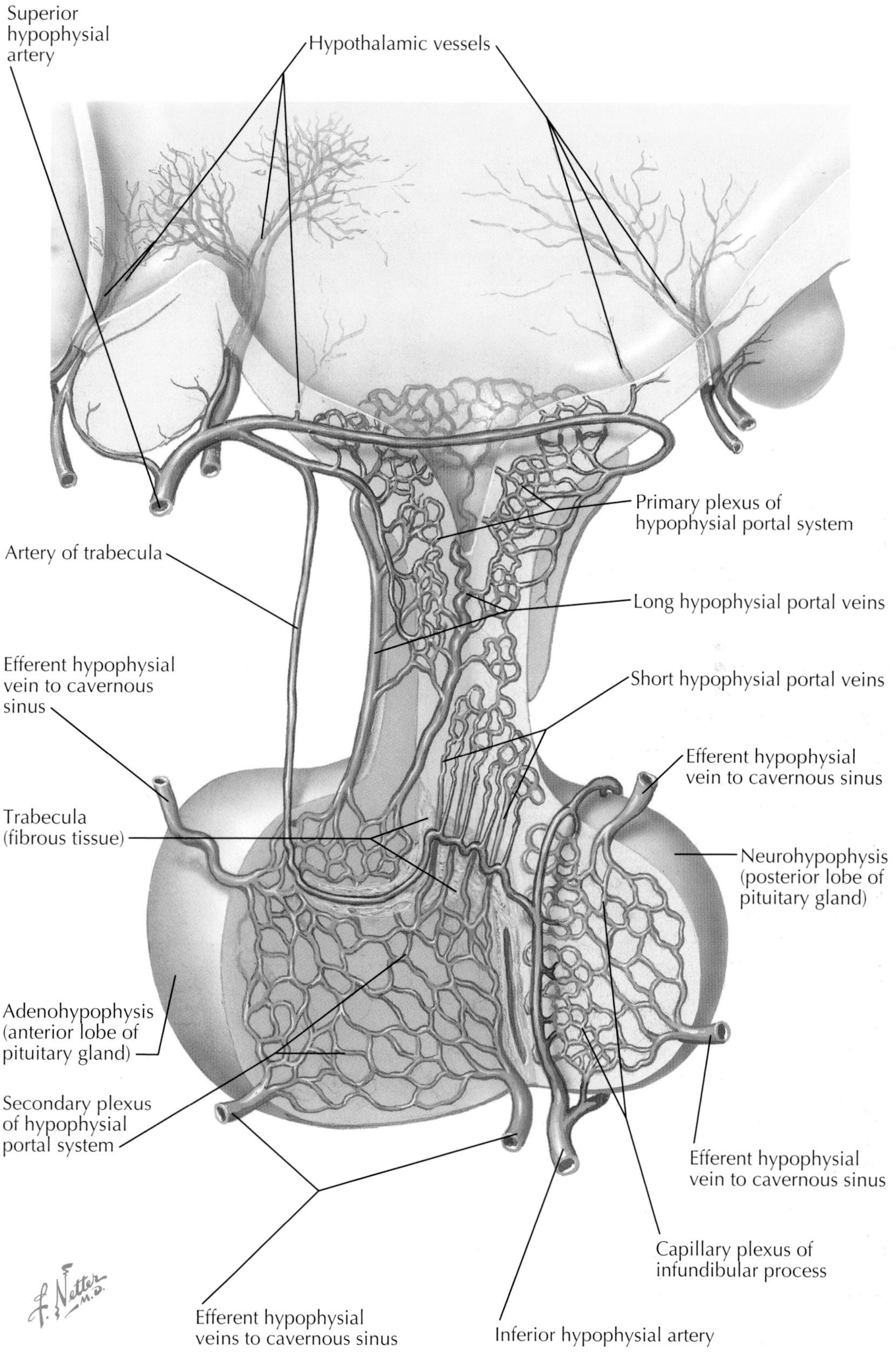

The pituitary gland receives its arterial blood supply from two paired systems of vessels: from above come the right and left superior hypophysial arteries, and from below arise the right and left inferior hypophysial arteries. Each superior hypophysial artery divides into two main branches—the anterior and posterior hypophysial arteries passing to the hypophysial stalk. Communicating branches between these anterior and posterior superior hypophysial arteries run on the lateral aspects of the hypophysial stalk; numerous branches arise from this arterial circle. Some pass upward to supply the optic chiasm and the hypothalamus. Other branches, called *infundibular arteries*, pass either superiorly to penetrate the stalk in its upper part or inferiorly to enter the stalk at a lower level. Another important branch of the anterior superior hypophysial artery on each side is the artery of the trabecula, which passes downward to enter the pars distalis. The trabecula is a prominent, compact band of connective tissue and blood vessels lying within the pars distalis on either side of the midline. At its central end the trabecula is contiguous with the mass of connective tissue, which is interposed between the pars distalis and the lower infundibular stem. Peripherally, the components of the trabecula spread out to form a fibrovascular tuft. On approaching the lower infundibular stem, the artery of the trabecula gives off numerous straight parallel vessels to the superior portion of this area and thus constitutes the "superior artery of the lower infundibular stem." The "inferior artery of the lower infundibular stem" is derived from the inferior hypophysial arterial system. The artery of the trabecula is of large caliber throughout its course; it gives off no branches to the epithelial tissue through which it passes. It is markedly tortuous and is always surrounded by connective tissue.

The inferior hypophysial arteries arise as a single branch from each internal carotid artery in its intracavernous segment. Near the junction of the anterior and posterior lobes of the pituitary, the artery gives off one or more tortuous vessels to the dural covering of the pars distalis and finally divides into two main branches—a medial and a lateral inferior hypophysial artery. The infundibular process is surrounded by an arterial ring formed by the medial and lateral branches of the paired inferior hypophysial arteries. From this arterial ring, branches are given off to the posterior lobe and to the lower infundibular stem. Components of the superior and inferior hypophysial arterial systems anastomose freely.

The epithelial tissue of the pars distalis receives no direct arterial blood. The sinusoids of the anterior lobe receive their blood supply from the hypophysial portal vessels, which arise from the capillary beds within the median eminence and the upper and lower portions of the infundibular stem. Blood is conveyed from this primary capillary network through hypophysial portal veins to the epithelial tissue of the anterior lobe. Here, a secondary plexus of the pituitary portal system is formed, leading to the venous dural sinuses, which surround the pituitary, and to the general circulation. Some of the long hypophysial portal veins run along the surface of the stalk, chiefly on its anterior and lateral aspects. Most of the long hypophysial portal vessels leave the neural tissue to run down within the pars tuberalis, but a few remain deep within the stalk until they reach the pars distalis. The short hypophysial

portal veins are embedded in the tissue surrounding the lower infundibular stem. They supply the sinusoidal bed of the posterior part of the pars distalis, and the long portal veins supply its anterior and lateral regions.

Vascular tufts, comprising the primary capillary network in the median eminence and infundibular stem, are intimately related to the great mass of nerve fibers of the hypothalamo-hypophysial tract running in this region. On excitation, these nerve fibers liberate into the portal vessels, releasing hormones (e.g., growth hormone–releasing hormone, corticotropin-releasing hormone, gonadotropin-releasing hormone, thyrotropin-releasing hormone) and inhibitory factors (e.g., somatostatin, prolactin-inhibitory factor [dopamine]), which are conveyed to the sinusoids of the pars distalis. Extensive occlusion of the hypophysial portal vessels or of the capillary beds of the hypophysial stalk may lead to ischemic necrosis of the anterior pituitary because these hypophysial portal vessels are the only afferent channels to the sinusoids of the pars distalis.

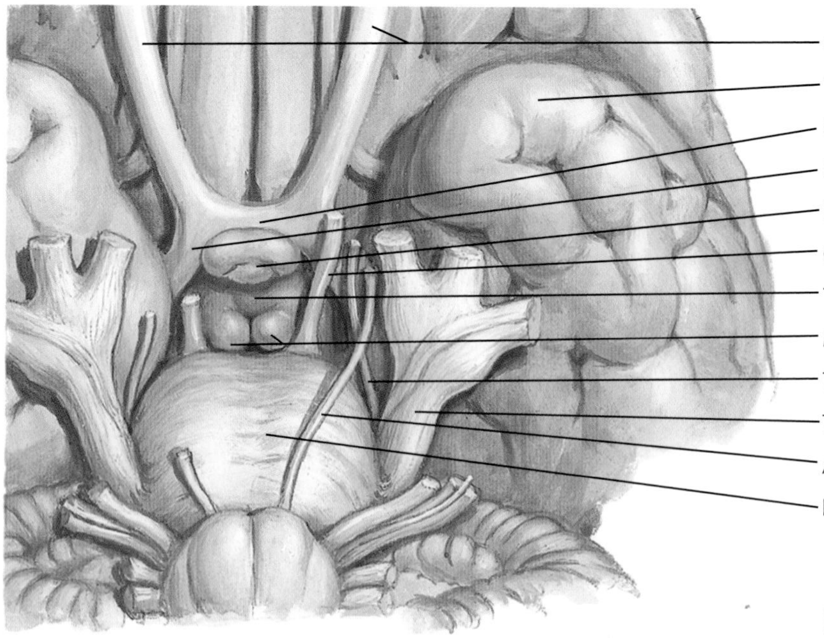

Plate 1-4

Endocrine System

Optic nerves
Temporal pole of brain
Optic chiasm
Right optic tract
Pituitary gland
Oculomotor nerve (III)
Tuber cinereum
Mamillary bodies
Trochlear nerve (IV)
Trigeminal nerve (V)
Abducens nerve (VI)
Pons

ANATOMY AND RELATIONSHIPS OF THE PITUITARY GLAND

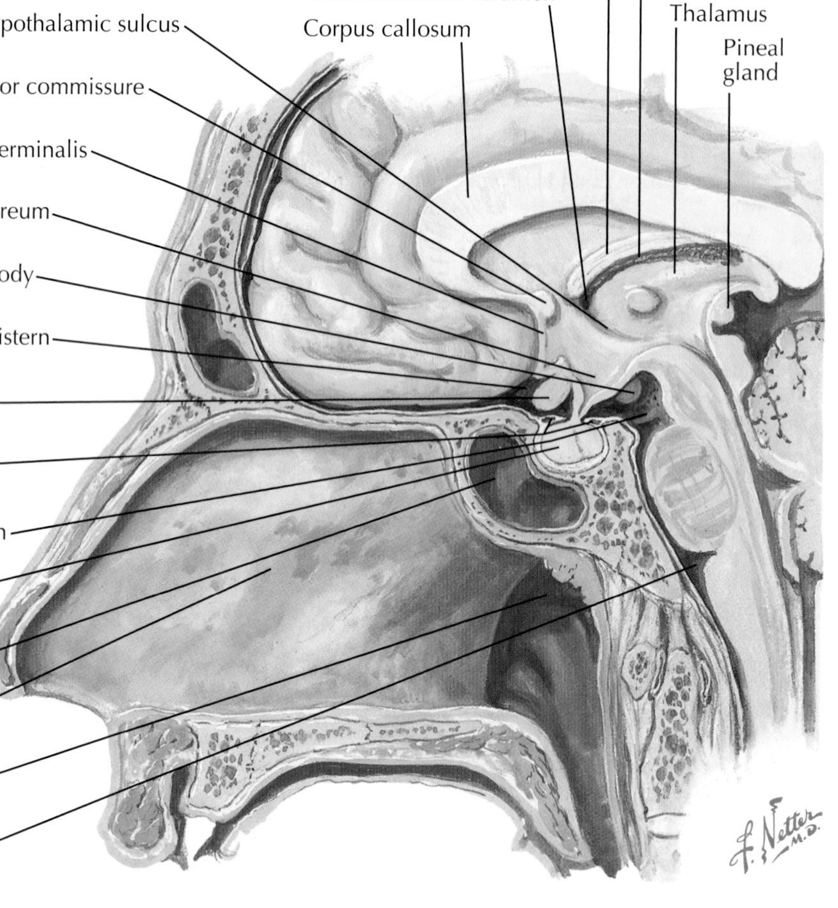

The pituitary gland is reddish-gray and ovoid, measuring about 12 mm transversely, 8 mm in its anterior-posterior diameter, and 6 mm in its vertical dimension. It weighs approximately 500 mg in men and 600 mg in women. It is contiguous with the end of the infundibulum and is situated in the hypophysial fossa of the sphenoid bone. A circular fold of dura mater, the diaphragma sellae, forms the roof of this fossa. In turn, the floor of the hypophysial fossa forms part of the roof of the sphenoid sinus. The diaphragma sellae is pierced by a small central aperture through which the pituitary stalk passes, and it separates the anterior part of the upper surface of the gland from the optic chiasm. The hypophysis is bound on each side by the cavernous sinuses and the structures that they contain. Inferiorly, it is separated from the floor of the fossa by a large, partially vacuolated venous sinus, which communicates freely with the circular sinus. The meninges blend with the capsule of the gland and cannot be identified as separate layers of the fossa. However, the subarachnoid space often extends a variable distance into the sella, particularly anteriorly, and may be referred to as a "partially empty sella" when seen on magnetic resonance imaging (MRI) (see Plate 1-12). In some cases of subarachnoid hemorrhage, the dorsal third of the gland may be covered with blood that has extended down into this space.

The hypothalamus is an important relation of the pituitary gland, both anatomically and functionally. This designation refers to the structures contained in the anterior part of the floor of the third ventricle and to those comprising the lateral wall of the third ventricle below and in front of the hypothalamic sulcus. The mamillary bodies are two round, white, pea-sized masses located side by side below the gray matter of the floor of the third ventricle in front of the posterior perforated substance. They form the posterior limits of the hypothalamus. At certain sites at the base of the brain, the arachnoid is separated from the pia mater by wide intervals that communicate freely with one another; these are called *subarachnoid cisterns*. As the arachnoid extends across between the two temporal lobes, it is separated from the cerebral peduncles by the interpeduncular cistern. Anteriorly, this space is continued in front of the optic chiasm as the chiasmatic cistern. Space-occupying lesions distort these cisterns.

The optic chiasm is an extremely important superior relation of the pituitary gland. It is a flat, somewhat quadrilateral bundle of optic nerve fibers situated at the junction of the anterior wall of the third ventricle with its floor. Its anterolateral angles are contiguous with the

Fornix
Choroid plexus of 3rd ventricle
Interventricular foramen
Corpus callosum
Thalamus
Pineal gland
Hypothalamic sulcus
Anterior commissure
Lamina terminalis
Tuber cinereum
Mamillary body
Chiasmatic cistern
Optic chiasm
Diaphragma sellae
Interpeduncular cistern
Pituitary gland
Sphenoidal sinus
Nasal septum
Nasopharynx
Pontine cistern

optic nerves, and its posterolateral angles are contiguous with the optic tracts. The lamina terminalis, which represents the cephalic end of the primitive neural tube, forms a thin layer of gray matter stretching from the upper surface of the chiasm to the rostrum of the corpus callosum. Inferiorly, the chiasm rests on the diaphragma sellae just behind the optic groove of the sphenoid bone. A small recess of the third ventricle, called the *optic recess*, passes downward and forward over its upper surface as far as the lamina terminalis. A more distant relationship is the pineal gland, which is a small, conical, reddish-gray body lying below the splenium of the corpus callosum. Rarely, ectopic pineal tissue occurs in the floor of the third ventricle and gives rise to tumors of that region. Compression of neighboring cranial nerves, other than the optic nerves, may occur if there is extensive cavernous sinus extension from a pituitary neoplasm (see Plate 1-24).

Plate 1-5

Pituitary and Hypothalamus

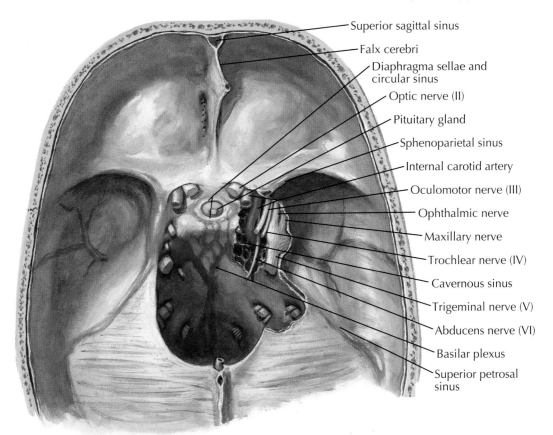

Superior sagittal sinus
Falx cerebri
Diaphragma sellae and circular sinus
Optic nerve (II)
Pituitary gland
Sphenoparietal sinus
Internal carotid artery
Oculomotor nerve (III)
Ophthalmic nerve
Maxillary nerve
Trochlear nerve (IV)
Cavernous sinus
Trigeminal nerve (V)
Abducens nerve (VI)
Basilar plexus
Superior petrosal sinus

RELATIONSHIP OF THE PITUITARY GLAND TO THE CAVERNOUS SINUS

The sinuses of the dura mater are venous channels that drain the blood from the brain. The cavernous sinuses are so named because of their reticulated structure, being traversed by numerous interlacing filaments that radiate out from the internal carotid artery extending anteroposteriorly in the center of the sinuses. They are located astride and on either side of the body of the sphenoid bone and adjacent to the pituitary gland. Each opens behind into the superior and inferior petrosal sinuses (see Plate 3-10). On the medial wall of each cavernous sinus, the internal carotid artery is in close contact with the abducens nerve (VI). On the lateral wall are the oculomotor (III) and trochlear (IV) nerves and the ophthalmic and maxillary divisions of the trigeminal nerve (V). These structures are separated from the blood flowing along the sinus by the endothelial lining membrane. The two cavernous sinuses communicate with each other by means of two intercavernous sinuses. The anterior sinus passes in front of the pituitary gland and the posterior behind it. Together they form a circular sinus around the hypophysis. These channels are found between the two layers of dura mater that comprise the diaphragma sellae and are responsible for copious bleeding when this structure is incised when a transcranial surgical approach to the pituitary gland is used. Sometimes profuse bleeding from an inferior circular sinus is encountered in the transsphenoidal approach to the pituitary gland (see Plate 1-31).

The superior petrosal sinus is a small, narrow channel that connects the cavernous sinus with the transverse sinus. It runs backward and laterally from the posterior end of the cavernous sinus over the trigeminal nerve (V) and lies in the attached margin of the tentorium cerebelli and in the superior petrosal sulcus of the temporal bone. The cavernous sinus also receives the small sphenoparietal sinus, which runs anteriorly along the undersurface of the lesser wing of the sphenoid.

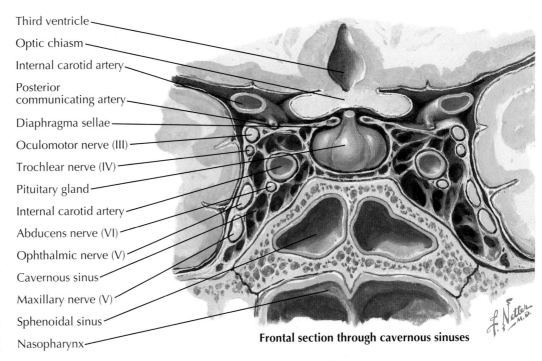

Third ventricle
Optic chiasm
Internal carotid artery
Posterior communicating artery
Diaphragma sellae
Oculomotor nerve (III)
Trochlear nerve (IV)
Pituitary gland
Internal carotid artery
Abducens nerve (VI)
Ophthalmic nerve (V)
Cavernous sinus
Maxillary nerve (V)
Sphenoidal sinus
Nasopharynx

Frontal section through cavernous sinuses

The intercavernous portion of the internal carotid artery runs a complicated course. At first, it ascends toward the posterior clinoid process; then it passes forward alongside the body of the sphenoid bone and again curves upward on the medial side of the anterior clinoid process. It perforates the dura mater that forms the roof of the sinus. This portion of the artery is surrounded by filaments of sympathetic nerves as it passes between the optic and oculomotor nerves. The hypophysial arteries are branches of the intercavernous segment of the internal carotid artery. The inferior branch supplies the posterior lobe of the pituitary gland, and the superior branch leads into the median eminence to start the hypophysial portal system to the anterior lobe.

The surgical approaches to the pituitary gland are designed to circumvent the major vascular channels and to avoid injury to the optic nerves and to the optic chiasm (see Plate 1-31).

Plate 1-6

Endocrine System

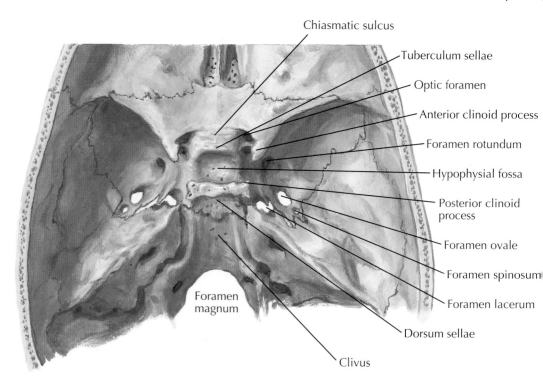

Chiasmatic sulcus
Tuberculum sellae
Optic foramen
Anterior clinoid process
Foramen rotundum
Hypophysial fossa
Posterior clinoid process
Foramen ovale
Foramen spinosum
Foramen lacerum
Dorsum sellae
Clivus
Foramen magnum

RELATIONSHIPS OF THE SELLA TURCICA

The sella turcica—where the pituitary gland is located—is the deep depression in the body of the sphenoid bone. In adults, the normal mean anterior-posterior length is less than 14 mm, and the height from the floor to a line between the tuberculum sellae and the tip of the posterior clinoid is less than 12 mm.

To understand its relations, a more general description of the sphenoid bone is needed. Situated at the base of the skull in front of the temporal bones and the basilar part of the occipital bone, the sphenoid bone somewhat resembles a bat with its wings extended. It is divided into a median portion, or body, two great and two small wings extending outward from the sides of the body, and two pterygoid processes projecting below. The cubical body is hollowed out to form two large cavities, the sphenoidal air sinuses, which are separated from each other by a septum that is often oblique. The superior surface of the body articulates anteriorly with the cribriform plate of the ethmoid and laterally with the frontal bones. Most of the frontal articulation is with the small wing of the sphenoid bone. Behind the ethmoidal articulation is a smooth surface, slightly raised in the midline and grooved on either side, for the olfactory lobes of the brain. This surface is bound behind by a ridge, which forms the anterior border of a narrow transverse groove, the chiasmatic sulcus, above and behind which lies the optic chiasm. The groove ends on either side in the optic foramen, through which the optic nerve and ophthalmic artery enter into the orbital cavity.

Behind the chiasmatic sulcus is an elevation, the tuberculum sellae. Immediately posterior there is a deep depression, the sella turcica, the deepest part of which is called the hypophysial fossa. The anterior boundary of the sella turcica is completed by two small prominences, one on each side, called the middle clinoid processes. The posterior boundary of the sella is formed by an elongated plate of bone, the dorsum sellae, which ends at its superior angles as two tubercles, the posterior clinoid processes.

Behind the dorsum sellae is a shallow depression, the clivus, which slopes obliquely backward to continue as a groove on the basilar portion of the occipital bone. The lateral surfaces of the sphenoid body are united with the great wings and the medial pterygoid plates. Above the attachment of each great wing is a broad

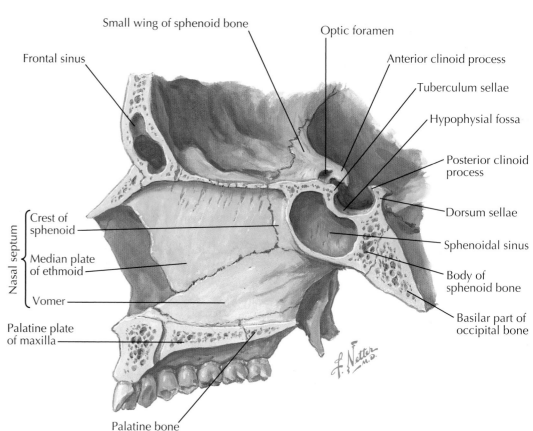

Small wing of sphenoid bone
Optic foramen
Frontal sinus
Anterior clinoid process
Tuberculum sellae
Hypophysial fossa
Posterior clinoid process
Dorsum sellae
Sphenoidal sinus
Body of sphenoid bone
Basilar part of occipital bone
Nasal septum
Crest of sphenoid
Median plate of ethmoid
Vomer
Palatine plate of maxilla
Palatine bone

groove that contains the internal carotid artery and the cavernous sinus. The superior surface of each great wing forms part of the middle fossa of the skull. The internal carotid artery passes through the foramen lacerum, a large, somewhat triangular aperture bound in the front by the great wing of the sphenoid, behind by the apex of the petrous portion of the temporal bone, and medially by the body of the sphenoid and the basilar portion of the occipital bone. The nasal relations

of the pituitary fossa are the crest of the sphenoid bone and the median, or perpendicular, plate of the ethmoid.

Since the introduction of the operating microscope in 1969 by Jules Hardy, the sublabial transseptal transsphenoidal approach to the pituitary has been the standard in the treatment of pituitary adenomas. However, improved endoscopes have led to development of endoscopic transnasal applications in many pituitary surgical centers (see Plate 1-31).

Plate 1-7

Pituitary and Hypothalamus

ANTERIOR PITUITARY HORMONES AND FEEDBACK CONTROL

The quantitative and temporal secretion of the pituitary trophic hormones is tightly regulated and controlled at three levels: (1) Adenohypophysiotropic hormones from the hypothalamus are secreted into the portal system and act on pituitary G-protein–linked cell surface membrane binding sites, resulting in either positive or negative signals mediating pituitary hormone gene transcription and secretion. (2) Circulating hormones from the target glands provide negative feedback regulation of their trophic hormones. (3) Intrapituitary autocrine and paracrine cytokines and growth factors act locally to regulate cell development and function. The hypothalamic-releasing hormones include growth hormone–releasing hormone (GHRH), corticotropin-releasing hormone (CRH), thyrotropin-releasing hormone (TRH), and gonadotropin-releasing hormone (GnRH). The two hypothalamic inhibitory regulatory factors are somatostatin and dopamine, which suppress the secretion of growth hormone (GH) and prolactin, respectively. The six anterior pituitary trophic hormones—corticotropin (adrenocorticotropic hormone [ACTH]), GH, thyrotropin (thyroid-stimulating hormone [TSH]), follicle-stimulating hormone (FSH), luteinizing hormone (LH), and prolactin—are secreted in a pulsatile fashion into the cavernous sinuses and circulate systemically.

Hypothalamic–pituitary–target gland hormonal systems function in a feedback loop, where the target gland blood hormone concentration—or a biochemical surrogate—determines the rate of secretion of the hypothalamic factor and pituitary trophic hormone. The feedback system may be "negative," in which the target gland hormone inhibits the hypothalamic–pituitary unit, or "positive," in which the target gland hormone or surrogate increases the hypothalamic–pituitary unit secretion. These two feedback control systems may be closed loop (regulation is restricted to the interacting trophic and target gland hormones) or open loop (the nervous system or other factors influence the feedback loop). All hypothalamic–pituitary–target gland feedback loops are in part open loop—they have some degree of nervous system (emotional and exteroceptive influences) inputs that either alter the setpoint of the feedback control system or can override the closed-loop controls. Feedback inhibition to the hypothalamus and pituitary is also provided by other target gland factors. For example, inhibin, a heterodimeric glycoprotein product of the Sertoli cell of the testes and the ovarian granulosa cell, provides negative feedback on the secretion of FSH from the pituitary. Synthesis and secretion of gonadal inhibin is induced by FSH.

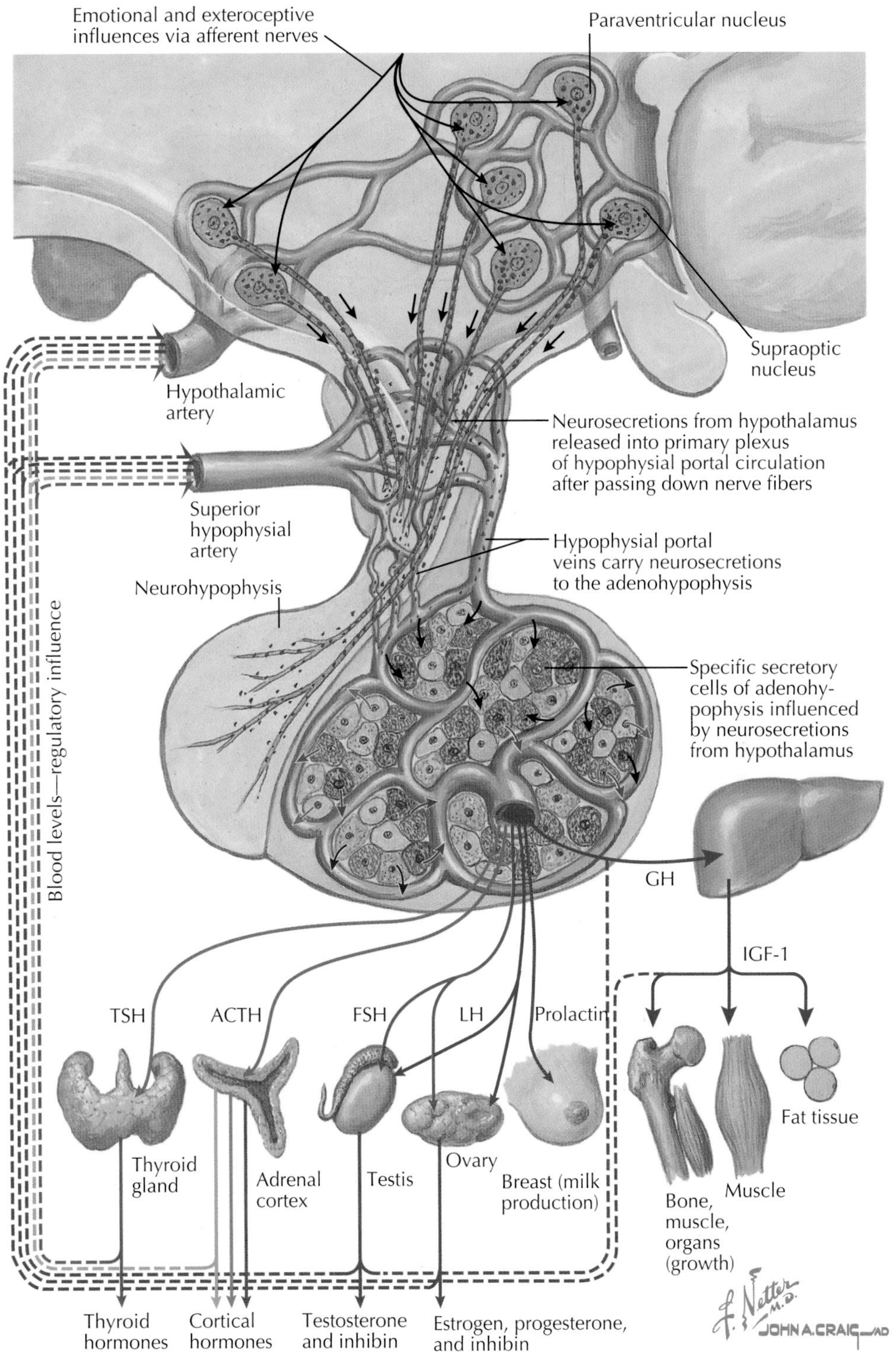

Blood levels of trophic and target gland hormones are also affected by endogenous secretory rhythms. Most hormonal axes have an endogenous secretory rhythm of 24 hours—termed *circadian* or *diurnal rhythms*—and are regulated by retinal inputs and hypothalamic nuclei. The retinohypothalamic tract affects the circadian pulse generators in the hypothalamic suprachiasmatic nuclei. Rhythms that occur more frequently than once a day are termed *ultradian rhythms*, and those that have a period longer than a day are termed *infradian rhythms* (e.g., menstrual cycle). Examples of circadian rhythms of pituitary and target gland hormones include the following: GH and prolactin secretion is highest shortly after the onset of sleep;

cortisol secretion is lowest at 11 PM and highest between 2 and 6 AM; and testosterone secretion is highest in the morning. In addition, GH, ACTH, and prolactin are also secreted in brief regular pulses, reflecting the pulsatile release of their respective hypothalamic releasing factors.

The circadian and pulsatile secretion of pituitary and target gland hormones must be considered when assessing endocrine function. For example, because of pulsatile secretion, a single blood GH measurement is not a good assessment of either hyperfunction or hypofunction of pituitary somatotropes; the serum concentration of the GH-dependent peptide insulinlike growth factor 1 (IGF-1)—because of its much longer serum

half-life—provides a better assessment of GH secretory status. Circulating hormone concentrations are a function of circadian rhythms and hormone clearance rates; laboratories standardize the reference ranges for hormones based on the time of day. For example, the reference range for cortisol changes depending on whether it is measured in the morning or afternoon. Normal serum testosterone concentrations are standardized based on samples obtained from morning venipuncture. Disrupted circadian rhythms should clue the clinician to possible endocrine dysfunction—thus, the loss of circadian ACTH secretion with high midnight concentrations of cortisol in the blood and saliva is consistent with ACTH-dependent Cushing syndrome.

Plate 1-8   Endocrine System

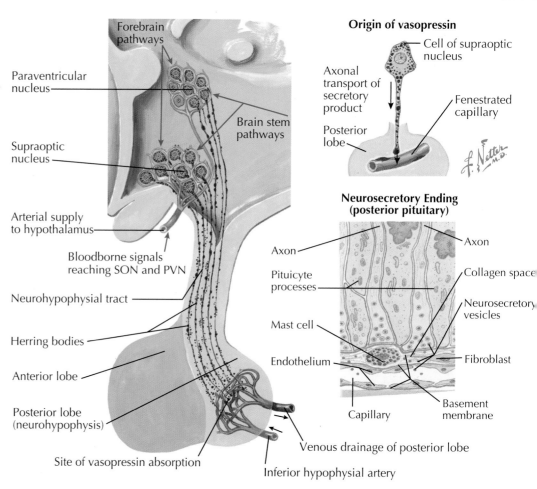

Forebrain pathways

Paraventricular nucleus

Supraoptic nucleus

Arterial supply to hypothalamus

Bloodborne signals reaching SON and PVN

Neurohypophysial tract

Herring bodies

Anterior lobe

Posterior lobe (neurohypophysis)

Site of vasopressin absorption

Brain stem pathways

Origin of vasopressin

Cell of supraoptic nucleus

Axonal transport of secretory product

Fenestrated capillary

Posterior lobe

Neurosecretory Ending (posterior pituitary)

Axon

Pituicyte processes

Mast cell

Endothelium

Axon

Collagen space

Neurosecretory vesicles

Fibroblast

Capillary

Basement membrane

Venous drainage of posterior lobe

Inferior hypophysial artery

POSTERIOR PITUITARY GLAND

The posterior pituitary is neural tissue and is formed by the distal axons of the supraoptic nucleus (SON) and the paraventricular nucleus (PVN) of the hypothalamus. The axon terminals store neurosecretory granules that contain vasopressin and oxytocin—both are non-apeptides consisting of a six–amino acid ring with a cysteine-to-cysteine bridge and a three–amino acid tail. In embryogenesis, neuroepithelial cells of the lining of the third ventricle migrate laterally to and above the optic chiasm to form the SON and to the walls of the third ventricle to form the PVN. The blood supply for the posterior pituitary is from the inferior hypophysial arteries, and the venous drainage is into the cavernous sinus and internal jugular vein.

The posterior pituitary serves to store and release vasopressin and oxytocin. The posterior pituitary stores enough vasopressin to sustain basal release for approximately 30 days and to sustain maximum release for approximately 5 days. Whereas approximately 90% of the SON neurons produce vasopressin, and all its axons end in the posterior pituitary, the PVN has five subnuclei that synthesize other peptides in addition to vasopressin (e.g., somatostatin, corticotropin-releasing hormone, thyrotropin-releasing hormone, and opioids). The neurons of the PVN subnuclei project to the median eminence, brainstem, and spinal cord. The major stimulatory input for vasopressin and oxytocin secretion is glutamate, and the major inhibitory input is γ-aminobutyric acid (GABA). When a stimulus for secretion of vasopressin or oxytocin acts on the SON or PVN, an action potential is generated that propagates down the long axon to the posterior pituitary. The action potential triggers an influx of calcium that causes the neurosecretory granules to fuse with the cell membrane and release the contents of the neurosecretory

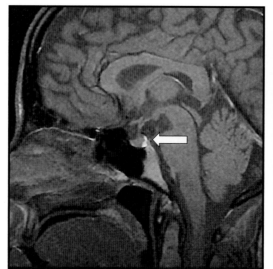

Posterior pituitary bright spot. Sagittal T1-MRI image showing hyperintensity (arrow) in the posterior aspect of the sella turcica.

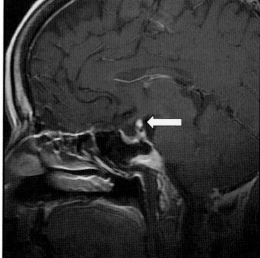

Ectopic posterior pituitary. Sagittal T1-MRI image showing hyperintensity (arrow) along the posterior aspect of the pituitary infundibulum.

granule into the perivascular space and subsequently into the fenestrated capillary system of the posterior pituitary.

The stored vasopressin in neurosecretory granules in the posterior pituitary produces a bright signal on T1-weighted magnetic resonance imaging (MRI)—the "posterior pituitary bright spot." The posterior pituitary bright spot is present in most healthy individuals and is absent in individuals with central diabetes

insipidus. In addition, this bright spot may be located elsewhere in individuals with congenital abnormalities such that the posterior pituitary is undescended—it may appear at the base of the hypothalamus or along the pituitary stalk. Although posterior pituitary function is usually intact, this "ectopic posterior pituitary" may be associated with a hypoplastic anterior pituitary gland and with varying degrees of anterior pituitary dysfunction.

Plate 1-9   Pituitary and Hypothalamus

MANIFESTATIONS OF SUPRASELLAR DISEASE

Suprasellar lesions that may lead to hypothalamic dysfunction include craniopharyngioma, dysgerminoma, granulomatous diseases (e.g., sarcoidosis, tuberculosis, Langerhans cell histiocytosis), lymphocytic hypophysitis, metastatic neoplasm, suprasellar extension of a pituitary tumor, glioma (e.g., hypothalamic, third ventricle, optic nerve), sellar chordoma, meningioma, hamartoma, gangliocytoma, suprasellar arachnoid cyst, and ependymoma.

Endocrine and nonendocrine sequelae are related to hypothalamic mass lesions. Because of the proximity to the optic chiasm, hypothalamic lesions are frequently associated with vision loss. An enlarging hypothalamic mass may also cause headaches and recurrent emesis. The hypothalamus is responsible for many homeostatic functions such as appetite control, the sleep–wake cycle, water metabolism, temperature regulation, anterior pituitary function, circadian rhythms, and inputs to the parasympathetic and sympathetic nervous systems. The clinical presentation is more dependent on the location within the hypothalamus than on the pathologic process. Mass lesions may affect only one or all of the four regions of the hypothalamus (from anterior to posterior: preoptic, supraoptic, tuberal, and mammary regions) or one or all of the three zones (from midline to lateral: periventricular, medial, and lateral zones). For example, hypersomnolence is a symptom associated with damage to the posterior hypothalamus (mammary region) where the rostral portion of the ascending reticular activating system is located. Patients with lesions in the anterior (preoptic) hypothalamus may present with hyperactivity and insomnia, alterations in the sleep–wake cycle (e.g., nighttime hyperactivity and daytime sleepiness), or dysthermia (acute hyperthermia or chronic hypothermia).

The appetite center is located in the ventromedial hypothalamus, and the satiety center is localized to the medial hypothalamus. Destructive lesions involving the more centrally located satiety center lead to hyperphagia and obesity, a relatively common presentation for patients with a hypothalamic mass. Destructive lesions of both of the more laterally located feeding centers may lead to hypophagia, weight loss, and cachexia.

Destruction of the vasopressin-producing magnocellular neurons in the supraoptic and paraventricular nuclei in the tuberal region of the hypothalamus results in central diabetes insipidus (DI) (see Plate 1-27). In addition, DI may be caused by lesions (e.g., high pituitary stalk lesions) that interrupt the transport of vasopressin through the magnocellular axons that terminate in the pituitary stalk and posterior pituitary. Polydipsia and hypodipsia are associated with damage to central osmoreceptors located in anterior medial and anterior lateral preoptic regions. The impaired thirst mechanism results in dehydration and hypernatremia.

Anterior pituitary function control emanates primarily from the arcuate nucleus in the tuberal region of the hypothalamus. Thus, lesions that involve the floor of the third ventricle and median eminence frequently result in varying degrees of anterior pituitary dysfunction (e.g., secondary hypothyroidism, secondary adrenal

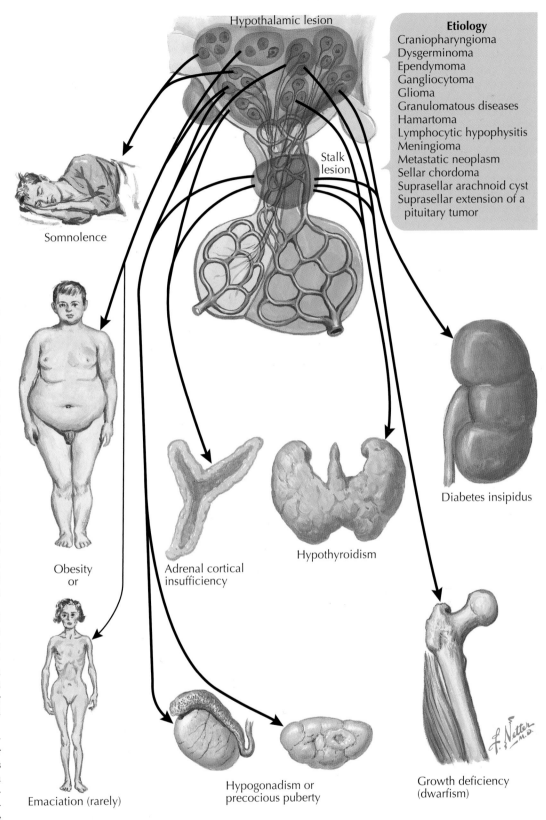

Hypothalamic lesion

Stalk lesion

Somnolence

Diabetes insipidus

Hypothyroidism

Obesity or

Adrenal cortical insufficiency

Growth deficiency (dwarfism)

Emaciation (rarely)

Hypogonadism or precocious puberty

insufficiency, secondary hypogonadism, and growth hormone deficiency).

Hypothalamic hamartomas, gangliocytomas, and germ cell tumors may produce peptides normally secreted by the hypothalamus. Thus, patients may present with endocrine hyperfunction syndromes such as precocious puberty with gonadotropin-releasing hormone expression by hamartomas; acromegaly or Cushing syndrome with growth hormone–releasing hormone expression or corticotropin-releasing hormone expression, respectively, by hypothalamic gangliocytomas; and precocious puberty with β-human chorionic gonadotropin (β-hCG) expression by suprasellar germ cell tumors.

Because of the close microanatomic continuity of the hypothalamic regions and zones, patients with suprasellar disease typically present with not one but many of the dysfunction syndromes discussed.

Plate 1-10

Endocrine System

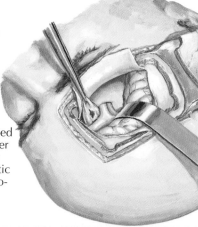

Large cystic suprasellar craniopharyngioma compressing optic chiasm and hypothalamus, filling third ventricle up to interventricular foramen (of Monro), thus causing visual impairment, diabetes insipidus, and hydrocephalus

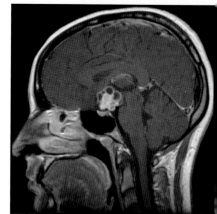

Tumor gently teased forward from under optic chiasm after evacuation of cystic contents via fronto-temporal flap

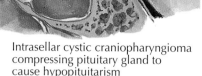

CRANIOPHARYNGIOMA

Craniopharyngioma is the most common tumor found in the region of the pituitary gland in children and adolescents and constitutes about 3% of all intracranial tumors and up to 10% of all childhood brain tumors. Craniopharyngiomas—histologically benign epithelioid tumors arising from embryonic squamous remnants of Rathke pouch—may be large (e.g., >6 cm in diameter) and invade the third ventricle and associated brain structures. This tumorous process is usually located above the sella turcica, depressing the optic chiasm and extending up into the third ventricle. Less frequently, craniopharyngiomas are located within the sella, causing compression of the pituitary gland and frequently eroding the boney confines of the sella turcica. Signs and symptoms—primarily caused by mass effect—typically occur in the adolescent years and rarely after age 40 years. The mass effect symptoms include vision loss by compression of the optic chiasm; diabetes insipidus by invasion or disruption of the hypothalamus or pituitary stalk; hypothalamic dysfunction (e.g., obesity with hyperphagia, hypersomnolence, disturbance in temperature regulation); various degrees of anterior pituitary insufficiency (e.g., growth hormone deficiency with short stature in childhood, hypogonadism, adrenal insufficiency, hypothyroidism); hyperprolactinemia caused by compression of the pituitary stalk or damage to the dopaminergic neurons in the hypothalamus; signs and symptoms of increased intracranial pressure (e.g., headache, projectile emesis, papilledema, optic atrophy); symptoms of hydrocephalus (e.g., mental dullness and confusion) when large tumors obstruct the flow of cerebrospinal fluid; and cranial nerve palsies caused by cavernous sinus invasion.

The findings on radiologic imaging are quite characteristic. Plain skull radiographs and computed tomography (CT) show irregular calcification in the suprasellar region. Magnetic resonance imaging (MRI) typically shows a multilobulated cystic structure that is usually suprasellar in location, but it may also appear to arise

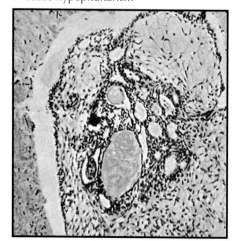

Intrasellar cystic craniopharyngioma compressing pituitary gland to cause hypopituitarism

Histologic section: craniopharyngioma (H & E stain, ×125)

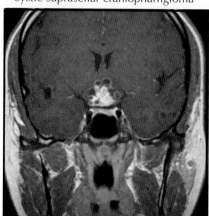

MRI (sagittal view) showing cystic suprasellar craniopharngioma

MRI (coronal view) showing suprasellar craniopharngioma

from the sella. The cystic regions are usually filled with a turbid, cholesterol-rich, viscous fluid. The walls of the cystic and solid components are composed of whorls and cords of epithelial cells separated by a loose network of stellate cells. If there are intercellular epithelial bridges and keratohyalin, the tumor is classified as an adamantinoma.

Treatment options for patients with craniopharyngiomas include observation, endonasal transsphenoidal surgery for smaller intrasellar tumors, craniotomy for larger suprasellar tumors, stereotactic radiotherapy, or a combination of these modalities. Most of these treatment approaches result in varying degrees of anterior or posterior pituitary hormone deficits (or both). In addition, recurrent disease after treatment is common (~40%) because of tumor adherence to surrounding structures, and long-term follow-up is indicated.

Plate 1-11

Pituitary and Hypothalamus

EFFECTS OF PITUITARY TUMORS ON THE VISUAL APPARATUS

The optic chiasm lies above the diaphragma sellae. The most common sign that a pituitary tumor has extended beyond the confines of the sella turcica is a visual defect caused by the growth pressing on the optic chiasm. The most frequent disturbance is a bitemporal hemianopsia, which is produced by the tumor pressing on the crossing central fibers of the chiasm and sparing the uncrossed lateral fibers. The earliest changes are usually enlargement of the blind spot; loss of color vision, especially for red; and a wedge-shaped area of defective vision in the upper-temporal quadrants, which gradually enlarges to occupy the whole quadrant and subsequently extends to include the lower temporal quadrant as well.

The type of visual defect produced depends on the position of the chiasm in relation to the pituitary gland and the direction of tumor growth. In about 10% of the cases, the chiasm may be found almost entirely anterior or posterior to the diaphragma sellae instead of in its usual position, which is directly above the diaphragma. There are also lateral displacements of the chiasm, which may cause either its right or its left branch to lie above the diaphragma. If the chiasm is abnormally fixed, the adenoma may grow upward for a long time before it seriously disturbs vision. Bilateral central scotomas are caused by damage to the posterior part of the chiasm, and their occurrence suggests that the chiasm is prefixed and that the tumor is large. In other cases of prefixed chiasm, the tumor may extend in such a direction as to compress the optic tract rather than the chiasm, thus producing a homonymous hemianopsia. However, homonymous defects do not always indicate a prefixed chiasm; they may also be produced by lateral extension into the temporal lobe below a normally placed chiasm. Other visual defects that may occur include unilateral central scotoma; dimness of vision (amblyopia) in one eye caused by compression of one optic nerve; and an inferior quadrantal hemianopsia, presumably resulting from a large tumor causing the anterior cerebral arteries to cut into the dorsal surface of a normally placed chiasm.

Primary optic atrophy is present in most cases, but it may be absent when the lesion is behind the chiasm. Although papilledema is rare, it may occur with large tumors that cause increased intracranial pressure. If pressure on the visual pathway is relieved (e.g., with surgery or pharmacotherapy), the visual fields may return to normal. However, vision recovery is caused partly by the degree and duration of the optic tract deformation. Field defects can be detected on gross examination by observing the angle at which an object, such as the examiner's finger, becomes visible when the patient looks straight ahead. Quantitative perimetry is

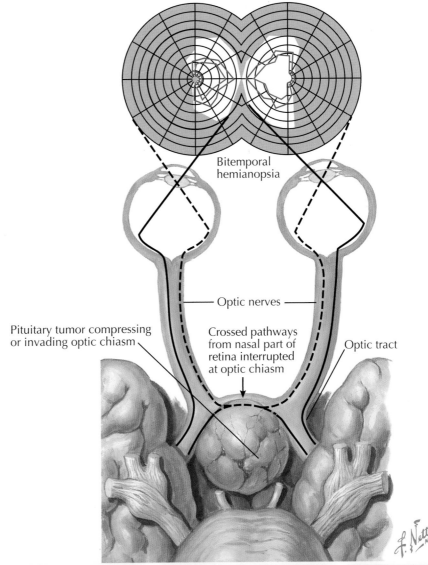

Bitemporal hemianopsia

Optic nerves

Pituitary tumor compressing or invading optic chiasm

Crossed pathways from nasal part of retina interrupted at optic chiasm

Optic tract

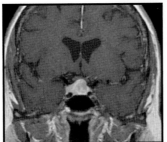

MRI showing pituitary macroadenoma with suprasellar and right cavernous sinus extension. Optic chiasm is raised slightly, but visual fields are normal.

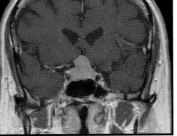

MRI showing pituitary macroadenoma with suprasellar and bilateral cavernous sinus extension. The optic chiasm is compressed, causing bitemporal superior quadrant vision loss.

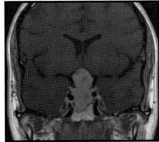

MRI showing pituitary macroadenoma with suprasellar, bilateral cavernous, and sphenoid extensions. The optic chiasm is markedly compressed, causing complete bitemporal hemianopsia.

necessary for exact plotting of the size and shape of the field defect.

In some cases of pituitary tumor showing expansive growth sufficient to enlarge the sella, the visual pathway escapes damage because the sellar diaphragm is tough and prevents expansion toward the chiasm. In these cases, the pituitary tumor may extend laterally into the cavernous sinus or inferiorly into the sphenoid sinus. This structure shows considerable variation, from a

dense, closely knit membrane to a small rim with a wide infundibular opening. In most cases, the diaphragm does yield to pressure from below. Usually, the chiasm lies directly on the diaphragm and is separated from it by only a potential cleft. Frequently, particularly where there is a well-developed chiasmatic cistern, the optic chiasm may be as high as 1 cm above the diaphragm, which allows an invading tumor considerable room for expansion before it presses on the visual pathway.

Plate 1-12

Endocrine System

NONTUMOROUS LESIONS OF THE PITUITARY GLAND AND PITUITARY STALK

The nontumorous lesions of the pituitary gland that can affect function include lymphocytic hypophysitis, granulomatous disorders (e.g., sarcoidosis, tuberculosis, Langerhans cell histiocytosis, Wegener granulomatosis), head trauma with skull base fracture, iron overload states (e.g., hemochromatosis, hemosiderosis), intrasellar carotid artery aneurysm, primary empty sella, pituitary cyst infection (e.g., encephalitis, pituitary abscess), mutations in genes encoding pituitary transcription factors, and developmental midline anomalies.

Lymphocytic hypophysitis is an autoimmune disorder characterized by lymphocytic infiltration and enlargement of the pituitary gland followed by selective destruction of pituitary cells. The most common clinical setting is in late pregnancy or in the postpartum period. Patients typically present with headaches and signs and symptoms of deficiency of one or more pituitary hormones. Frequently, there is a curious preferential destruction of corticotrophs. However, these patients may have panhypopituitarism (including diabetes insipidus [DI]). Magnetic resonance imaging (MRI) usually shows a homogeneous, contrast-enhancing sellar mass with pituitary stalk involvement. The pituitary hormone deficits are usually permanent, but recovery of both anterior and posterior pituitary function may occur.

Granulomatous hypophysitis can be caused by sarcoidosis, tuberculosis, Langerhans cell histiocytosis, or Wegener granulomatosis. The granulomatous inflammation may involve the hypothalamus, pituitary stalk, and pituitary gland and cause hypopituitarism, including DI.

Head trauma that results in a skull base fracture may cause hypothalamic hormone deficiencies, resulting in deficient secretion of anterior and posterior pituitary hormones. Head trauma may lead to direct pituitary damage by a sella turcica fracture, pituitary stalk section, trauma-induced vasospasm, or ischemic infarction after blunt trauma.

Iron overload states of hemochromatosis and hemosiderosis of thalassemia may involve the pituitary, resulting in iron deposition (siderosis) in pituitary cells. Iron overload most commonly results in selective gonadotropin deficiency.

The term *empty sella* refers to an enlarged sella turcica that is not entirely filled with pituitary tissue. A secondary empty sella occurs when a pituitary adenoma enlarges the sella but is then surgically removed or damaged by radiation or infarction. In a primary empty sella, a defect in the sellar diaphragm allows cerebrospinal fluid to enter and enlarge the sella (≤50% of patients with a primary empty sella have benign increased intracranial pressure). With a primary empty sella, pituitary function is usually intact. On MRI, demonstrable pituitary tissue is usually compressed against the sellar floor.

Hypopituitarism is also associated with mutations in genes that encode the transcription factors whose expression is necessary for the differentiation of anterior pituitary cells (e.g., HESX1, LHX3, LHX4, PROP1, POU1F1 [formerly PIT1], TBX19 [also known as TPIT]). Mutations in PROP1 are the most common cause of familial and sporadic congenital hypopituitarism. PROP1 is necessary for the differentiation of a cell type that is a precursor of somatotroph, lactotroph, thyrotroph, and gonadotroph cells. The protein

encoded by POU1F1, which acts temporally just after the protein encoded by PROP1, is necessary for the differentiation of a cell type that is a precursor of somatotroph, lactotroph, and to a lesser degree, thyrotroph cells. TBX19 is required for specific differentiation of the corticotroph cells. Because the proteins encoded by HEXS1, LHX3, and LHX4 act early in pituicyte differentiation, mutations in these genes cause combined pituitary hormone deficiency, which refers to deficiencies of growth hormone (GH), prolactin, thyrotropin (thyroid-stimulating hormone [TSH]),

luteinizing hormone (LH), and follicle-stimulating hormone (FSH) (see Plate 1-13).

Developmental midline anomalies may lead to structural pituitary anomalies (e.g., pituitary aplasia or hypoplasia). Craniofacial developmental anomalies may result in cleft lip and palate, basal encephalocele, hypertelorism, and optic nerve hypoplasia, with varying degrees of pituitary dysplasia and aplasia. Congenital basal encephalocele may cause the pituitary to herniate through the sphenoid sinus roof, resulting in pituitary failure and DI.

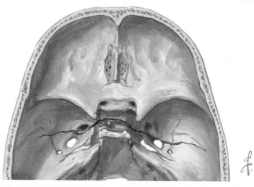

Suprasellar	Intrasellar anterior lobe	Intrasellar posterior lobe
↓	↓	↓
Hypothalamic manifestations (obesity, somnolence) with or without hypopituitarism and/or diabetes insipidus	Anterior lobe hypofunction of variable degree	Diabetes insipidus

Lymphocytic hypophysitis and granulomatous disorders
Degree and type of hypopituitarism depend on size and location of involvement

Trauma Skull fracture, hemorrhage → Hypopituitarism of variable degree

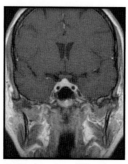

MRI showing diffusely enhancing lymphocytic hypophysitis filling the sella and extending toward the optic chiasm

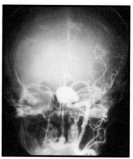

Angiogram showing intrasellar carotid artery aneurysm

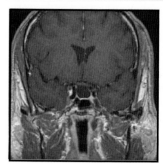

MRI showing a primary empty sella

Imaging is key in the diagnosis of and in determining the type of nontumorous sellar process

Plate 1-19

Pituitary and Hypothalamus

MRI (coronal view) shows a large GH-secreting pituitary tumor in a 16-year-old adolescent boy with gigantism.

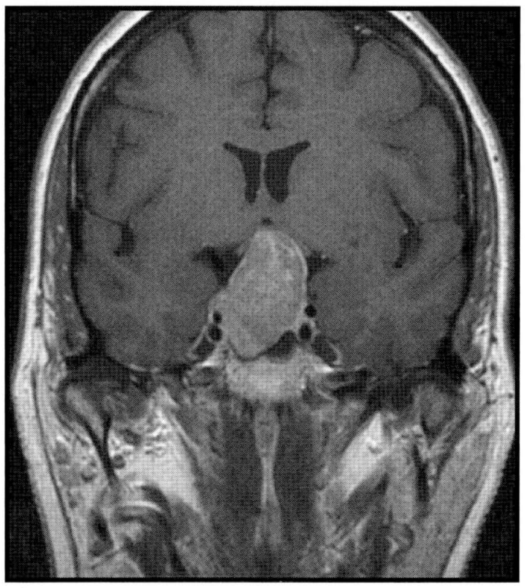

PITUITARY GIGANTISM

Pituitary gigantism occurs when a growth hormone (GH)–secreting pituitary tumor develops before fusion of the epiphyseal growth plates in a child or adolescent. In contrast, when GH-secreting pituitary tumors develop in an adult (after complete epiphyseal fusion), there is no linear growth, but there are acral changes, and the condition is termed *acromegaly* (see Plate 1-20).

Pituitary gigantism is rare. When it starts in infancy, it may lead to exceptional height. The tallest well-documented person with pituitary gigantism measured 8 ft, 11 in (272 cm). When untreated, pituitary giants are typically taller than 7 ft. The GH-secreting pituitary tumors in individuals with pituitary gigantism are usually sporadic, but they may arise as part of a syndrome such as multiple endocrine neoplasia type 1 (see Plate 8-1), McCune-Albright syndrome (see Plate 4-11), and the Carney complex (see Plate 3-12).

Although usually caused by a pituitary GH-secreting adenoma, pituitary gigantism may also be caused by an ectopic tumor secreting GH-releasing hormone (GHRH) or by hypothalamic dysfunction with hypersecretion of GHRH.

In addition to the accelerated linear growth, patients with pituitary gigantism may slowly develop many of those features seen in adults with acromegaly—for example, soft tissue overgrowth, progressive dental malocclusion (underbite), a low-pitched voice, headaches, malodorous hyperhidrosis, oily skin, proximal muscle weakness, diabetes mellitus, hypertension, obstructive sleep apnea, and cardiac dysfunction. The mass effects of GH-producing pituitary macroadenomas (>10 mm) are similar to those of other pituitary macroadenomas—they include visual field defects, oculomotor pareses, headaches, and pituitary insufficiency.

It is important to note that most children with accelerated linear growth do not have pituitary gigantism. More common causes of tall stature include precocious puberty, genetic tall stature, and hyperthyroidism.

High plasma GH levels are not diagnostic of pituitary gigantism. The diagnosis of pituitary gigantism should be considered in patients after other causes of accelerated linear growth have been excluded. The biochemical diagnosis is based on two criteria: a GH level that is not suppressed to less than 0.4 ng/dL after an oral glucose load (75–100 g) and an increased serum concentration (based on normal range adjusted for age and gender) of insulinlike growth factor 1 (IGF-1). Serum prolactin concentrations should also be measured because the pituitary neoplasm in children frequently arises from the mammosomatotroph, so cohypersecretion of prolactin may occur. The laboratory assessment of pituitary gigantism is supplemented with magnetic

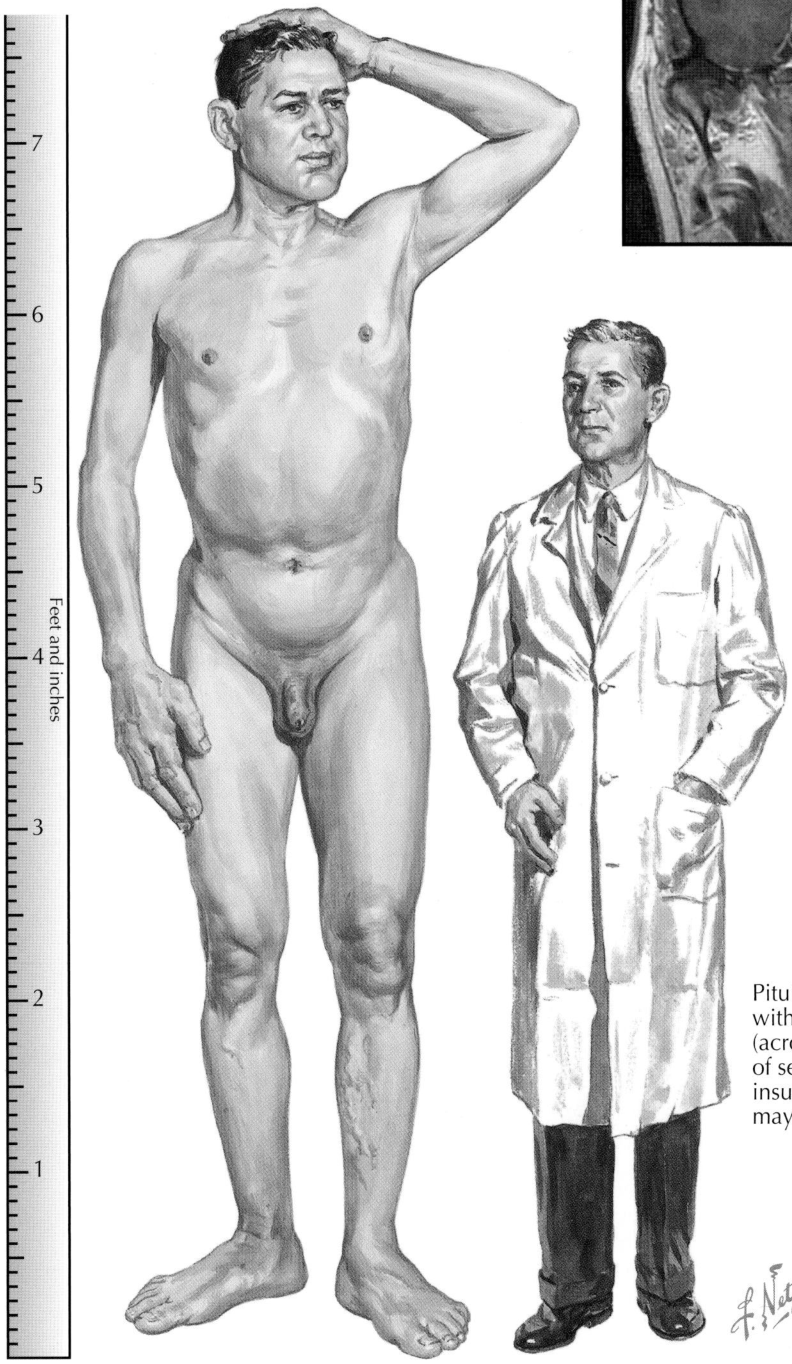

Pituitary giant contrasted with average-size man (acromegaly and signs of secondary pituitary insufficiency may or may not be present)

resonance imaging (MRI) of the pituitary and visual field examination by quantitative perimetry. If imaging of the pituitary fails to detect an adenoma, then plasma GHRH concentration and CT of the chest and abdomen are indicated in search of an ectopic GHRH-producing tumor (e.g., pancreatic or small cell lung neoplasm).

Treatment is indicated for all patients with confirmed pituitary gigantism. The goals of treatment are

to prevent the long-term consequences of GH excess, remove the sellar mass, and preserve normal pituitary tissue and function. Treatment options include surgery, targeted irradiation, and medical therapy. Surgery—transsphenoidal adenectomy by an experienced neurosurgeon—is the treatment of choice and should be supplemented, if necessary, with Gamma knife radiotherapy, pharmacotherapy, or both.

Plate 1-20

Endocrine System

ACROMEGALY

Chronic growth hormone (GH) excess from a GH-producing pituitary tumor results in the clinical syndrome of acromegaly. Acromegaly was the first pituitary syndrome to be recognized, described by Pierre Marie in 1886. If untreated, this syndrome is associated with increased morbidity and mortality. Although the annual incidence is estimated to be only three per 1 million persons in the general population, a GH-secreting pituitary adenoma is the second most common hormone-secreting pituitary tumor. The effects of the chronic GH excess include acral and soft tissue overgrowth, progressive dental malocclusion (underbite), degenerative arthritis related to chondral and synovial tissue overgrowth within joints, a low-pitched sonorous voice, headaches, malodorous hyperhidrosis, oily skin, perineural hypertrophy leading to nerve entrapment (e.g., carpal tunnel syndrome), proximal muscle weakness, carbohydrate intolerance (the initial presentation may be diabetes mellitus), hypertension, colonic neoplasia, obstructive sleep apnea, and cardiac dysfunction. The mass effects of GH-producing pituitary macroadenomas (>10 mm) are similar to those of other pituitary macroadenomas and include visual field defects, oculomotor pareses, headaches, and pituitary insufficiency.

Patients with acromegaly have a characteristic appearance with coarsening of the facial features, prognathism, frontal bossing, spadelike hands, and wide feet. Often there is a history of progressive increase in shoe, glove, ring, or hat size. These changes may occur slowly and may go unrecognized by the patient, family, and physician. The average delay in diagnosis from the onset of the first symptoms to the eventual diagnosis is 8.5 years. Comparison with earlier photographs of the patient is helpful in confirming the clinical suspicion of acromegaly.

High plasma GH levels are not diagnostic of acromegaly. Basal plasma GH levels are increased in patients with poorly controlled diabetes mellitus, chronic hepatic or renal failure, or conditions characterized by protein-calorie malnutrition such as anorexia nervosa. The diagnosis of acromegaly depends on two criteria: a GH level that is not suppressed to less than 0.4 ng/dL after an oral glucose load (75–100 g) and an increased serum concentration (based on normal range adjusted for age and gender) of insulinlike growth factor 1 (IGF-1, a GH-dependent growth factor responsible for many of the effects of GH and previously known as somatomedin C). Serum IGF-1 levels are rarely falsely elevated. IGF-1 levels do rise in pregnancy two- to threefold above the upper limit of gender- and age-adjusted normal values. The laboratory assessment of acromegaly is supplemented with magnetic resonance imaging of the pituitary and visual field examination by quantitative perimetry. If imaging of the pituitary fails to detect an adenoma, then plasma GH-releasing hormone (GHRH) concentration and CT of the chest and abdomen are indicated in search of an ectopic GHRH-producing tumor (e.g., pancreatic or small cell lung neoplasm).

Treatment is indicated for all patients with acromegaly. The goals of treatment are to prevent the long-term consequences of GH excess, remove the sellar mass, and preserve normal pituitary tissue and function. Treatment options include surgery, targeted irradiation, and medical therapy. Surgery—transsphenoidal adenectomy by an experienced neurosurgeon—is the treatment of choice and should be supplemented, if necessary, with Gamma knife radiotherapy, pharmacotherapy, or both.

After successful surgical treatment, there is a marked regression of the soft tissue excess, but the bone changes are permanent. After the soft tissue changes have stabilized, combined oral and plastic surgery may be indicated (e.g., mandibular osteotomies, recession of the supraorbital ridges, rhinoplasties, and reduction of tongue size). Disabling hypertrophic osteoarthropathy of the hip or other large joints may require joint replacement. Because of the increased risk of colorectal adenomas and cancer, patients with acromegaly should be offered regular colonoscopic screening.

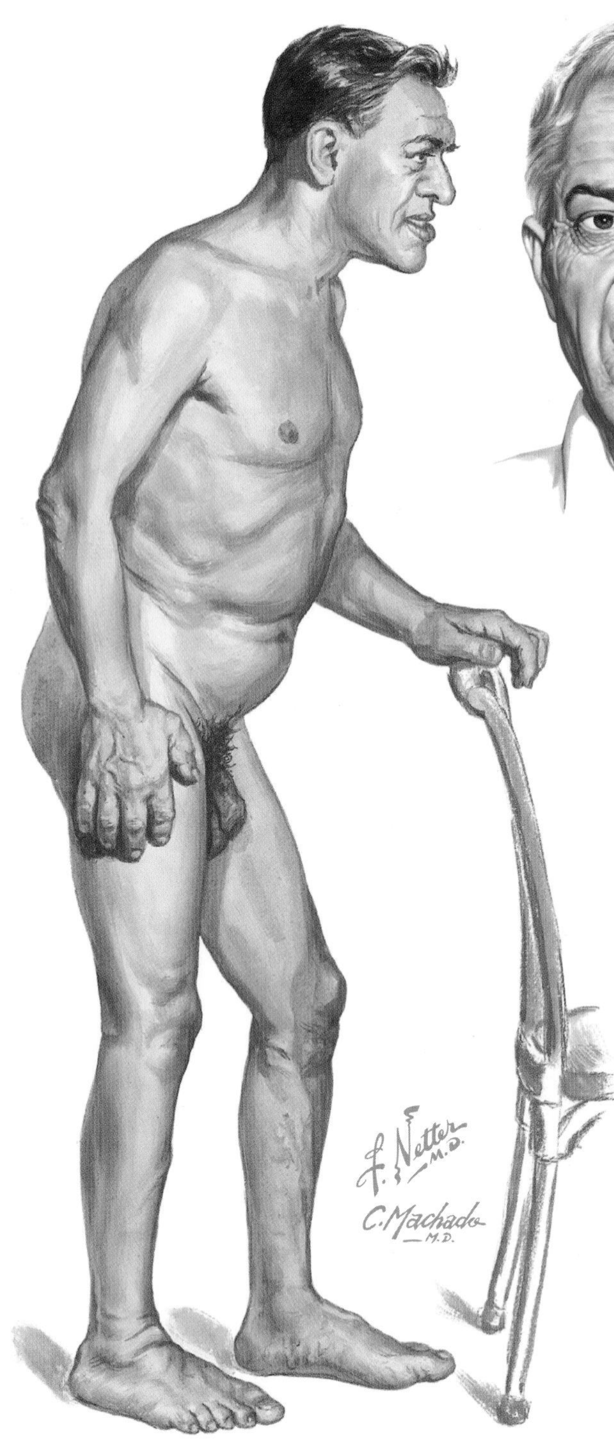

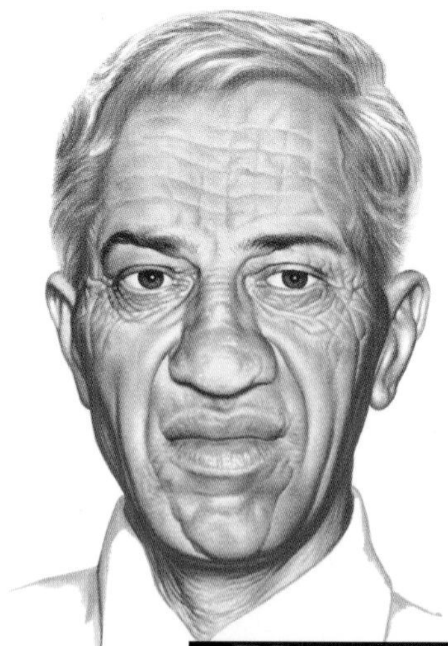

The effects of the chronic GH excess include acral and soft tissue overgrowth, coarsening of facial features, prognathism, frontal bossing, and progressive dental malocclusion (underbite).

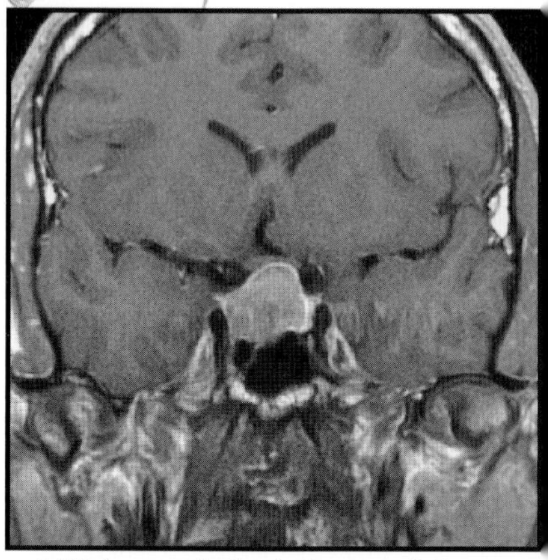

MRI (coronal view) shows a 2.1-cm pituitary macroadenoma eroding the sellar floor on the right, extending into the right cavernous sinus, and extending to the optic chiasm above the sella turcica.

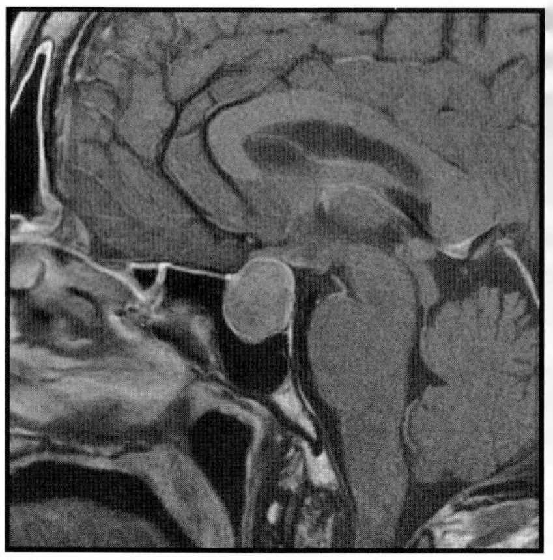

MRI (midline sagittal view) shows pituitary macroadenoma extending into the sphenoid sinus and suprasellar region.

Plate 1-21   Pituitary and Hypothalamus

PROLACTIN-SECRETING PITUITARY TUMOR

Prolactin-secreting pituitary tumors (prolactinomas) are the most common hormone-secreting pituitary tumor. They are monoclonal lactotroph cell adenomas that appear to result from sporadic mutations. Although most prolactinomas are sporadic, they are the most frequent pituitary tumor in persons with multiple endocrine neoplasia type 1 (see Plate 8-1). In addition, more than 99% of prolactinomas are benign. Approximately 10% of prolactin-secreting pituitary tumors cosecrete growth hormone because of a somatotroph or mammosomatotroph component.

In women, the typical clinical presentation of a prolactin-secreting microadenoma (≤10 mm in largest diameter) is secondary amenorrhea with or without galactorrhea. But in men, because of the lack of symptoms related to small prolactinomas, a prolactinoma is not usually diagnosed until the tumor has enlarged enough to cause mass-effect symptoms. This late diagnosis is also the typical clinical scenario in postmenopausal women. Mass-effect symptoms of prolactin-secreting macroadenomas include visual field defects with suprasellar extension, cranial nerve palsies with lateral (cavernous sinus) extension (e.g., diplopia, ptosis), headaches, and varying degrees of hypopituitarism with compression of the normal pituitary tissue.

Hyperprolactinemia results in decreased gonadotropin secretion in men and women. In men, hypogonadotropic hypogonadism causes testicular atrophy, low serum testosterone concentrations, decreased libido, sexual dysfunction, decreased facial hair growth, and decreased muscle mass. Because men lack the estrogen needed to prepare breast glandular tissues, they rarely present with galactorrhea. In premenopausal women, however, hyperprolactinemia may cause bilateral spontaneous or expressible galactorrhea (see Plate 4-26). In addition, prolactin-dependent hypogonadotropic hypogonadism in women results in secondary amenorrhea and estrogen deficiency symptoms. Long-standing hypogonadism in both men and women may lead to osteopenia and osteoporosis.

In general, the blood concentration of prolactin is proportionate to the size of the prolactinoma. For example, a 5-mm prolactinoma is associated with serum prolactin concentrations of 50 to 250 ng/mL (reference range, 4-30 ng/mL), but prolactinomas larger than 2 cm in diameter are associated with serum prolactin concentrations greater than 1000 ng/mL. However, there are exceptional cases of small prolactinomas that have extremely efficient prolactin secretory capacity (e.g., serum prolactin concentration >1000 ng/mL) and cases of the converse—very inefficient prolactin-secreting macroadenomas (e.g., serum prolactin concentrations <200 ng/mL).

Treatment decisions in patients with prolactin-secreting pituitary tumors are guided by the signs and symptoms related to hyperprolactinemia and mass-effect symptoms related to the sellar mass. For example, a 4-mm prolactin-secreting microadenoma detected incidentally in an asymptomatic postmenopausal woman may be observed without treatment. However, because prolactin-secreting pituitary macroadenomas grow over time, treatment is almost always indicated for macroprolactinomas even if the patient lacks tumor-related symptomatology. When treatment is indicated (e.g., if secondary hypogonadism is present in men or in premenopausal women or if a

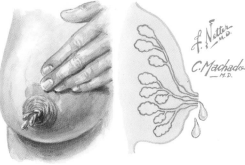
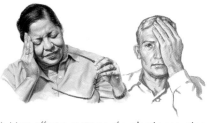

In premenopausal women, hyperprolactinemia causes bilateral spontaneous galactorrhea

▲ Mass-effect symptoms of prolactin-secreting macroadenomas include visual field defects with suprasellar extension, cranial nerve palsies with lateral (cavernous sinus) extension (e.g., diplopia, ptosis), headaches, and varying degrees of hypopituitarism

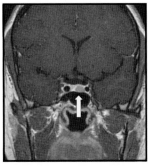
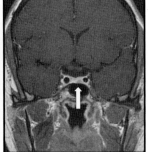

◄ Serial head MRI scans (coronal views) from a patient with a 9-mm prolactin-secreting pituitary microadenoma (arrows). At the time of diagnosis (image on left), the serum prolactin concentration was 280 ng/mL. The image on the right was obtained 6 months after normalizing the serum prolactin concentration with a dopamine agonist. The size of the prolactinoma decreased more than 50% (image on right).

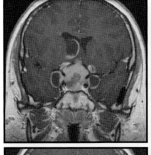
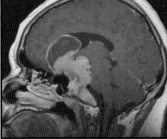
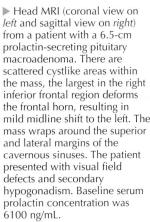
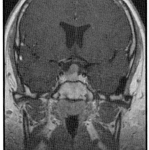
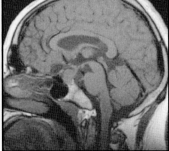

▶ Head MRI (coronal view on left and sagittal view on right) from a patient with a 6.5-cm prolactin-secreting pituitary macroadenoma. There are scattered cystlike areas within the mass, the largest in the right inferior frontal region deforms the frontal horn, resulting in mild midline shift to the left. The mass wraps around the superior and lateral margins of the cavernous sinuses. The patient presented with visual field defects and secondary hypogonadism. Baseline serum prolactin concentration was 6100 ng/mL.

▶ Head MRI (coronal view on left and sagittal view on right) from the same patient 6 months after normalizing the serum prolactin concentration with a dopamine agonist. Dramatic shrinkage on the MRI is evident. Visual field defects resolved, and pituitary function returned to normal.

macroadenoma is present), an orally administered dopamine agonist (e.g., cabergoline or bromocriptine) is the treatment of choice. Dopamine agonists are very effective in promptly normalizing the serum prolactin concentration and reducing the size of the lactotroph adenoma. After initiating a dopamine agonist, the serum prolactin concentration should be monitored every 2 weeks, and the dosage of bromocriptine or cabergoline should be increased until the prolactin levels decrease into the reference range. Approximately 3 to 6 months after achieving a normal serum prolactin concentration, pituitary-directed magnetic resonance imaging (MRI) should be performed to document tumor shrinkage. The minimal dosage of the dopamine agonist that results in normoprolactinemia should be continued indefinitely. In a small percentage of patients,

prolactin-secreting adenomas may be cured with long-term dopamine agonist therapy. Thus, a periodic (e.g., every 2 years) 2-month holiday off the dopamine agonist is indicated to determine whether hyperprolactinemia recurs. Patients with macroprolactinomas that have sphenoid sinus extension should be cautioned about the potential for cerebrospinal fluid (CSF) rhinorrhea that may occur as the tumor shrinks. CSF rhinorrhea requires an urgent neurosurgical procedure to prevent the development of pneumocephalus and bacterial meningitis. When patients are intolerant of the dopamine agonist (e.g., nausea, lightheadedness, mental fogginess, or vivid dreams) or if the tumor is resistant to this form of therapy, transsphenoidal surgery or gamma knife radiation therapy may be considered.

Plate 1-22

Endocrine System

CORTICOTROPIN-SECRETING PITUITARY TUMOR

Corticotropin (adrenocorticotropic hormone [ACTH])-secreting pituitary adenomas stimulate excess adrenal secretion of cortisol, resulting in the signs and symptoms characteristic of Cushing syndrome (see Plate 3-9). ACTH-secreting pituitary tumors are typically benign microadenomas (≤10 mm in largest diameter); occasionally, they are macroadenomas, and very rarely they are carcinomas. Treatment of choice for an ACTH-secreting pituitary adenoma is transsphenoidal selective adenectomy. Surgical success is defined as cure of Cushing syndrome and intact anterior and posterior pituitary function.

The most common operative approach is an endonasal approach (with use of an endoscope), traversing the sphenoid sinus (transsphenoidal) and through the floor of the sella (see Plate 1-31). Corticotroph adenomas are basophilic and stain positively for ACTH on immunohistochemistry. Tissue adjacent to the adenoma usually shows Crooke hyaline change, a result of atrophy of normal corticotrophs. Cure rates are 80% to 90% when a microadenoma can be localized preoperatively with either magnetic resonance imaging (MRI) or inferior petrosal sinus sampling (see Plate 3-10). A lack of cure in patients with microadenomas is attributable to either their small size, so they cannot be seen at surgery, or to an inaccessible location (e.g., cavernous sinus). MRI should be performed with a high-strength magnet (e.g., 3 tesla) and gadolinium enhancement. Only about half of ACTH-secreting pituitary tumors are large enough to be detected by MRI. In addition, approximately 10% of healthy individuals have an apparent microadenoma on MRI; thus, in a patient with Cushing syndrome, an apparent small sellar adenoma on MRI is not specific for a corticotroph adenoma. The lower cure rate (~60%) for macroadenomas is usually because of cavernous sinus involvement that prevents complete resection.

On the day of surgery, these patients should receive an intravenous dose of glucocorticoid (e.g., hydrocortisone, 100 mg). The serum cortisol concentration should be measured the morning after surgery (before additional exogenous glucocorticoid administration) to document a short-term cure, defined as a low serum cortisol concentration (e.g., <1.8 μg/dL). If the patient develops symptoms of acute glucocorticoid withdrawal before the serum cortisol laboratory result is available, stress dosages of glucocorticoids should be administered (e.g., hydrocortisone, 100 mg intravenously twice daily). The glucocorticoid dosage is then decreased daily, and patients are typically discharged from the hospital on dosages of exogenous orally administered glucocorticoids twofold above the standard replacement therapy dosage (e.g., prednisone, 10 mg in the morning and 5 mg at 4 PM daily). However, this dosage should be adjusted according to the severity of hypercortisolism preoperatively to prevent severe steroid withdrawal symptoms. Then the dosage of exogenous glucocorticoid is slowly tapered to a standard replacement dosage over 4 to 6 weeks after operation. The hypothalamic corticotropin-releasing hormone neurons and the atrophic anterior pituitary corticotrophs take months to recover from chronic suppression. Most patients tolerate a single dose of a short-acting glucocorticoid (e.g., 15-20 mg of hydrocortisone every morning) starting 8 to 12 weeks after surgical cure. The 8 AM serum cortisol concentration should be measured

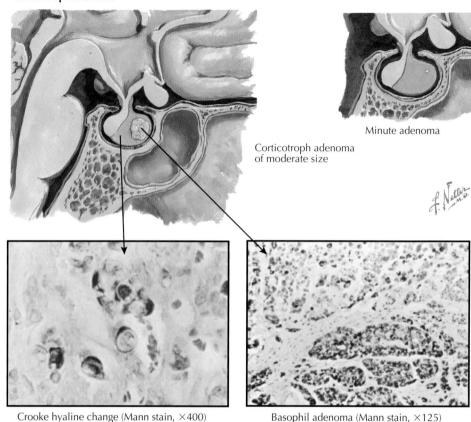

Corticotroph adenoma

Corticotroph adenoma of moderate size

Minute adenoma

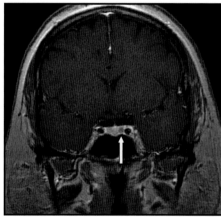

Crooke hyaline change (Mann stain, ×400)

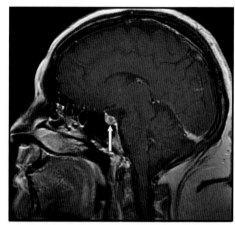

Basophil adenoma (Mann stain, ×125)

Head MRI (coronal view) with a 4-mm corticotroph adenoma (*arrow*) seen as a rounded, hypodense nodule on left side of the sella

Head MRI (sagittal view) with a 4-mm corticotroph adenoma (*arrow*) located between the anterior and posterior lobes of the pituitary gland

every 6 weeks; venipuncture should be performed before taking a morning dose of hydrocortisone. The serum cortisol concentration will slowly increase from undetectable levels to a concentration higher than 10 μg/dL; when this occurs, the hydrocortisone dosage can be tapered and discontinued over 2 weeks. With this postoperative management protocol, the patient with typical pituitary-dependent Cushing syndrome requires exogenous administration of glucocorticoids for approximately 12 months after curative pituitary surgery. The signs and symptoms related to Cushing syndrome resolve very slowly over the first 6 months after surgery.

However, even when the postoperative serum cortisol concentration is low, a risk for recurrent disease remains—if a small number of viable adenomatous corticotroph cells are not resected at surgery, they multiply

over time and eventually have the ACTH secretory mass to cause recurrent Cushing syndrome. The average time to clinically evident recurrence is 3 to 4 years. Thus, all patients should be followed up annually and assessed for recurrent disease.

Patients with Cushing syndrome are at increased thromboembolic risk perioperatively, and prophylactic measures to prevent deep venous thrombosis (including starting ambulation the day after surgery) are encouraged.

When transsphenoidal surgery fails to cure a patient with pituitary-dependent Cushing syndrome, the two main treatment options are to perform another transsphenoidal surgery or to perform bilateral laparoscopic adrenalectomy. Less frequently used options are radiation therapy to the sella or pharmacotherapy to decrease adrenal cortisol production.

Plate 1-23

Pituitary and Hypothalamus

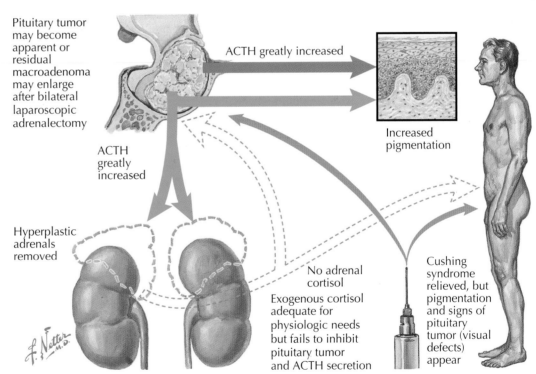

NELSON SYNDROME

Nelson syndrome is progressive pituitary corticotroph tumor enlargement after bilateral adrenalectomy is performed for the treatment of pituitary-dependent Cushing syndrome. Although the treatment of choice for a corticotroph adenoma is selective adenectomy at the time of transsphenoidal surgery (see Plate 1-22), bilateral laparoscopic adrenalectomy is indicated when pituitary surgery is not successful. When bilateral adrenalectomy cures hypercortisolism, there is less negative feedback on the corticotroph tumor cells with physiologic glucocorticoid replacement, and the adenoma may grow. Nelson syndrome occurs in a minority of patients who follow the treatment sequence of failed transsphenoidal surgery and bilateral adrenalectomy. Most corticotroph microadenomas do not enlarge over time in this setting. However, when pituitary-dependent Cushing syndrome is caused by a corticotroph macroadenoma (>10 mm in largest diameter), the risk of tumor enlargement after bilateral adrenalectomy is high.

The clinical features of Nelson syndrome are skin hyperpigmentation related to the markedly increased blood levels of pro-opiomelanocortin and corticotropin (adrenocorticotropic hormone [ACTH]) and symptoms related to mass effects of an enlarging pituitary tumor (e.g., visual field defects, oculomotor nerve palsies, hypopituitarism, and headaches). As in Addison disease (see Plate 3-22), generalized hyperpigmentation is caused by ACTH-driven increased melanin production in the epidermal melanocytes. The extensor surfaces (e.g., knees, knuckles, elbows) and other friction areas (e.g., belt line, bra straps) tend to be even more hyperpigmented. Other sites of prominent hyperpigmentation include the inner surface of the lips, buccal mucosa, gums, hard palate, recent surgical scars, areolae, freckles, and palmar creases (the latter may be a normal finding in darker-skinned individuals). The fingernails may show linear bands of darkening arising from the nail beds. Suspected Nelson syndrome can be confirmed by magnetic resonance imaging (MRI) of the sella that demonstrates an enlarging sellar mass. In addition, blood ACTH concentrations are markedly increased in this setting (e.g., >1000 pg/mL; reference range, 10–60 pg/mL).

Patients with pituitary-dependent Cushing syndrome who are treated with bilateral adrenalectomy should be monitored annually with pituitary MRI for approximately 10 years. Tumor-directed radiation therapy should be considered if tumor growth is documented on serial MRI. If feasible, gamma knife radiosurgery is the treatment of choice for Nelson corticotroph tumors. However, unlike most pituitary adenomas, these neoplasms may demonstrate aggressive growth despite radiotherapy. Extensive cavernous sinus involvement may result in multiple cranial nerve palsies. No effective pharmacologic options are available to treat this locally aggressive neoplasm. Temozolomide is being investigated as a potential treatment option for aggressive pituitary tumors or carcinoma.

Despite the concern about potential development of Nelson syndrome, clinicians should never hesitate to cure Cushing syndrome with bilateral laparoscopic adrenalectomy when transsphenoidal surgery has not been curative. Untreated Cushing syndrome can be fatal, but Nelson syndrome is usually manageable.

Plate 1-24

Endocrine System

CLINICALLY NONFUNCTIONING PITUITARY TUMOR

Clinically nonfunctioning pituitary tumors are identified either incidentally (e.g., on head magnetic resonance imaging [MRI] to evaluate unrelated symptoms) or because of sellar mass–related symptoms (e.g., visual field defect). On the basis of autopsy studies, pituitary microadenomas (≤10 mm in largest dimension) are relatively common, present in approximately 11% of all pituitary glands examined. However, pituitary macroadenomas (>10 mm in largest dimension) are uncommon. Immunohistochemical studies on resected pituitary adenomas can determine the adenohypophyseal cell of origin. The most frequent type of pituitary macroadenoma is the gonadotroph cell adenoma; most do not hypersecrete gonadotropins; thus, affected patients do not present with a hormone excess syndrome. The second most common clinically nonfunctioning pituitary macroadenoma is the null cell adenoma that is not basophilic or acidophilic (chromophobe adenoma); this is a benign neoplasm of adenohypophyseal cells that stains negatively for any anterior pituitary hormone on immunohistochemistry. Rarely, lactotroph, somatotroph, and corticotroph pituitary adenomas may be clinically silent.

The mass-effect symptoms in patients with clinically nonfunctioning pituitary macroadenomas usually prompt evaluation with head MRI. Suprasellar extension of the pituitary adenoma causes compression of the optic chiasm, resulting in the gradual onset of superior bitemporal quadrantopia that may progress to complete bitemporal hemianopsia (see Plate 1-11). Because the onset is gradual, patients may not recognize vision loss until it becomes marked. Additional mass-effect symptoms from an enlarging sellar mass include diplopia (with cavernous sinus extension and oculomotor nerve compression), varying degrees of pituitary insufficiency (related to compression of the normal pituitary gland by the macroadenoma), and headaches.

MRI is the imaging of choice to evaluate the sella and surrounding structures. MRI clearly shows the degree of suprasellar and parasellar extension of pituitary macroadenomas. All patients with pituitary macroadenomas should be assessed for tumoral hyperfunction, compression-related hypopituitarism, and visual field defects. Nonfunctioning pituitary macroadenomas are often associated with mild hyperprolactinemia (e.g., serum prolactin concentration between 30 and 200 ng/mL) because of pituitary stalk compression and prevention of hypothalamic dopamine (prolactin inhibitory factor) from reaching all of the anterior pituitary lactotrophs. Pituitary lactotrophs are the only anterior pituitary cells that are under continuous inhibitory control from the hypothalamus. Additional pituitary-related hormones that should be measured in all patients with pituitary macroadenomas include luteinizing hormone, follicle-stimulating hormone, α-subunit of glycoprotein hormones, target gonadal hormone (estrogen in women and testosterone in men), insulinlike growth factor 1, corticotropin, cortisol, thyrotropin, and free thyroxine. Diabetes insipidus is rare in patients with benign tumors of the adenohypophysis.

The goals of treatment are to correct mass-effect symptoms (e.g., vision loss) and to preserve pituitary

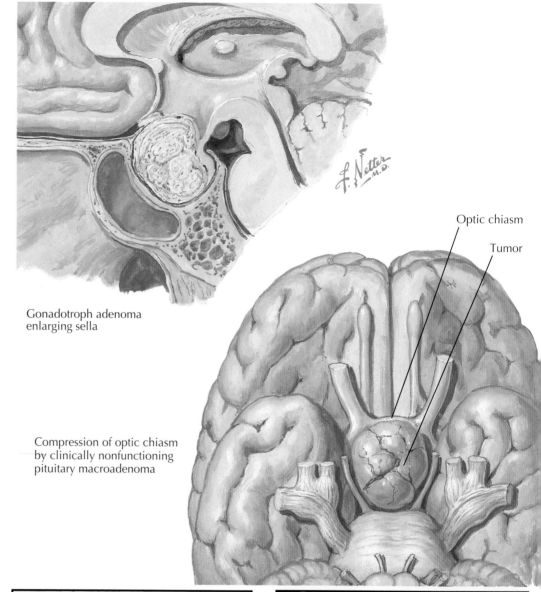

Gonadotroph adenoma enlarging sella

Compression of optic chiasm by clinically nonfunctioning pituitary macroadenoma

Optic chiasm

Tumor

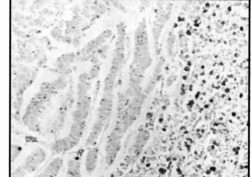

Null cell adenoma (Mann stain, ×100)

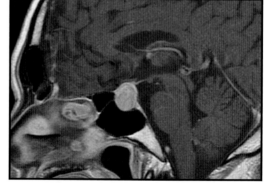

MRI (sagittal view) showing suprasellar extension of a clinically nonfunctioning pituitary macroadenoma

function. Currently, no effective pharmacologic options are available to treat patients with clinically nonfunctioning pituitary tumors. Observation is a reasonable management approach in elderly patients who have normal visual fields. However, intervention should be considered in all patients with vision loss. Transsphenoidal surgery (see Plate 1-31) can provide prompt resolution of visual field defects and a permanent cure. If present preoperatively, pituitary insufficiency may

recover in some patients after operation. Effectiveness of transsphenoidal surgery is assessed by the findings on postoperative MRI (typically performed 3 months after surgery) and by blood levels of adenoma secretory products that may have been increased before surgery (e.g., α-subunit of glycoprotein hormones). Recurrence of the pituitary adenoma after transsphenoidal surgery can be treated with stereotactic Gamma knife radiotherapy.

Plate 1-29

Pituitary and Hypothalamus

LANGERHANS CELL HISTIOCYTOSIS IN ADULTS

Langerhans cell histiocytosis (LCH)—previously known as histiocytosis-X, eosinophilic granuloma, Hand-Schüller-Christian disease, or Letterer-Siwe disease—is a disorder of the Langerhans cell, a bone marrow–derived dendritic cell that has a key role in antigen processing. Normal Langerhans cells—located in the epidermis, lymph nodes, thymic epithelium, and bronchial mucosa—process antigens and then migrate to lymphoid tissues where they function as effector cells stimulating T-cell responses. Although the cause of the defect in LCH is unknown, it is a result of immunologic dysfunction. In LCH, the Langerhans cell loses its ability to present antigens.

LCH in adults is rare, affecting one to two persons per million each year. The mean age at the time of diagnosis is 32 years. The most common presentation is dermatologic symptomatology (rash) followed by pulmonary symptoms (e.g., cough, dyspnea, tachypnea), pain (e.g., bone pain), diabetes insipidus (DI), systemic symptoms (e.g., fever, weight loss), lymphadenopathy, ataxia, and gingival hypertrophy. Because of the diverse presentation and the rarity of this disorder, LCH may not be accurately diagnosed for many years. In some cases, apparent isolated DI is diagnosed in childhood, and the other sites of involvement and associated symptoms do not develop until later in life. DI, caused by Langerhans cell infiltration of the hypothalamus and pituitary stalk, occurs in approximately 25% of patients with LCH and is irreversible.

The skin rash of LCH is papular and pigmented (red, brown). Papule size ranges from 1 mm to 1 cm. Some of the skin lesions may become ulcerated, especially in intertriginous areas.

The most common sites of bone involvement in LCH are the mandible, skull, long bones, pelvic bones, scapula, vertebral bodies, and ribs. Thus, the initial presenting symptoms in a patient with LCH may be jaw pain and loose teeth. Dental radiographs may show erosion of the lamina dura and the appearance of "floating teeth." Solitary or polyostotic eosinophilic granuloma, representing 75% of all cases of LCH, typically occur in children or young adults. These lesions present as areas of tenderness and swelling. Radiographs show round lesions with a beveled edge.

Isolated pulmonary involvement may present with pneumothorax. Pulmonary LCH is exacerbated by cigarette smoking. Chest radiographs show a diffuse infiltrate with a "honeycomb lung" appearance. Computed tomography (CT) shows typical nodules and cysts of LCH.

The diagnosis of LCH should be confirmed with a biopsy of a lesion. Pathologic examination shows a mixed cellular infiltrate with proliferation of immature clonal Langerhans cells. Other inflammatory cells (e.g., eosinophils, macrophages, granulocytes, and lymphocytes) are frequently seen in the specimen. Multinucleated giant cells may be present. The macrophages and multinucleated giant cells are phagocytic and can accumulate cholesterol and have the appearance of "foam cells." Immunohistochemical studies are confirmatory with positive staining for S100 protein, vimentin, CD1a, and antilangerin.

A full laboratory and imaging evaluation is indicated to determine the extent of disease in newly diagnosed patients. Typical laboratory tests include a complete blood cell count, liver function tests, coagulation studies, and simultaneous fasting urine and serum

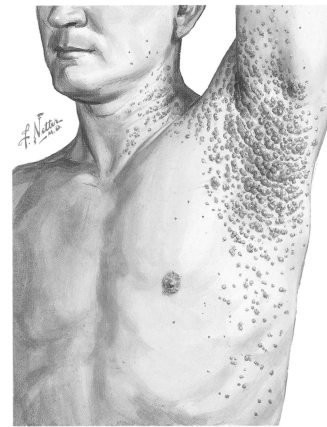

Disseminated LCH lesions in axilla and on neck and trunk

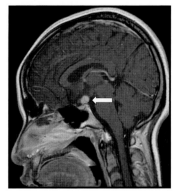

Sagittal head MRI showing a 1-cm enhancing suprasellar lesion (*arrow*) of LCH. Also note the lack of the posterior pituitary bright spot in this patient with diabetes insipidus.

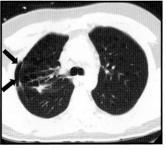

Chest CT showing multiple pulmonary cysts typical of pulmonary LCH. Also note the small pneumothorax on the right lateral chest (*arrows*).

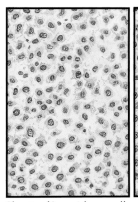
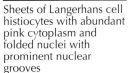

Sheets of Langerhans cell histiocytes with abundant pink cytoplasm and folded nuclei with prominent nuclear grooves

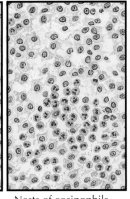

Nests of eosinophils among Langerhans cell

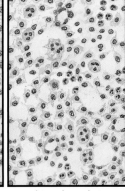

Multinucleated giant cells in granulation tissue

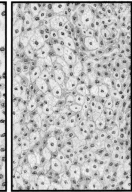

Lipid accumulation within macrophages and giant cells

osmolalities. Imaging should include a skeletal survey, skull radiography, and chest radiography. Signs and symptoms should guide whether additional tests are needed (e.g., dental radiographs, head magnetic resonance imaging [MRI], chest CT, pulmonary function tests, bone marrow biopsy).

The prognosis for patients with LCH can be predicted in part by the age of onset, number of organs involved, and degree of organ dysfunction (e.g., hyperbilirubinemia). For example, whereas an adult with a solitary bone lesion (eosinophilic granuloma) has an excellent prognosis, an infant with marked multiorgan involvement has a worse prognosis. Thus, in general, a better prognosis is associated with an age of onset older than 2 years and involvement of fewer than four organ systems.

Treatment based on prognosis stratification may include cladribine (2-chlorodeoxyadenosine) or a combination of chemotherapeutic agents (e.g., vinblastine, etoposide, methotrexate, and 6-mercaptopurine), corticosteroids (topical or systemic), and radiotherapy. Solitary bone lesions may be treated with surgical curettage, localized radiation therapy, or both. Anticytokine-based therapies are under investigation. Bone marrow transplantation may be considered for patients whose disease does not respond to standard therapies.

Plate 1-30

Endocrine System

TUMORS METASTATIC TO THE PITUITARY

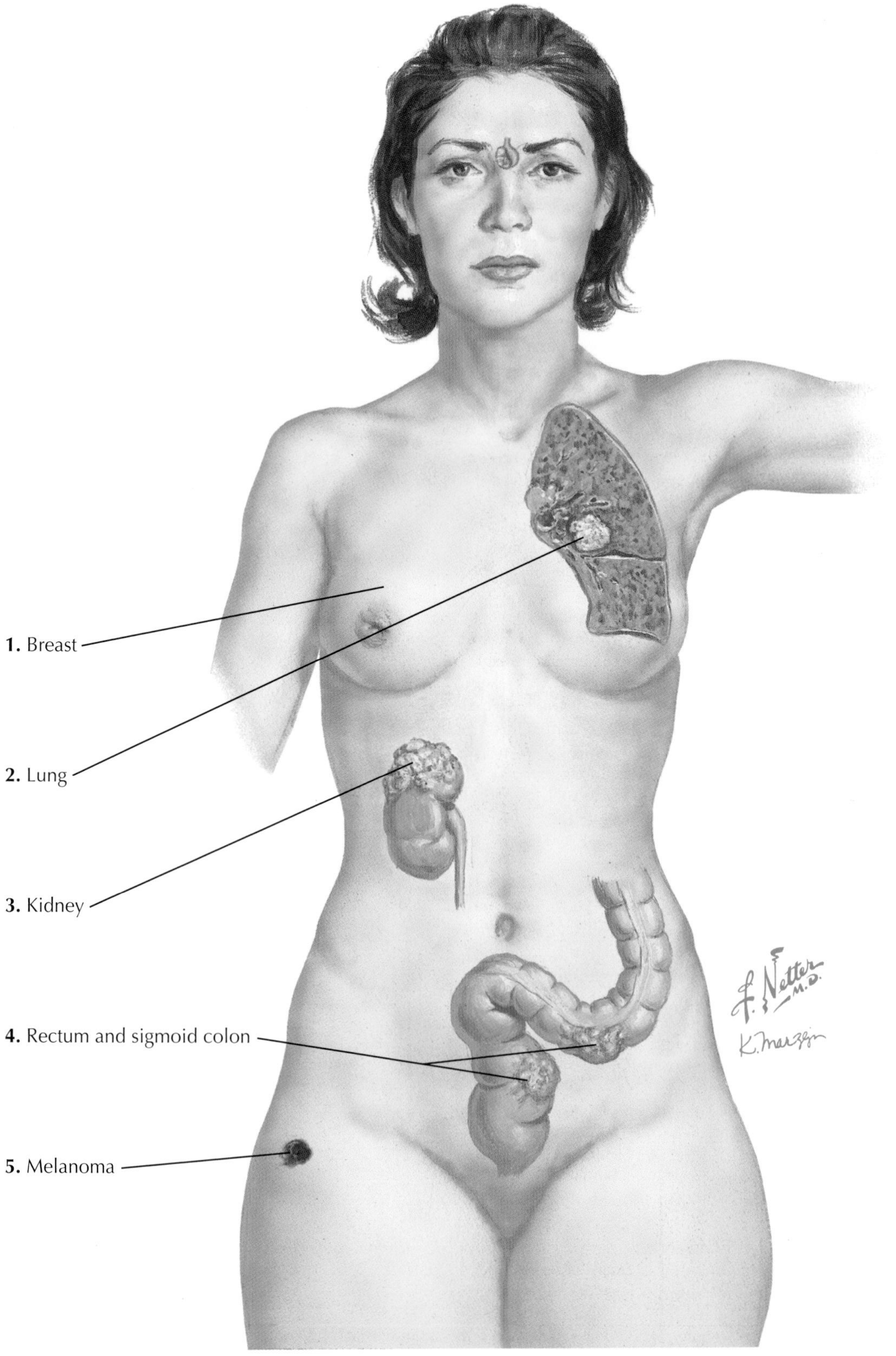

Metastasis to the pituitary gland is a rare cause of an intrasellar mass discovered during life. When the pituitary gland of patients with cancer is examined at autopsy, pituitary metastases are found in about 3.5% of patients. Most metastases to the pituitary are clinically silent and may be too small to be detected on computed imaging. When detected during life, the most common clinical presentations are diabetes insipidus (DI), visual impairment (e.g., bitemporal hemianopsia), headaches, cranial nerve deficits (e.g., palsies of cranial nerves III or IV), and varying degrees of hypopituitarism. Mild hyperprolactinemia (i.e., serum prolactin concentrations are usually <200 ng/mL) may be present and associated with an interruption of the pituitary stalk delivery of dopamine to suppress normal lactotroph production of prolactin. The most common locations for the primary malignancy (in order of frequency) are the breast, lung, kidney, colon, skin (melanoma), prostate, thyroid, stomach, pancreas, nasopharynx, lymph nodes, uterus, and liver. Breast and lung cancer account for most metastases to the pituitary. In approximately 80% of cases, the pituitary metastasis is discovered after or concurrent with the primary malignancy—the average interval is 3 years. The longest interval between the diagnosis of primary cancer and the discovery of the pituitary metastasis is found in patients with breast cancer, and the shortest interval is found in those with lung cancer. Most of these patients have metastatic disease to five or more sites in addition to the sellar region. The most common sites of extrapituitary metastases are the lymph nodes, lung, and bone.

The routes by which metastases reach the pituitary include hematogenous spread, spread from a hypothalamo–hypophyseal metastasis though the portal vessels, direct extension from parasellar sites or skull base, or meningeal spread from the suprasellar cistern. Most metastases involve the posterior lobe, presumably because of its direct arterial blood supply from the hypophyseal arteries. Because the anterior lobe does not have a direct arterial supply (see Plate 1-3), metastases that involve the anterior lobe are usually attributable to direct extension from the posterior lobe nidus.

A pituitary metastasis may closely mimic pituitary adenoma. Indeed, the clinical presentation and the neuroimaging and endocrinologic data usually suggest a nonfunctioning pituitary adenoma. Thus, metastatic disease should always be considered in the differential diagnosis of a pituitary mass. Because DI is a very unusual (<1%) component of the presentation of benign pituitary adenomas, sellar metastasis should be highly suspected when patients present with DI and a rapidly growing pituitary mass. Tissue diagnosis is required to confirm metastatic disease.

Metastatic disease to the pituitary is a poor prognostic sign; the 1-year mortality rate is 70%. Because of the poor prognosis associated with sellar metastases, the most reasonable therapeutic approaches are palliative radiotherapy, pituitary target hormone replacement therapy when indicated, and primary tumor–directed chemotherapy. Total resection is usually not possible because metastases are usually diffuse, invasive, vascular, and hemorrhagic. Surgical debulking of the sellar metastasis may be beneficial in patients with visual field defects caused by compression of the optic chiasm.

1. Breast
2. Lung
3. Kidney
4. Rectum and sigmoid colon
5. Melanoma

Plate 1-31

Pituitary and Hypothalamus

SURGICAL APPROACHES TO THE PITUITARY

The three primary goals of pituitary surgery are to (1) completely resect the pituitary adenoma so that visual field defects are corrected and the hormone excess syndrome (e.g., acromegaly, Cushing disease) is cured, (2) avoid complications (e.g., cerebrospinal fluid rhinorrhea, neurologic damage), and (3) preserve viable pituitary tissue and avoid hypopituitarism. The ability to meet these three objectives depends on the expertise of the pituitary surgeon and on the size, location, and consistency of the pituitary tumor. For example, whereas the cure rate for pituitary microadenomas (≤10 mm in diameter) is 80% to 90%, the cure rate for pituitary macroadenomas (>10 mm in diameter) is 50% to 60%. When pituitary tumors are larger than 20 mm in diameter, the surgical cure rate decreases to 20%. In addition, the location of the pituitary tumor is an important determinant of the cure rate; invasion of the cavernous sinuses usually prevents complete removal. Some tumors with marked suprasellar extension may adhere to the optic chiasm, the hypothalamus, or both, and attempting complete removal risks vision loss or hypothalamic damage. Most pituitary adenomas are soft in consistency and can be easily curetted. However, when very fibrous, complete resection is difficult.

The sublabial transseptal transsphenoidal surgical approach to the pituitary was developed in the early 1900s but was abandoned because of the high mortality rate related to infection. Up until 1969, the most common surgical approach to the sella was transfrontal craniotomy, an approach associated with clinically significant morbidity and mortality. With the development of the operative microscope and the availability of antibiotics, the sublabial transseptal transsphenoidal surgical approach to the pituitary was reintroduced in the 1970s. This approach to the sphenoid sinus involved making a sublabial incision for access to the nasal cavity and then removing the nasal septum. The sphenoid sinus was entered, allowing access to the sella turcica. After resection of the tumor, the nasal septum was replaced, requiring nasal packing postoperatively. Complications included nasal septal perforation and permanent numbness of the front teeth and upper lip. The sublabial transseptal transsphenoidal surgical approach to the sella has been replaced by the direct transnasal approaches.

The direct transnasal transsphenoidal approach—introduced in the 1990s—requires no external incision. This surgical approach can be completed with an operating microscope or with an endoscope. With the microscope-based procedure, a long, narrow speculum is placed directly into the nostril and extended to the sphenoid ostia. The mucosal incision is made at the posterior aspect of the nasal airway passage, and there is no disruption of the nasal septum. On entering the sphenoid sinus, the anterior wall of the sella is seen and opened under microscopic vision. The tumor is removed under direct microscopic view. The transnasal technique may also be completed with an endoscope. The nasal endoscope is advanced through a nostril to the anterior wall of the sphenoid sinus. The sphenoid ostium is enlarged, and the posterior portion of the vomer is removed, allowing access to the sphenoid sinus. After placement of a self-retaining nasal speculum, the sella turcica is entered, and the neurosurgical portion of the procedure is undertaken as with the sublabial transseptal approach. After resection of the

tumor, the nasal speculum is withdrawn, the nasal septum is adjusted to midline if necessary, and a mustache nasal dressing is applied. The operative time, anesthesia time, and hospital length of stay are shorter in patients who undergo the endoscopic transnasal approach to pituitary surgery than in those who undergo the sublabial transseptal procedure. Most patients are in the hospital for 1 night.

Although intraoperative complications are rare, they can be serious, and they include injury to the cavernous

carotid artery; injury to the optic pathways; injury to cranial nerves III, IV, V, and VI; and cerebrospinal fluid (CSF) leakage. Postoperatively, the potential complications include sellar hematoma, CSF rhinorrhea, meningitis, and hypopituitarism.

More than 90% of sellar and parasellar tumors can be removed with the transnasal approach. The transcranial approach is reserved for lesions that extend into the middle fossa or have a large, complex suprasellar component.

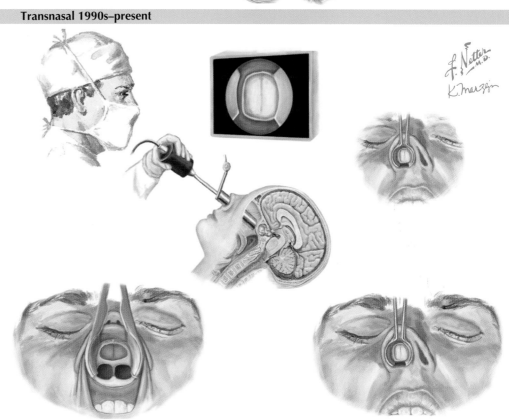

Craniotomy 1930–1960s

Transseptal 1969–1990s

Transnasal 1990s–present

Sublabial transseptal transsphenoidal surgical approach

Endoscopic transnasal transsphenoidal surgical approach

Plate 2-4

Thyroid

DEVELOPMENT OF THE THYROID AND PARATHYROID GLANDS

(Continued)

The variably occurring "pyramidal lobe of the thyroid" results from the retention and growth of the lower end of the stalk. A ligament or a band of muscle, usually located to the left of the midline, may connect the pyramidal lobe either to the thyroid cartilage or to the hyoid bone. The pyramidal lobe undergoes gradual atrophy; therefore, it is found more often in children than in adults.

Other variations of the thyroid gland are found. For example, the isthmus may be voluminous, rudimentary, or absent. The lateral lobes may be of different sizes, or both may be absent, with only the isthmic portion present. The shape of the gland may be more like that of an "H" than that of a "horseshoe." Rarely, the gland may be located at the base of the tongue (lingual thyroid) or deep to the sternum. Complete absence of the gland or failure of the gland to function is seldom noticed until a few weeks after birth because fetuses are supplied, through the placenta, with sufficient maternal thyroid hormone to permit normal development. If proper hormonal treatment is not instituted after birth, the result is congenital hypothyroidism

PARATHYROID AND THYMUS GLANDS

During the fifth and sixth weeks of development, the entodermal epithelium of the dorsal portions of the distal ends of the third and fourth pharyngeal pouches differentiates into the primordia of the parathyroid glands. At the same time, the ventral portions of the distal ends of the third pouches differentiate into the primordia of the thymus gland (see Plate 2-3C). The ventral portions of the distal ends of the fourth pouches may give rise to thymic primordia, which soon disappear without contributing to the adult thymus.

Usually, two pairs of parathyroid glands are formed. By the end of the sixth gestational week, the primordia of the parathyroids and thymus lose their connection with the pouches. At this time, the lumen of the third and fourth pouches becomes obliterated. Parathyroid tissue from the third pouch and thymic primordia migrate, during the seventh week, in a caudomedial direction. During the eighth week, the lower ends of the thymic primordia enlarge and become superficially fused together in the midline. This bilobated lower end continues to descend, to be located in the superior mediastinum of the thorax, posterior to the manubrium. During this descent, the upper ends of the thymic primordia are drawn out into tail-like extensions that usually disappear. Occasionally, they persist as fragments embedded in the thyroid gland or as isolated thymic nests or cords.

The parathyroids from the third pouch migrates with the thymic primordia and usually comes to rest at the caudal level of the thyroid gland to become the inferior parathyroid glands of the adult. Situated within the cervical fascial sheath of the thyroid, the glands are attached to the back of the proper capsule of each lateral thyroid lobe; however, each has its own proper capsule. Occasionally, parathyroid tissue descends with the thymic primordia to a lower level, being located in the thorax, close to the thymus.

The parathyroids from the fourth pouch do not shift their position appreciably; therefore, parathyroids from the third pouch pass them in their caudal migration to

a lower level. Thus, parathyroids from the fourth pouch become the superior parathyroid glands of the adult, located within the fascial sheath of the thyroid, attached to the back of the proper capsule of each lateral thyroid lobe at the level of the lower border of the cricoid cartilage. Variations in the number, size, and location of the parathyroids are common. Both the regularly occurring and accessory glands may be situated at some distance from the thyroid. The parathyroids produce

parathyroid hormone, which maintains the normal calcium and phosphorus balance.

The thymus gland is a conspicuous organ in infants. At about 2 years of age, it attains its largest relative size, continuing to grow until puberty. It undergoes a gradual involution after puberty as the thymic tissue is replaced by fat. Therefore, in adults, the thymus is of approximately the same form and size as during the earlier years, but it now consists chiefly of adipose tissue.

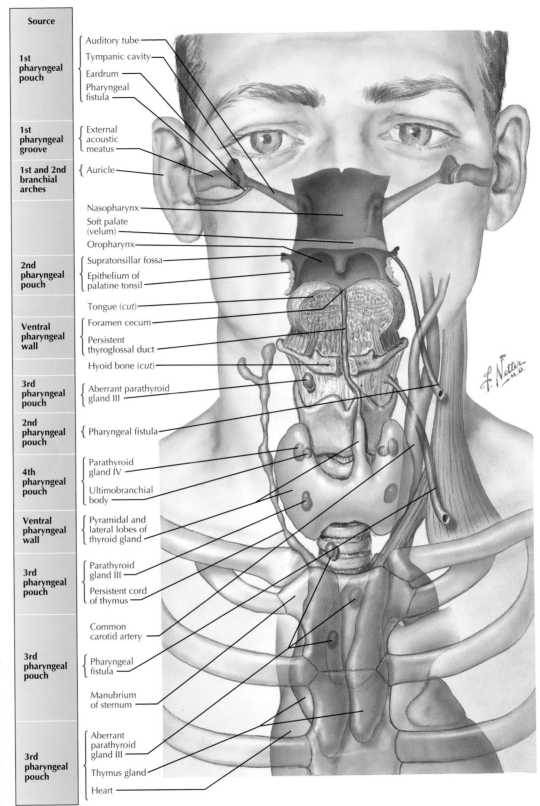

Source
1st pharyngeal pouch
1st pharyngeal groove
1st and 2nd branchial arches
2nd pharyngeal pouch
Ventral pharyngeal wall
3rd pharyngeal pouch
2nd pharyngeal pouch
4th pharyngeal pouch
Ventral pharyngeal wall
3rd pharyngeal pouch
3rd pharyngeal pouch
3rd pharyngeal pouch

Auditory tube
Tympanic cavity
Eardrum
Pharyngeal fistula
External acoustic meatus
Auricle
Nasopharynx
Soft palate (velum)
Oropharynx
Supratonsillar fossa
Epithelium of palatine tonsil
Tongue *(cut)*
Foramen cecum
Persistent thyroglossal duct
Hyoid bone *(cut)*
Aberrant parathyroid gland III
Pharyngeal fistula
Parathyroid gland IV
Ultimobranchial body
Pyramidal and lateral lobes of thyroid gland
Parathyroid gland III
Persistent cord of thymus
Common carotid artery
Pharyngeal fistula
Manubrium of sternum
Aberrant parathyroid gland III
Thymus gland
Heart

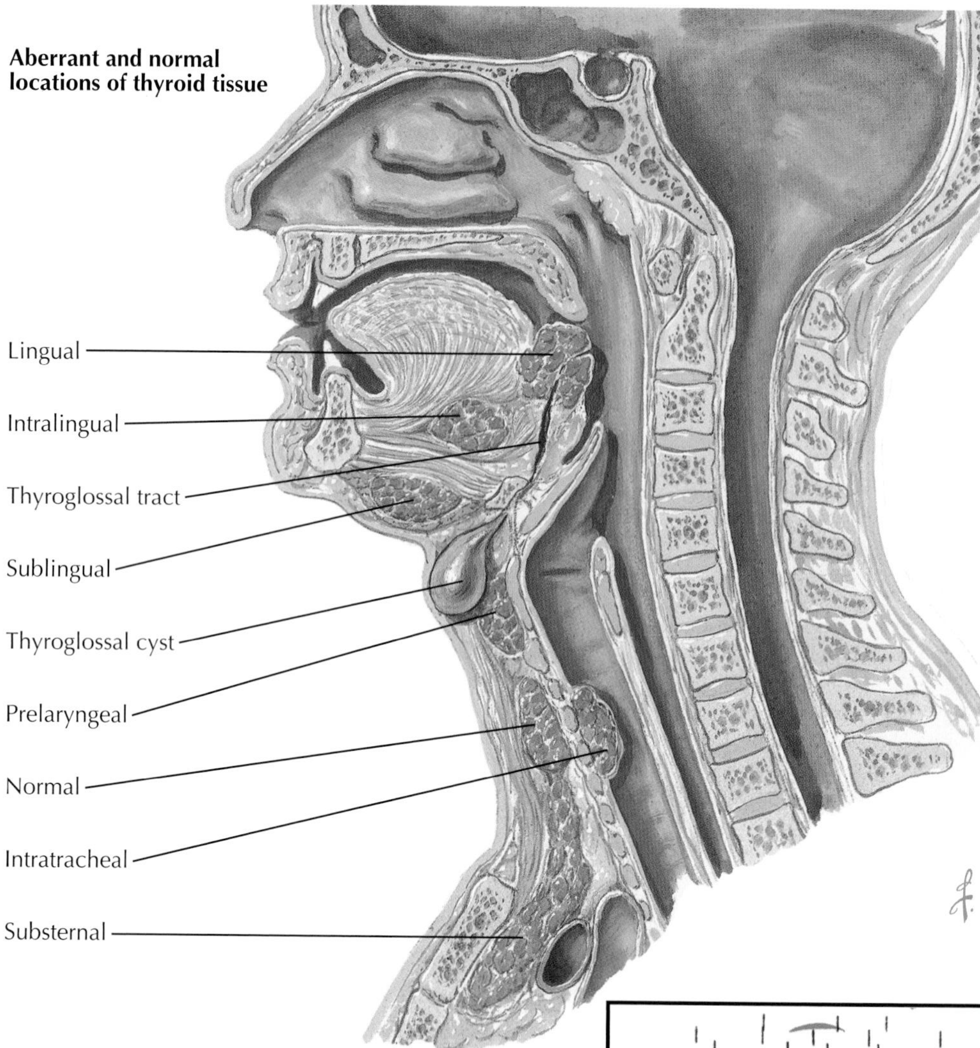

Plate 2-5   Endocrine System

Aberrant and normal
locations of thyroid tissue

Lingual
Intralingual
Thyroglossal tract
Sublingual
Thyroglossal cyst
Prelaryngeal
Normal
Intratracheal
Substernal

CONGENITAL ANOMALIES OF THE THYROID GLAND

Aberrant, or abnormal, locations of thyroid tissue may be explained on the basis of abnormal embryologic migration of the thyroid and of its close association with lateral thyroid anlagen. These abnormal settings of thyroid tissue can better be understood if one considers the embryology of the thyroid gland, which, in humans, arises about the seventeenth day of gestation and is derived from the alimentary tract. The median part of the thyroid is formed from the ventral evagination of the floor of the pharynx at the level of the first and second pharyngeal pouches. The lateral thyroid anlage, from the area of the fourth pouch, becomes incorporated into the median thyroid anlage to contribute a small proportion of the final thyroid parenchyma. The thyroid anlage becomes elongated and enlarges laterally, with the pharyngeal region contracting to become a narrow stalk—the thyroglossal tract or duct. This subsequently atrophies, leaving at its point of origin on the tongue a depression known as the foramen cecum. Normally, the thyroid continues to grow and simultaneously migrates caudally.

The anatomic sites for the location of anomalously formed thyroid tissue range from the posterior tongue down into the region of the heart, within the mediastinum. Persistence of thyroid tissue on the posterior tongue is a fairly uncommon anomaly known as lingual thyroid. This may be the only source of thyroid tissue in the individual. It can often be demonstrated with radioactive iodine scintigraphy, revealing the localization of radioiodine only within the lingual thyroid without any thyroid tissue being demonstrated in the neck.

Intralingual and sublingual rests of thyroid tissue have been described, but these are quite uncommon. The thyroglossal tract that persists usually atrophies completely. However, it may fail to atrophy, remaining as a cystic mass in the midline of the neck, somewhere between the base of the tongue and the hyoid bone. A thyroglossal cyst should therefore be considered in any individual presenting with an enlarging cystic mass immediately beneath the chin in the midline. Occasionally, such cysts may be associated with thyroid tissue capable of concentrating radioactive iodine.

Substernal aberrant thyroid, tissue in the mediastinum, is rarely the consequence of abnormal development, representing glandular rests remaining from the

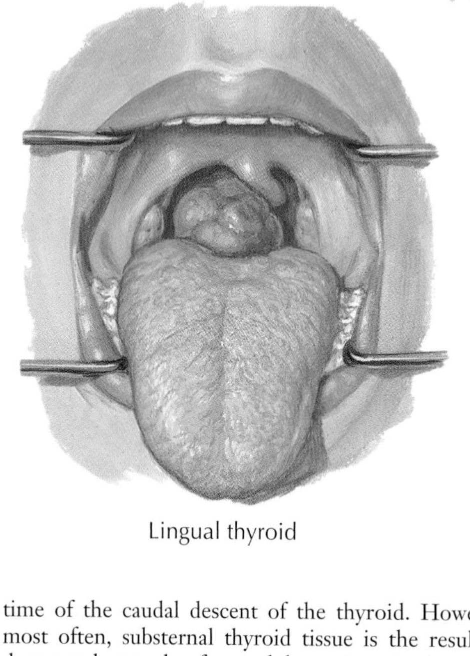

Lingual thyroid

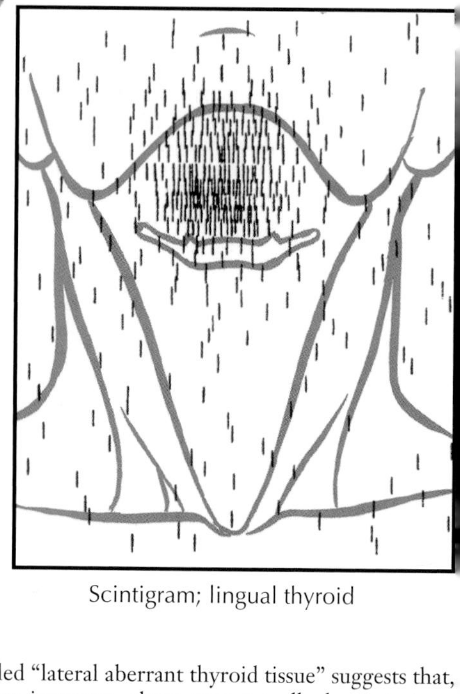

Scintigram; lingual thyroid

time of the caudal descent of the thyroid. However, most often, substernal thyroid tissue is the result of downward growth of a nodular goiter. Prelaryngeal thyroid tissue may exist, being attached to a very long pyramidal lobe or to a thyroglossal cyst. Intratracheal thyroid rests have also been reported, although infrequently. The "lateral aberrant thyroid" may represent original branchial tissue that did not fuse with the median thyroid. However, the demonstration of microscopic carcinoma in the thyroids of some patients with

so-called "lateral aberrant thyroid tissue" suggests that, in most instances, these may actually be metastases from a low-grade, well-differentiated thyroid papillary thyroid carcinoma.

The medical significance of aberrant thyroid tissue is quite limited. Occasionally, an inflammatory change or, rarely, enlargement and consequent thyrotoxicity will call for surgical or radiotherapeutic intervention. The exact interpretation of these lesions necessitates an understanding of their embryologic derivation.

Plate 2-6

Thyroid

Effects of Thyrotropin on the Thyroid Gland

The hypothalamic–pituitary unit has an indispensable role in the regulation of thyroid function. Hypothalamic dysfunction or anterior pituitary failure leads to diminished thyroid mass and decreased production and secretion of thyroid hormones. The pituitary hormone that targets the thyroid gland is the glycoprotein thyrotropin (thyroid-stimulating hormone [TSH]), which is secreted by pituitary thyrotrophs. TSH is the main regulator of the structure and function of the thyroid gland. TSH is composed of an α subunit and a β subunit. The α subunit consists of 92 amino acids, and it is identical to the α subunit of luteinizing hormone, follicle-stimulating hormone, and human chorionic gonadotropin. The β subunit of glycoprotein hormones confers specificity. The β subunit synthesized in thyrotrophs is an 112-amino acid protein. Hypothalamic thyrotropin-releasing hormone (TRH) is a modified tripeptide (pyroglutamyl-histidyl-proline-amide) that increases the transcription of both subunits, and thyroid hormones (thyroxine [T_4] and triiodothyronine [T_3]) suppress the transcription of both subunits. In healthy persons, the serum TSH concentration is between 0.3 and 5.0 mIU/L. TSH concentrations are increased in primary hypothyroidism, increased in secondary hyperthyroidism (e.g., TSH-secreting pituitary tumor), and decreased in primary hyperthyroidism. Blood TSH concentrations vary in both a pulsatile and a circadian manner—a nocturnal surge precedes the onset of sleep.

Both T_4 and T_3 mediate feedback regulation of TRH and TSH secretion. A linear inverse relationship exists between the serum free T_4 concentration and the log of the TSH. Thus, the serum TSH concentration is a very sensitive indicator of the thyroid state of patients with intact hypothalamic-pituitary function.

A TSH receptor is expressed on thyroid cells. The TSH receptor is a member of the glycoprotein G protein–coupled receptor family. The TSH receptor couples to Gs and induces a signal via the phospholipase C and intracellular calcium pathways that regulate iodide efflux, H_2O_2 production, and thyroglobulin iodination. Signaling by the protein kinase A pathways mediated by cyclic adenosine monophosphate regulates iodine uptake and transcription of thyroglobulin, thyroperoxidase, and the sodium-iodide symporter mRNAs, leading to thyroid hormone production. In addition to TSH, the TSH receptor also binds thyroid-stimulating antibody (increased in the setting of Graves disease) and thyroid-blocking antibodies (increased in the setting of Hashimoto thyroiditis). At high concentrations, the closely related glycoprotein hormones—luteinizing hormone and chorionic gonadotropin—also bind to and activate TSH receptor signaling and can cause physiologic hyperthyroidism of early pregnancy.

With an intact hypothalamic–pituitary–thyroid axis, the thyroid gland mass is normal, thyroid follicle cells

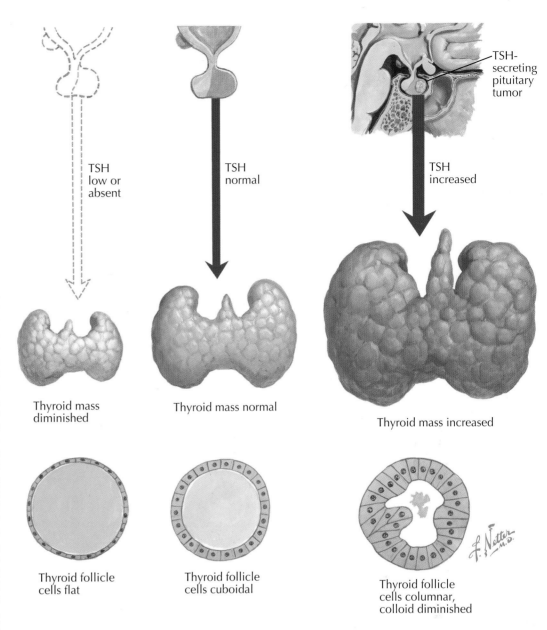

Thyroid mass diminished

Thyroid mass normal

Thyroid mass increased

Thyroid follicle cells flat

Thyroid follicle cells cuboidal

Thyroid follicle cells columnar, colloid diminished

TSH low or absent

TSH normal

TSH increased

TSH-secreting pituitary tumor

TSH: low	TSH: normal	TSH: high
Free T_4: low	Free T_4: normal	Free T_4: high
Total T_3: low	Total T_3: normal	Total T_3: high
^{131}I-uptake: low	^{131}I-uptake: normal	^{131}I-uptake: high

appear cuboidal, TSH concentration is in the reference range, free T_4 and total T_3 concentrations are in the reference range, and radioactive iodine uptake is normal. In the setting of hypothalamic or pituitary dysfunction, secondary hypothyroidism is manifest by decreased thyroid gland mass (which may not be palpable on physical examination), flat-appearing thyroid follicle cells, low TSH concentration (or inappropriately low for the low thyroid hormone levels), free T_4 and total T_3 concentrations below the reference range,

and low radioactive iodine uptake. However, in a patient with a TSH-secreting pituitary tumor, the thyroid gland mass is increased and is usually evident as a firm goiter on physical examination, thyroid follicle cells appear columnar and the colloid is diminished, TSH concentration is inappropriately within or slightly above the reference range, free T_4 and total T_3 concentrations are above the reference range, and radioactive iodine uptake is increased.

Plate 2-7

Endocrine System

PHYSIOLOGY OF THYROID HORMONES

The role of the thyroid gland in the total body economy comprises the synthesis, storage, and secretion of thyroid hormones, which are necessary for growth, development, and normal body metabolism. These thyroid functions can be considered almost synonymous with iodine metabolism. Iodination of the tyrosine molecule leads to synthesis of thyroxine (tetraiodothyronine [T_4]) and triiodothyronine (T_3).

Inorganic iodine (I^-) is rapidly absorbed in the gastrointestinal (GI) tract and circulates as iodide, until it is either trapped by the thyroid or salivary glands or excreted by the urinary tract. The thyroid extracts iodine from the plasma, against a 25-fold concentration gradient, by virtue of the sodium–iodide symporter (NIS). The function of NIS requires a sodium gradient across the basolateral membrane—the transport of 2 Na^+ ions allows the transport of 1 iodide atom. NIS also transports TcO_4^-, which is used clinically for thyroid scintigraphy, and potassium perchlorate ($KClO_4^-$), which can block thyroid iodide uptake. NIS gene transcription and protein half-life are enhanced by thyrotropin (thyroid-stimulating hormone [TSH]). Intrafollicular cell iodide is also generated by the action of iodotyrosine dehalogenase 1 isoenzyme (Dhal-1) that deiodinates monoiodotyrosine (MIT) and diiodotyrosine (DIT).

Pendrin is a glycoprotein expressed on the apical border of the thyroid follicular cell, where it facilitates the transfer of iodide into the follicular colloid. After the pendrin-facilitated iodide transfer to the colloid, iodide is oxidized by thyroid peroxidase (TPO) to facilitate the iodination of tyrosine to MIT and DIT. Antithyroid drugs (e.g., propylthiouracil, methimazole, carbimazole) inhibit the function of TPO. TPO requires H_2O_2 that is generated by thyroid oxidase 2 (THOX2), a step that is inhibited by iodide excess. The organic compounds of iodine are stored in the thyroid as part of thyroglobulin (Tg; molecular weight, 660 kDa). TPO also serves to catalyze the coupling of 2 molecules of DIT to form T_4 and 1 molecule of MIT and 1 molecule of DIT to form T_3. T_4 and T_3 are stored in the colloid as part of the Tg molecule—there are 3 to 4 T_4 molecules in each molecule of Tg. TSH stimulates the retrieval of Tg from the colloid by micropinocytosis to form phagolysosomes, where proteases free T_4, T_3, DIT, and MIT within the phagolysosome. T_4 and T_3 are then transported from the phagolysosome across the basolateral cell membrane and into the circulation. This action is inhibited by large amounts of iodine, a finding that can be used therapeutically in the treatment of patients with hyperthyroidism caused by Graves disease. DIT and MIT are deiodinated by Dhal-1, and the iodide is returned to the follicular lumen.

The ratio of T_4 to T_3 in Tg is approximately 15 to one, and when released from the follicular cell, it is approximately 10 to one (the difference reflecting the action of a 5′-deiodination). The deiodination step can be inhibited by propylthiouracil. T_4 is produced only in the thyroid gland. Although T_3 is released from the thyroid, 75% of T_3 in the body is derived from peripheral 5′-deiodination of one of the outer ring iodine atoms in T_4. T_4 and T_3 can be inactivated by inner ring (5-deiodination) to form reverse T_3 and diiodothyronine (T_2), respectively. The presence of these deiodinases in various cell types provides for local regulation of thyroid hormone effect.

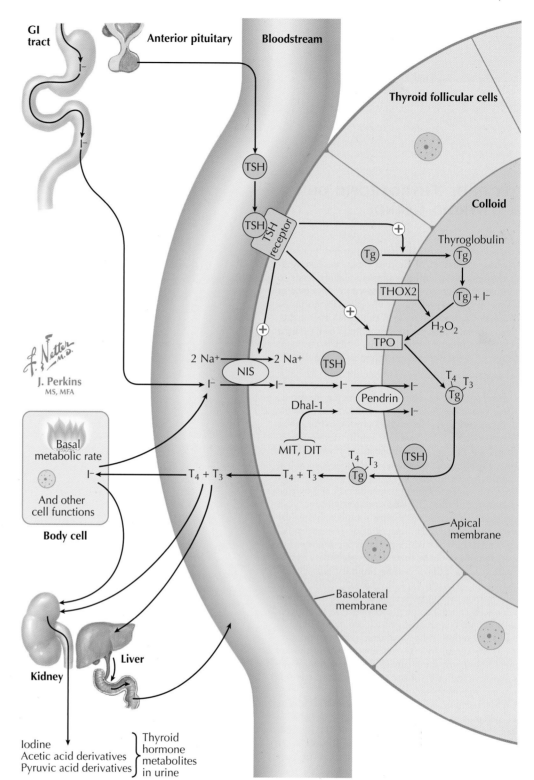

T_4 and T_3 are poorly water soluble and circulate bound to plasma proteins—thyroxine-binding globulin (TBG), T_4-binding prealbumin (transthyretin), and albumin. TBG has one iodothyronine binding site per molecule. The affinity of TBG for T_3 is 20-fold less than that for T_4.

From the thyroxine-binding proteins, T_4 and T_3 enter the body cells, where they exert their metabolic actions, which are, predominantly, calorigenic (raising the basal metabolic rate). Thyroid hormones act by binding to the thyroid hormone receptor, which, in turn, binds to DNA. T_3 has a 15-fold higher binding affinity for the thyroid hormone receptor than does T_4.

Both T_4 and T_3 are metabolized by kidney and liver tissue to their pyruvic acid and acetic acid derivatives and, eventually, to iodide. These metabolites are concentrated and conjugated in the liver to glucuronic acid, excreted with the bile, hydrolyzed in the small bowel, and reabsorbed.

The thyroid gland is unique with regard to the amount of stored hormone. There is approximately 250 µg of T_4 for every gram of thyroid gland—approximately 5 mg of T_4 in a 20-g thyroid. Thus, it is not surprising that thyrotoxicosis is common when the thyroid gland is acutely damaged by inflammation (e.g., subacute thyroiditis).

Plate 2-8

Thyroid

GRAVES DISEASE

Graves disease is an eponym that describes a thyroid autoimmune syndrome characterized by hyperthyroidism, goiter, ophthalmopathy, and occasionally an infiltrative dermopathy (pretibial or localized myxedema). Graves disease and hyperthyroidism are not synonymous because some patients with Graves disease have ophthalmopathy but not hyperthyroidism. Also, in addition to Graves disease, hyperthyroidism has several other causes. The hyperthyroidism in Graves disease is caused by autoantibodies to the thyrotropin (thyroid-stimulating hormone [TSH]) receptor that activate the receptor and stimulate the synthesis and secretion of thyroid hormones (thyroxine [T_4] and triiodothyronine [T_3]) and thyroid gland growth.

Graves disease occurs more commonly in females than in males (8:1) and more frequently during the childbearing years, although it may occur as early as in infancy and in extreme old age. Although this malady's primary signs are an enlarged thyroid gland and prominent eyes, along with cardiovascular symptoms, it actually involves most systems of the body and is thus a systemic disease. The thyroid is diffusely enlarged (goiter) and is anywhere from two to several times its normal size. Some asymmetry may be observed, the right lobe being somewhat larger than the left. The pyramidal lobe is usually enlarged. Rarely in a patient with Graves disease, there is no palpable enlargement of the thyroid gland. The gland has an increased vascularity, as evidenced by a bruit that can be heard with a stethoscope and sometimes by a thrill felt on palpation, which may be demonstrated over the upper poles. Histologically, the gland shows follicular hyperplasia with a marked loss of colloid from the follicles and an increased cell height, with high columnar acinar cells that may demonstrate papillary infolding into the follicles. Late in the disease, there may be multifocal lymphocytic (primarily T cells) infiltration throughout the thyroid gland, and, occasionally, even lymph follicles (primarily B cells) may be seen within the thyroid parenchyma.

The hyperplastic thyroid functions at a markedly accelerated pace, evidenced by an increased uptake and turnover of radioactive iodine and increased levels of T_4 and T_3, which cause an increased rate of oxygen consumption or increased basal metabolic rate and decreased serum total and high-density lipoprotein cholesterol concentrations. The increased levels of T_4 and T_3 cause a variety of physical and psychologic manifestations. Patients with this malady are usually nervous; agitated; restless; and experience insomnia, personality changes, and emotional lability. Behavioral findings include difficulty concentrating, confusion, and poor immediate recall.

On physical examination, patients with Graves disease present a fine tremor that may not be obvious but is best demonstrated by placing a paper towel on the extended fingers. The increased levels of T_4 and T_3 and the increased levels of oxygen consumption, with concomitant generalized vasodilatation, result in increased cardiac output, presenting with palpitation and sinus tachycardia. The increased stimulus to the heart action may result in atrial fibrillation and heart failure.

The skin of patients with this disease is warm and velvety (because of a decrease in the keratin layer); it may also be flushed and is often associated with marked perspiration caused by increased calorigenesis. Occasionally, vitiligo—another autoimmune manifestation—is

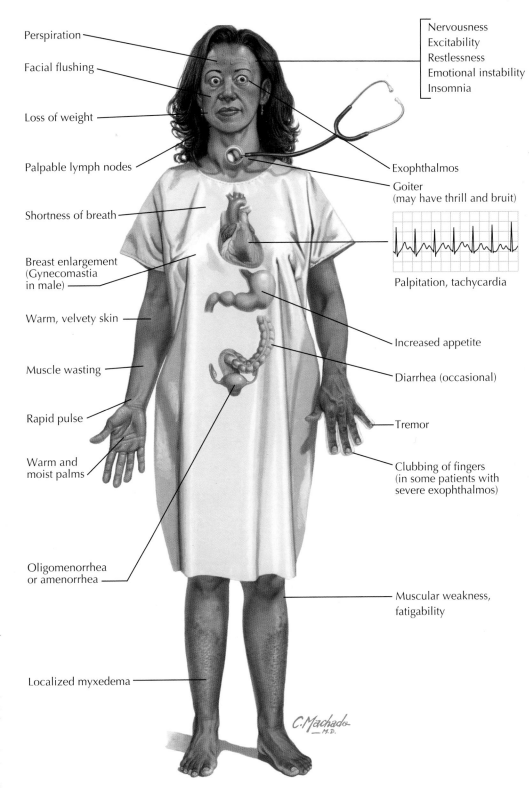

Perspiration

Facial flushing

Loss of weight

Palpable lymph nodes

Shortness of breath

Breast enlargement (Gynecomastia in male)

Warm, velvety skin

Muscle wasting

Rapid pulse

Warm and moist palms

Oligomenorrhea or amenorrhea

Localized myxedema

Nervousness
Excitability
Restlessness
Emotional instability
Insomnia

Exophthalmos

Goiter (may have thrill and bruit)

Palpitation, tachycardia

Increased appetite

Diarrhea (occasional)

Tremor

Clubbing of fingers (in some patients with severe exophthalmos)

Muscular weakness, fatigability

C. Machado M.D.

observed. Onycholysis (known as Plummer nails)—loosening of the nails from the nail bed and softening of the nails—occurs in a minority of patients with Graves disease. Infiltrative dermopathy (pretibial myxedema) is the skin change that sometimes occurs in the lower extremities or on the forearms in patients with severe progressive ophthalmopathy. This is associated with a brawny, nonpitting thickening of the skin. It presents as a rubbery, nonpitting swelling of the cutaneous and subcutaneous tissues, with a violaceous discoloration of the skin on the lower third of the legs. Usually, it is predominant in the outer half of the leg. Nodules (as large

as 1 cm in diameter) over the tibia, extending up as high as the knees, may be associated with classic localized pretibial myxedema. This lesion may also occur on the forearms, and it has been known to involve the feet and even the toes. Characteristically, hair does not grow in such myxedematous sites, but the occasional presence of hair follicles, producing hair at the site, does not exclude the diagnosis. When localized myxedema occurs, it is almost always in patients who have severe and progressive ophthalmopathy. Graves disease is also associated with clubbing of the fingers and of the toes (thyroid acropachy).

Plate 2-9

Endocrine System

GRAVES DISEASE (Continued)

Sympathetic overactivity results in a stare and eyelid lag in most patients with hyperthyroidism. Eyelid lag is demonstrated by having the patient follow the examiner's finger through a vertical arc—the sclera can usually be seen above the iris as the patient looks down. Unique to Graves disease is ophthalmopathy (see Plate 2-10).

The increased metabolic rate and calorigenesis of these patients leads to a loss of weight despite a good to increased appetite, and to wasting of certain muscles, which is associated with muscular weakness. Hyperthyroidism has mixed effects on glucose metabolism, but affected patients typically have fasting hyperglycemia. Severe hyperthyroidism may be associated with hyper-defecation and malabsorption.

In women, the total serum estradiol concentrations are increased because of increased serum sex hormone–binding globulin concentrations. However, free estradiol concentrations are low, and serum luteinizing hormone concentrations are increased—factors that lead to oligomenorrhea or even amenorrhea, which is corrected by restoring the euthyroid state. The increase in serum sex hormone–binding globulin concentrations is also observed in hyperthyroid men, reflected in high serum total testosterone concentrations, low serum free testosterone concentrations, and mild increases in serum luteinizing hormone concentrations. The aromatization of testosterone to estradiol is increased, frequently resulting in gynecomastia, decreased libido, and sexual dysfunction.

Patients with Graves disease manifest the symptoms and signs of profound muscle changes known as thyroid myopathy. Atrophy of the temporal muscles, the muscles of the shoulder girdle, and the muscles of the lower extremities—notably the quadriceps femoris group—is typical. Muscular weakness is present, and these patients are often unable to climb steps or to lift their own weight from a chair. The muscular weakness may also contribute to dyspnea. Characteristically, these patients have a tremor, and when asked to extend a leg, they manifest a marked trembling and are usually unable to hold the leg in the extended position for more than 1 minute.

Excess T_4 and T_3 stimulate bone resorption, which reduces trabecular bone volume and increases the porosity of cortical bone. The effect on cortical bone density is usually greater than that on trabecular bone density. The high bone turnover state can be confirmed by measurement of increased blood concentrations of osteocalcin and bone-specific alkaline phosphatase. In some patients, the increased bone resorption leads to hypercalcemia. The hypercalcemia inhibits parathyroid hormone secretion and the genesis of 1,25-dihydroxy-vitamin D, which leads to impaired calcium absorption and increased urinary calcium excretion. Thus, patients with long-standing hyperthyroidism are at increased risk for bone fracture and osteoporosis.

The earliest descriptions of Graves disease concerned patients who had goiters and some degree of heart failure. Characteristically, patients with hyperthyroidism report a variety of cardiac symptoms and signs. An increased heart rate is usually present. Cardiac output is increased, and those who develop heart failure present the manifestations of high-output failure characterized by a shorter than normal circulation time despite elevated venous pressure. Systolic hypertension is frequently present. Enlargement of the heart is

unusual except in a case of frank heart failure or in a patient with previous heart disease. The heart does not show any characteristic anatomic or microscopic changes that can be attributed to hyperthyroidism. The stimulus to cardiac output has been attributed to the elevated basal metabolic rate and the increased oxygen demands of the body. The usual cardiac effects of the catecholamines are accentuated by thyroid hormones, and all sympathetic activity is exaggerated in

hyperthyroidism. Atrial fibrillation occurs in approximately 15% of patients and is more common in patients older than age 60 years. In most patients, the atrial fibrillation spontaneously converts to normal sinus rhythm when euthyroidism is established. Thus, a peripheral β-adrenergic blocker will control most of the circulatory manifestations, reduce sweating, and diminish eyelid retraction—all independent of any effect on circulating levels of T_4 and T_3.

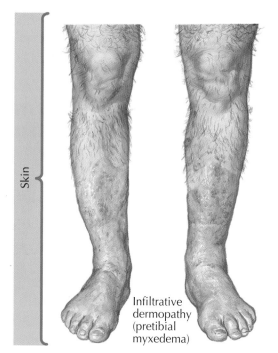

Muscles

Shoulder muscle atrophy

Temporal muscle atrophy

Eyelid lag

Tremor

Skin

Infiltrative dermopathy (pretibial myxedema)

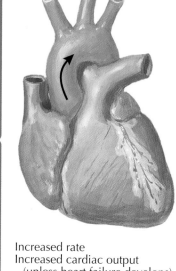

Heart

Increased rate
Increased cardiac output (unless heart failure develops)
Usually little or no enlargement

Plate 2-10

Thyroid

GRAVES OPHTHALMOPATHY

Graves ophthalmopathy is an autoimmune disease of the retro-orbital tissues, and the eye signs, of which proptosis and periorbital edema are the most common, vary in degree from mild to extremely severe and progressive.

Most patients with hyperthyroidism (regardless of the cause) have retraction of the eyelids (caused by contraction of the eyelid levator palpebrae muscles), which leads to widened palpebral fissures and a stare. Although the stare may give the appearance of proptosis, it must be confirmed with an exophthalmometer (see following text). Frequently, an eyelid lag can be demonstrated. This is a failure of the upper eyelid to maintain its position relative to the globe as the gaze is directed downward. There also may be globe lag—the eyelid moves upward more rapidly than does the globe as the patient looks upward. The eyelid retraction and eyelid lag regress after correction of the hyperthyroidism.

Graves ophthalmopathy includes varying degrees of additional findings such as true proptosis, conjunctival injection, conjunctival edema (chemosis), periorbital edema, weakness of convergence, and palsy of one or more extraocular muscles. Patients often report increased lacrimation (aggravated by bright light, wind, or cold air), a sandy feeling in the eyes, and an uncomfortable sense of fullness in the orbits. When the patient is requested to look in one direction or another, a significant weakness of one or more of the extraocular muscles may be noted. The patient may complain of blurred vision, or even of diplopia on looking either upward or to the side.

If the distance, measured with an exophthalmometer, from the canthus to the front of the cornea exceeds 20 mm in white patients and 22 mm in black patients, proptosis is present. The proptosis may be asymmetric, and it may be masked by periorbital edema. Testing the eye and the orbital contents for resiliency to pressure is also useful. This is done by applying the fingers to the eyeball over the closed eyelid and attempting to move the eyeball backward. Normally, the eyeball can be pushed back easily and without resistance; in patients with severe ophthalmopathy, however, a significant decrease in resiliency is evident, and in some patients, it is impossible to push the eyeball back at all—a poor prognostic sign of progressive ophthalmopathy. The progression may be so rapid and extensive that the eyelids cannot be closed over the eyes, so that ulcerations of the cornea may result. These ulcerations may become infected and may even lead to loss of the eye. Rarely, the optic nerve may be involved by papilledema, papillitis, or retrobulbar neuritis, causing blindness.

The pathogenesis of Graves ophthalmopathy is related to an increased volume in the retro-orbital space—the extraocular muscles and retro-orbital connective and adipose tissues—because of inflammation and the accumulation of hydrophilic glycosaminoglycans (GAGs) (e.g., hyaluronic acid). As GAGs accumulate in these tissues, a change in osmotic pressure and an increase in fluid content displace the globes forward and compromise the function of the extraocular muscles. The extraocular muscles are swollen and infiltrated with T lymphocytes—the latter also probably play a key role in the pathogenesis of this disorder. T cells appear to be activated by the thyrotropin (thyroid-stimulating hormone [TSH]) receptor antigen. There is a positive correlation between the severity of

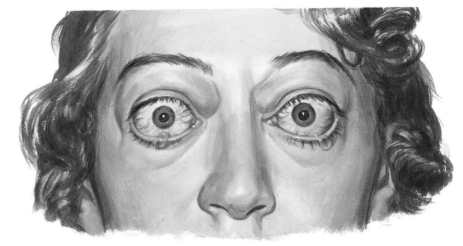

Moderately severe ophthalmopathy

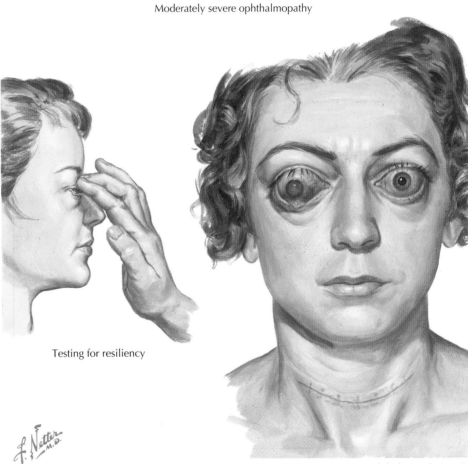

Testing for resiliency

Severe progressive ophthalmopathy

ophthalmopathy and serum TSH receptor antibody concentrations.

In addition to a high titer of TSH receptor antibodies, several other risk factors for the development of ophthalmopathy in patients with Graves disease have been identified. Graves eye disease is more common in women, as is hyperthyroidism. However, when present, men appear to have more severe ophthalmopathy than women. Cigarette smoking has been clearly shown to increase both the risk for and the severity of ophthalmopathy. Cigarette smoke appears to increase GAG production and adipogenesis. Radioiodine therapy for hyperthyroidism appears to trigger or worsen ophthalmopathy more than subtotal thyroidectomy or antithyroid drug therapy. Although treating hyperthyroidism decreases the eyelid retraction, it does not improve

Graves ophthalmopathy. Finally, there is a temporal relationship between the Graves eye disease and the onset of hyperthyroidism. Ophthalmopathy appears before the onset of hyperthyroidism in 20% of patients, concurrently in 40%, when hyperthyroidism is treated in 20%, and in the 6 months after diagnosis in 20%.

Most patients can be successfully treated by raising the head of the bed at night, using saline eye drops frequently through the day, and wearing sunglasses when outside. In patients with more severe symptoms (e.g., chemosis, diplopia), glucocorticoid therapy should be considered. Orbital decompression surgery should be considered if the ophthalmopathy progresses despite glucocorticoid therapy, if vision is threatened, or if there is a cosmetic reason in patients with severe proptosis.

Plate 2-11

Endocrine System

THYROID PATHOLOGY IN GRAVES DISEASE

In patients with Graves disease, the most dramatic anatomic changes are those found in the thyroid gland, although characteristic changes in organs other than the thyroid also occur. The thyroid, which in healthy adults weighs between 15 and 20 g, is usually two to four times its normal size in patients with Graves disease. In extreme situations, it may be as large as 10 times the normal size. Rarely, patients with Graves disease do not have any significant enlargement of the thyroid gland. Diffuse enlargement and engorgement of the thyroid occur in a more or less symmetric fashion. These features can very well be demonstrated by scintigraphy of the thyroid after the administration of a test dose of radioactive iodine. As shown here, the thyroids of such patients concentrate radioactive iodine very diffusely and evenly. Notwithstanding the diffuseness of the process and the apparent symmetry of the thyroid, some surgeons have called attention to the fact that one lobe may be somewhat larger, although minimally so, than the other. Characteristically, the pyramidal lobe, which extends above the isthmus on one or the other side of the trachea, is enlarged enough to be easily palpable. The enlarged thyroid gland is firm, smooth, and rubbery to palpation. Typically, it is very vascular, as evidenced by an audible bruit (which may be heard usually over the superior poles of either lobe) and, in some instances, by a palpable thrill over the lateral lobes. The untreated thyroid gland, being vascular and friable in this disease, can be a source of serious bleeding during surgery.

Histologic examination of the untreated thyroid reveals a very characteristic microscopic picture of diffuse hyperplasia. Usually, the colloid is completely lost from within the follicle. Any colloid that remains is pale-staining and demonstrates marginal scalloping and vacuolization. The thyroid cells are hypertrophied and hyperplastic. The acinar cells, which are normally low cuboidal, become high cuboidal or columnar and, by measurement, may be more than twice as high as those in the normal thyroid gland. In some instances, the hyperplasia of the acinar cells is so great that an intra-acinar papillary infolding takes place.

Along with the marked hyperplasia, there is a pronounced increase in avidity for radioactive iodine. Whereas the normal iodine uptake is 3% to 16% at 6 hours and 8% to 25% at 24 hours, in patients with Graves disease, it is nearly always more than 50% and may be as great as 80% or 90%.

In a small number of patients with long-standing Graves disease, hyperplasia is accompanied by significant to extensive lymphocytic infiltration (most are T lymphocytes) of the thyroid parenchyma, occasionally with large lymph follicles being present. The degree of lymphocytic infiltration may be decreased by antithyroid drug therapy. The size of the follicular epithelial

cells correlates with the intensity of the local lymphocytic infiltrate, implicating local thyroid cell stimulation by thyrotropin receptor antibodies.

Other anatomic and functional changes include those in the eyes, skin, skeletal muscles, nervous system, heart, liver, thymus, and lymphoid tissues. The eyes are frequently proptosed; associated with this condition are enlarged, edematous extraocular muscles with increased fluid and fat in the retro-orbital space (see Plate 2-10). These muscles and the skeletal muscles

show edema, round cell infiltration, hyalinization, fragmentation, and destruction. Hyperthyroidism can affect the central and peripheral nervous systems—most of these represent direct or indirect effects of thyrotoxicosis. Other nervous system effects are related to the autoimmune nature of Graves disease (e.g., myasthenia gravis). The heart may be somewhat enlarged, but it does not present any characteristic or classic pathologic changes. Characteristically, the thymus and lymphoid tissues are enlarged, displaying simple hypertrophy.

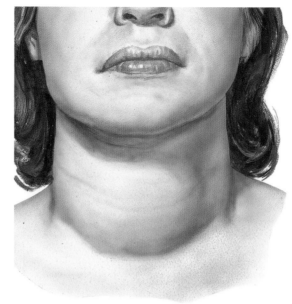

Diffuse goiter of moderate size

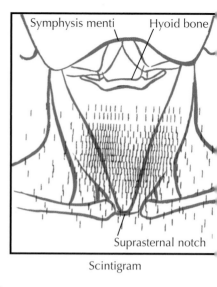

Scintigram

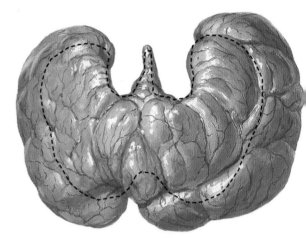

Diffuse enlargement and engorgement of thyroid gland (*broken line* indicates normal size of gland)

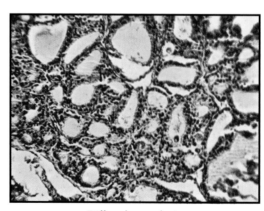

Diffuse hyperplasia

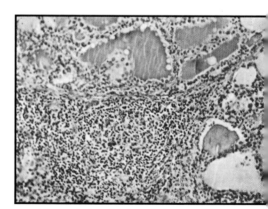

Hyperplasia with lymphocytic infiltration

Plate 2-12

Thyroid

CLINICAL MANIFESTATIONS OF TOXIC ADENOMA AND TOXIC MULTINODULAR GOITER

The hyperthyroidism associated with toxic adenomas and toxic multinodular goiters is caused by hyperfunctioning adenoma(s), which are the most common cause of hyperthyroidism after Graves disease. Hyperthyroidism is caused by nodular hyperplasia of thyroid follicular cells that is independent of thyrotropin (thyroid-stimulating hormone [TSH]) regulation. The clinical picture of this type of hyperthyroidism differs in important ways from that observed in patients with Graves disease. Patients with adenomatous goiters with hyperthyroidism are usually older than 40 years. They often give a history of having had either a multinodular thyroid or a single nodule in the thyroid for a long time. As a rule, they have cardiovascular symptoms, and frequently they have been referred to a cardiologist before being sent to an endocrinologist. They describe marked shortness of breath and have tachycardia, frequently with atrial fibrillation. When in heart failure, they may manifest all the signs and symptoms of this disease except that they usually do not have an increased circulation time, as in Graves disease. Characteristically, these patients do not have ophthalmopathy. Rarely, one may observe a minimal eyelid retraction or even a minimal eyelid lag. There is no thyroid acropachy or pretibial myxedema. Patients with this type of hyperthyroidism have less of the muscular weakness so characteristic of Graves disease. The basal metabolic rate is not as markedly elevated as it is in Graves disease, and these patients are not especially nervous or excitable. Typically, they do not show signs of marked weight loss or of muscle wasting, both of which are striking in Graves disease. Because a large percentage of affected female patients are postmenopausal, changes in the menstrual cycle, often seen in Graves disease, are not present.

The pathogenesis of a toxic adenoma and toxic multinodular goiter is frequently associated with activating somatic mutations in the gene encoding the TSH receptor. Toxic multinodular goiter tends to be more common in geographic areas where iodine intake is relatively low, but the incidence of solitary toxic thyroid adenomas does not seem to be affected by iodine intake.

Patients with this malady have a moderate elevation in serum free thyroxine (T_4) and total triiodothyronine (T_3) concentrations. The serum total and high-density lipoprotein (HDL) cholesterol concentrations are slightly decreased.

Studies with radioactive iodine are highly useful in examining these patients, especially if the site of radioactive iodine concentration is localized. Although the uptake of radioactive iodine may not be as great as is observed in classic Graves disease, in this malady, the radioactive iodine is usually concentrated primarily in the hyperfunctioning adenoma, with practically none in the remainder of the thyroid gland. However, in patients with toxic multinodular goiter, typically one or more focal areas of increased radioiodine uptake are found; nonfunctioning (or "cold") nodules are also evident in some of these patients.

Effective treatment of hyperthyroidism is aimed at both symptomatic relief and decreasing the excess production of thyroid hormone. β-Adrenergic blockers control many of the hypermetabolic-type symptoms of hyperthyroidism. The treatment options to normalize

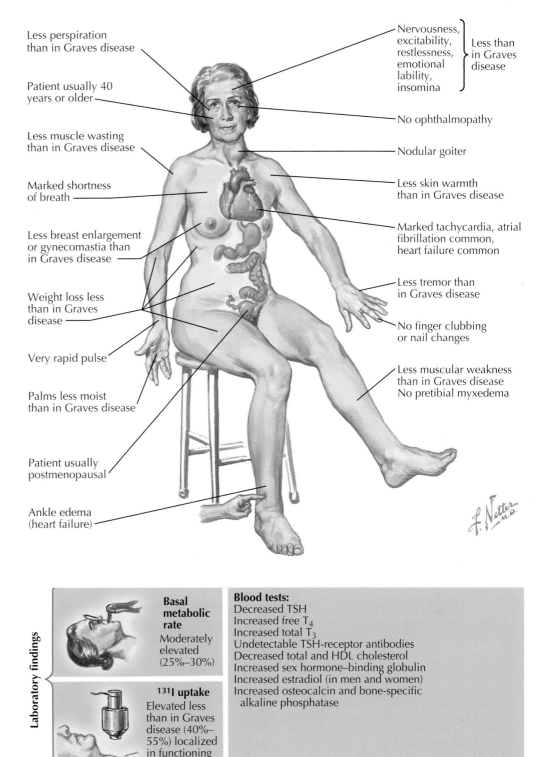

Less perspiration than in Graves disease

Patient usually 40 years or older

Less muscle wasting than in Graves disease

Marked shortness of breath

Less breast enlargement or gynecomastia than in Graves disease

Weight loss less than in Graves disease

Very rapid pulse

Palms less moist than in Graves disease

Patient usually postmenopausal

Ankle edema (heart failure)

Nervousness, excitability, restlessness, emotional lability, insomina } Less than in Graves disease

No ophthalmopathy

Nodular goiter

Less skin warmth than in Graves disease

Marked tachycardia, atrial fibrillation common, heart failure common

Less tremor than in Graves disease

No finger clubbing or nail changes

Less muscular weakness than in Graves disease. No pretibial myxedema

Laboratory findings

Basal metabolic rate
Moderately elevated (25%–30%)

131I uptake
Elevated less than in Graves disease (40%–55%) localized in functioning adenoma

Blood tests:
Decreased TSH
Increased free T_4
Increased total T_3
Undetectable TSH-receptor antibodies
Decreased total and HDL cholesterol
Increased sex hormone–binding globulin
Increased estradiol (in men and women)
Increased osteocalcin and bone-specific alkaline phosphatase

T_4 and T_3 excess include thionamide administration, radioiodine administration, or surgery.

Thionamides (methimazole and propylthiouracil) are frequently used as the initial treatment of choice in patients who are elderly and have underlying cardiovascular disease. However, unlike Graves hyperthyroidism, which may go into long-term remission after the thionamide is discontinued, hyperthyroidism associated with toxic nodules and toxic multinodular goiters recurs when thionamide therapy is discontinued. The goal of thionamide therapy is to achieve a euthyroid state before definitive therapy (e.g., radioiodine or surgery).

Patients who are young and healthy usually do not need thionamide treatment before definitive therapy. A permanent cure can be achieved with radioiodine; it causes extensive tissue damage and destroys the adenoma or autonomous foci within 2 to 4 months after treatment. However, because the radioiodine is taken up primarily by the hyperfunctioning nodules and intervening normal thyroid tissue is quiescent, most patients are euthyroid after radioiodine therapy. Because the cure rate of radioiodine therapy decreases with very large toxic multinodular goiters, surgery is the treatment of choice for this subset of patients.

Plate 2-13

Endocrine System

PATHOPHYSIOLOGY OF TOXIC ADENOMA AND TOXIC MULTINODULAR GOITER

Hyperthyroidism arising in a hyperfunctioning adenoma(s) of the thyroid is the second most common cause of hyperthyroidism. This syndrome usually occurs in patients who previously had nontoxic nodular goiters. In the most clear-cut and classic setting, the patient, usually a middle-aged woman, presents with cardiovascular symptoms varying from complaints of palpitation and dyspnea to the picture of chronic atrial fibrillation and frank heart failure. The heart failure of hyperthyroidism exhibits a few characteristic features that should direct the physician to an investigation of the thyroid. Such patients have high-output failure with a decreased circulation time despite an elevated venous pressure. Other extrathyroidal pathology in patients with hyperthyroidism arising from hyperfunctioning adenomas of the thyroid is uncommon. Patients do not develop the typical eye signs, thyroid acropachy, or pretibial myxedema of Graves disease. These patients do not have the muscle weakness so characteristic of Graves disease.

Pathologically, the most classic feature of this disease is that found in the patient with a rare "single" hyperfunctioning adenoma of the thyroid, which may be significantly enlarged while the rest of the thyroid gland remains uninvolved. No palpable nodules are present in the remainder of the gland, which may actually be smaller than normal. In such unique situations, the examiner may be impressed by the small size or the impalpability of the unaffected lobe, as contrasted with the large, single nodule in the opposite lobe. It is extremely uncommon to hear a bruit or to detect a thrill over a hyperfunctioning adenoma of the thyroid. If a test dose of radioactive iodine is administered to the patient and a scintigram is made over the neck at 24 hours, all the radioactive iodine will be found in the nodule, the remainder of the gland having concentrated none.

Grossly, whereas the nodule may be red, the rest of the gland is pale in color.

Histologic examination of the hyperfunctioning adenoma demonstrates a uniform hypertrophy and hyperplasia of the acinar cells. Some papillary infolding may be present, although this is much less common than in the diffusely hyperplastic gland of Graves disease. Lymphocytic infiltration is not found in this type of hyperplastic thyroid lesion. The remainder of the gland shows involution. If the acinar cells are measured, the cell height will be uniformly increased, averaging around 12 to 14 μm, whereas the cell height of the uninvolved tissue may be less than that of a normal thyroid, averaging around 5 to 6 μm.

The toxic adenoma is a true follicular adenoma that has one of several somatic point mutations in the gene encoding the thyrotropin (thyroid-stimulating hormone [TSH]) receptor, which lead to constitutive activation of the TSH receptor in the absence of TSH.

The more common type of hyperfunctioning adenomatous goiter, the "multinodular" type, occurs in patients who had a long-standing multinodular goiter before developing hyperthyroidism, with a number of adenomas within the gland. Some of these nodules may

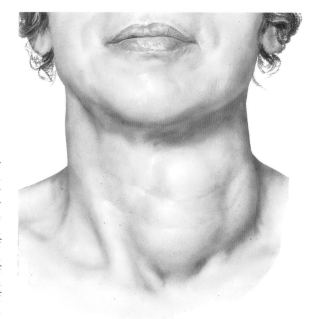

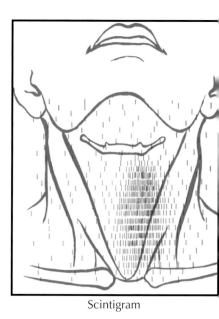

Hyperfunctioning adenoma

Scintigram

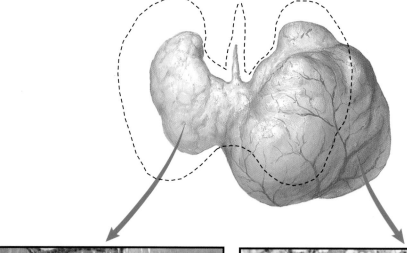

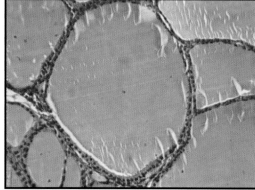

Remainder of gland—involution

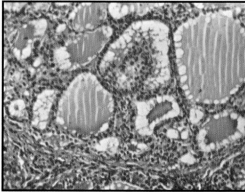

Adenoma—hyperplasia

be highly undifferentiated adenomas, and, rarely, even a cancerous lesion may be found within one of the nodules. If all multinodular thyroids could be examined, it is quite possible that in many of them, the structure of undifferentiated adenomas would be present; others would show varying degrees of differentiation; and a few would exhibit the structure of a well-differentiated, functional adenoma.

The somatic mutations in the TSH receptor gene found in solitary toxic nodules may also be seen in some cases of toxic multinodular goiter but may differ from one nodule to another. Radioiodine scans show localization of isotope in more than one of the nodules; iodine uptake in the rest of the gland is usually suppressed. Histopathologic examination shows that the functioning areas resemble adenomas and are distinct from the surrounding tissue. These multinodular thyroid glands contain multiple solitary hyperfunctioning and hypofunctioning adenomas in the midst of suppressed normal thyroid tissue.

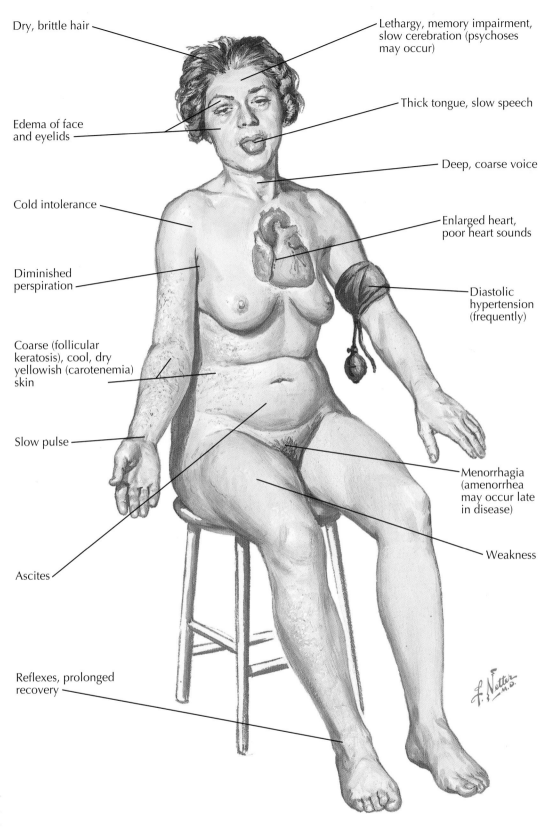

Dry, brittle hair

Lethargy, memory impairment, slow cerebration (psychoses may occur)

Thick tongue, slow speech

Edema of face and eyelids

Deep, coarse voice

Cold intolerance

Enlarged heart, poor heart sounds

Diminished perspiration

Diastolic hypertension (frequently)

Coarse (follicular keratosis), cool, dry yellowish (carotenemia) skin

Slow pulse

Menorrhagia (amenorrhea may occur late in disease)

Weakness

Ascites

Reflexes, prolonged recovery

CLINICAL MANIFESTATIONS OF HYPOTHYROIDISM IN ADULTS

SYMPTOMS AND SIGNS

Primary hypothyroidism, although not described until 1874, is a common endocrine disorder that occurs about seven or eight times more often in females than in males. The clinical presentation of hypothyroidism depends on the degree of thyroid hormone deficiency and the rapidity of the loss of the thyroid hormones, thyroxine (T_4) and triiodothyronine (T_3). Patients with gradual onset of hypothyroidism may not be diagnosed for many years—patients often attribute the signs and symptoms to aging. In addition, the clinical presentation of hypothyroidism may be affected by coexisting morbidities. For example, in patients with hypothyroidism caused by hypothalamic or pituitary disease, the presentation may be dominated by the signs and symptoms of secondary adrenal failure, hypogonadism, or diabetes insipidus.

The basis of the pathophysiology of hypothyroidism can be thought of as the "slowing down" of most metabolic processes. Patients may be lethargic with slow cerebration, slow speech patterns, cold intolerance, constipation, and bradycardia. These patients typically have dry, brittle hair, which, if previously curly, loses its curl. Individuals with profound hypothyroidism may actually manifest many psychotic features, which have been labeled "myxedema madness." The edema of the face and eyelids (periorbital edema) is associated with the subcutaneous accumulation of glycosaminoglycans. The tongue is thick, and the voice is deep and coarse, with a relative lack of inflection.

The skin is cool and dry because of diminished perspiration and may be coarse. Often, a sandpapery follicular hyperkeratosis occurs over the extensor surfaces of the arms and elbows, frequently on the lateral thoracic wall and over the lateral thighs, and occasionally over the shoulders. The skin of the hands or face frequently acquires a yellowish color, suggesting carotenemia. The fingernails may be brittle and chip easily. Loss of hair of the lateral third of the eyebrows is frequently observed. Vitiligo and alopecia may be present in patients with autoimmune polyglandular failure.

Patients with hypothyroidism generally have a slow pulse and diastolic hypertension; the latter is associated with increased peripheral vascular resistance. Cardiac output is decreased, and patients may note dyspnea on exertion. A typical feature in patients with marked and long-standing primary hypothyroidism is diffuse cardiac enlargement owing to myxedematous fluid in the myocardium and to pericardial effusions, which may also be associated with pleural effusions and even with ascites. Heart sounds are distant. There is a decreased rate of cholesterol metabolism that leads to hypercholesterolemia.

Respiratory muscle weakness may contribute to dyspnea on exertion. Some of these patients may have hypoxia and hypercapnia. Macroglossia may contribute to obstructive sleep apnea.

Younger female patients may have menorrhagia severe enough to require surgical curettage. Later in the disease, reversible secondary amenorrhea may occur. Hyperprolactinemia and galactorrhea may be seen in women with primary hypothyroidism, in whom increased hypothalamic thyrotropin (thyroid-stimulating hormone [TSH])–releasing hormone secretion can stimulate prolactin release from pituitary lactotrophs.

Plate 2-15

Endocrine System

CLINICAL MANIFESTATIONS OF HYPOTHYROIDISM IN ADULTS
(Continued)

Neurologic findings include a prolonged relaxation phase of the ankle jerk reflex and generalized weakness. Carpal tunnel syndrome is fairly common in these patients. Myxedema coma—a rare complication—should be considered in patients who have hyponatremia, hypercapnia, and hypothermia. Myxedema coma may be triggered in patients with severe hypothyroidism by the administration of opiates or by infection or trauma.

Hypochromic anemia, if present, may be of any type—microcytic or normocytic. Occasionally, normochromic macrocytic anemia is found. If the patient has polyglandular failure, pernicious anemia may be present. The menorrhagia seen in hypothyroid premenopausal women may lead to iron-deficiency anemia. Decreased free water clearance may result in hyponatremia.

Primary hypothyroidism (resulting from disease of the thyroid gland itself) must be distinguished from central hypothyroidism (resulting from disease of the pituitary gland or hypothalamus). Some signs and symptoms may provide clues as to the cause of hypothyroidism. The history of patients with the latter disease often includes severe postpartum hemorrhage followed by absence of lactation and failure of the menstrual cycle to return after recovery from the postpartum period. Usually, the picture of myxedema does not develop until some time after the first sign of pituitary insufficiency (e.g., amenorrhea without hot flushes). These individuals usually describe extreme weakness, somnolence, intolerance to the cold, impaired memory, and slow cerebration. On physical examination, they differ from patients with primary hypothyroidism if they lack other pituitary hormones. Thus, patients with central hypothyroidism may also have finer, softer hair; loss of axillary and pubic hair; a small heart (in contrast to the enlarged heart of patients with primary myxedema); some degree of hypotension; and skin that is less dry and not scaly.

Although findings on the history and physical examination provide the clinician with clues regarding primary vs central hypothyroidism, serum TSH and free T_4 concentrations are the key tests. In primary hypothyroidism, the serum TSH concentration is above the reference range, and the blood concentration of free T_4 is usually below the lower limit of the reference range. In central hypothyroidism caused by hypothalamic or pituitary dysfunction, the serum TSH concentration is inappropriately low for the low level of free T_4. Radioactive iodine uptake is low in both types of hypothyroidism.

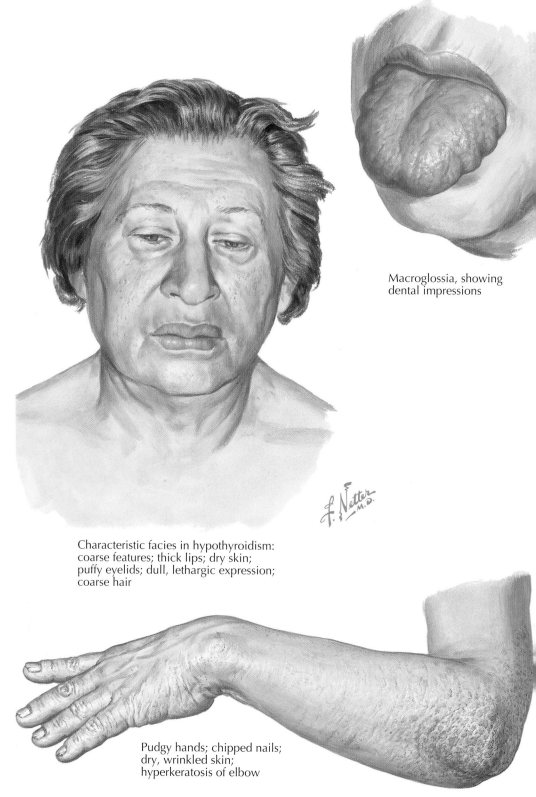

Macroglossia, showing dental impressions

Characteristic facies in hypothyroidism: coarse features; thick lips; dry skin; puffy eyelids; dull, lethargic expression; coarse hair

Pudgy hands; chipped nails; dry, wrinkled skin; hyperkeratosis of elbow

ETIOLOGY

Primary hypothyroidism, with deficient secretion of the thyroid hormones T_4 and T_3, is the most common cause of hypothyroidism. This may result from destruction or removal of the thyroid gland or from thyroid gland atrophy and subsequent replacement by fibrous tissue. Primary hypothyroidism may also develop with goiters, which are incapable of synthesizing thyroid hormone either because of the administration of some agent that inhibits the organification of iodine or because of some defect in the enzymes necessary for the synthesis of thyroid hormone. It may also result from autoimmune chronic thyroiditis, such as Hashimoto thyroiditis. Central hypothyroidism is caused by a process that inhibits release of TSH-releasing hormone from the hypothalamus or TSH release from the pituitary.

Plate 2-16

Thyroid

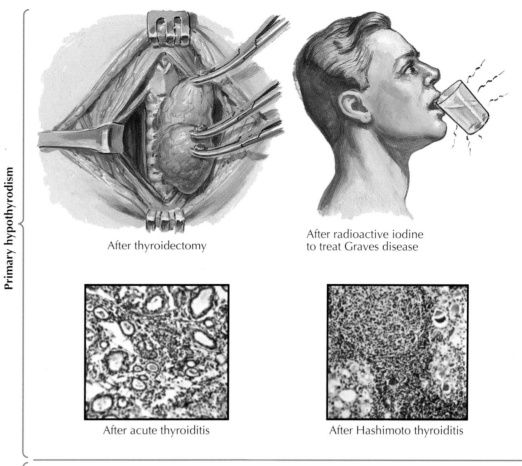

Primary hypothyroidism

After thyroidectomy

After radioactive iodine
to treat Graves disease

After acute thyroiditis

After Hashimoto thyroiditis

CLINICAL MANIFESTATIONS OF HYPOTHYROIDISM IN ADULTS
(Continued)

The most common cause of primary hypothyroidism is Hashimoto thyroiditis. The second most common cause is iatrogenic. For example, most patients who have undergone thyroidectomy in the treatment of nontoxic goiter or of Graves disease develop primary hypothyroidism. The most common treatment of Graves disease is radioactive iodine with the goals of total thyroid gland destruction and primary hypothyroidism.

Hashimoto thyroiditis is the most common spontaneous cause of primary hypothyroidism. Transient primary hypothyroidism may develop after subacute and acute thyroiditis (see Plate 2-22). A high serum thyroid peroxidase antibody concentration is consistent with Hashimoto thyroiditis.

Central hypothyroidism is the result of a variety of processes that affect the anterior pituitary gland, resulting in loss of TSH secretion. TSH deficiency may occur in isolation (e.g., with lymphocytic hypophysitis) or, more commonly, as part of complete anterior pituitary failure (see Plate 1-16). Complete anterior pituitary failure may be the result of inflammation, infarction (e.g., postpartum apoplexy), primary neoplasms, metastatic disease, infiltrative disorders (e.g., sarcoidosis, Langerhans cell histiocytosis, hemochromatosis), surgery, head trauma, or radiation therapy (see Plates 1-12 to 1-18). Pituitary-directed head magnetic resonance imaging is indicated in these patients to assist in differentiating among these multiple causes.

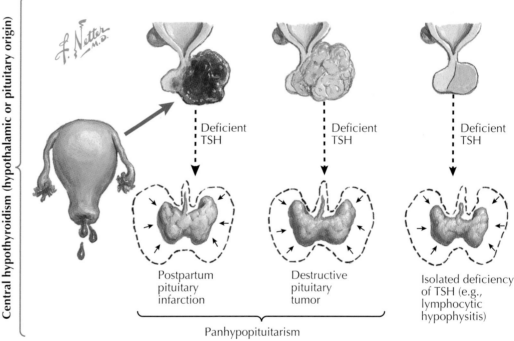

Central hypothyroidism (hypothalamic or pituitary origin)

Deficient TSH

Deficient TSH

Deficient TSH

Postpartum pituitary infarction

Destructive pituitary tumor

Isolated deficiency of TSH (e.g., lymphocytic hypophysitis)

Panhypopituitarism

TREATMENT

Whether primary or secondary in etiology, the treatment of hypothyroidism is daily levothyroxine administered orally. In patients with primary hypothyroidism, the serum TSH concentration is measured to guide the adjustment of the levothyroxine dosage; the goal is a TSH concentration in the middle of the reference range. In patients with central hypothyroidism, blood TSH measurement is useless, and the levothyroxine dosage is adjusted to a free T_4 concentration in the middle of the reference range. However, before starting levothyroxine therapy in patients with central hypothyroidism, it is essential to assess the hypothalamic–pituitary–adrenal axis. If levothyroxine, which can accelerate cortisol metabolism, is administered to a patient with concomitant untreated adrenal insufficiency, it may precipitate an adrenal crisis.

Plate 2-17

Endocrine System

CONGENITAL HYPOTHYROIDISM

Congenital hypothyroidism is the most common cause of mental retardation that can be prevented and treated. The intelligence quotient later in life is inversely related to the age at the time of diagnosis; thus, identifying congenital hypothyroidism as soon as possible after birth is critical. The most common cause is thyroid dysgenesis, including congenital absence (agenesis) of the thyroid gland itself, thyroid hypoplasia, or thyroid gland ectopy. Less commonly, congenital hypothyroidism is associated with nonfunctioning goiters or with goiters that have inborn errors of thyroid hormone biosynthesis (goitrous hypothyroidism). The synthetic defects are usually inherited in an autosomal recessive pattern and include deficits in impaired thyroid peroxidase activity, abnormal iodide transport, iodotyrosine deiodinase deficiency, and abnormal thyroglobulin molecules. This malady occurs most frequently in endemic goiter regions, but goitrous congenital hypothyroidism has been observed in areas where goiters are quite uncommon.

Central (hypothalamic or pituitary) hypothyroidism is a much less common cause of congenital hypothyroidism (one in 100,000 babies) and can be detected only by measuring the serum thyroxine (T_4) concentration. When present, it may occur in the setting of other midline developmental disorders (e.g., cleft lip and palate, septo-optic dysplasia) and be associated with other anterior pituitary gland hormone deficiencies.

The physical stigmata of congenital hypothyroidism may be mild or absent at the time of birth because some maternal T_4 crosses the placenta. Congenital hypothyroidism is sporadic more than 85% of the time and is thus unsuspected. In the mid-1970s, state-wide newborn screening programs in the United States were developed. These programs measure either thyrotropin (thyroid-stimulating hormone [TSH]), T_4, or both in blood samples collected by heel stick on filter paper cards 24 to 48 hours after delivery. On the basis of these data, the incidence of elevated TSH levels varies from one in 2000 to one in 32,000 babies; the variance depends on geographic location and ethnicity. The frequency of congenital hypothyroidism is approximately twofold higher in baby girls. Rapid institution of thyroid hormone replacement therapy can prevent subsequent irreversible disabilities.

When untreated, congenital hypothyroidism in infants has similar features to those seen in adults with hypothyroidism, but there are some important differences. There is a failure of skeletal growth and maturation and a marked retardation and deficiency in intellect. The development of centers of ossification is markedly delayed, and the epiphyses show a characteristic stippling. Delayed ossification of bone, of epiphysial union, and of dentition is observed. The skull base is usually short; there may be persistence of the cartilaginous junctions between the presphenoid and postsphenoid bones, which normally ossify in the eighth month of fetal life. Furthermore, because of a delay in ossification of the membranous bones, the frontal suture is usually wide, and the anterior fontanels are exceptionally large.

The face of a child with untreated congenital hypothyroidism is round, with a dull expression and yellowish color. The eyelids are puffy, and the palpebral fissures are generally narrowed but horizontal. The

Infant with only mild stigmata of congenital hypothyroidism

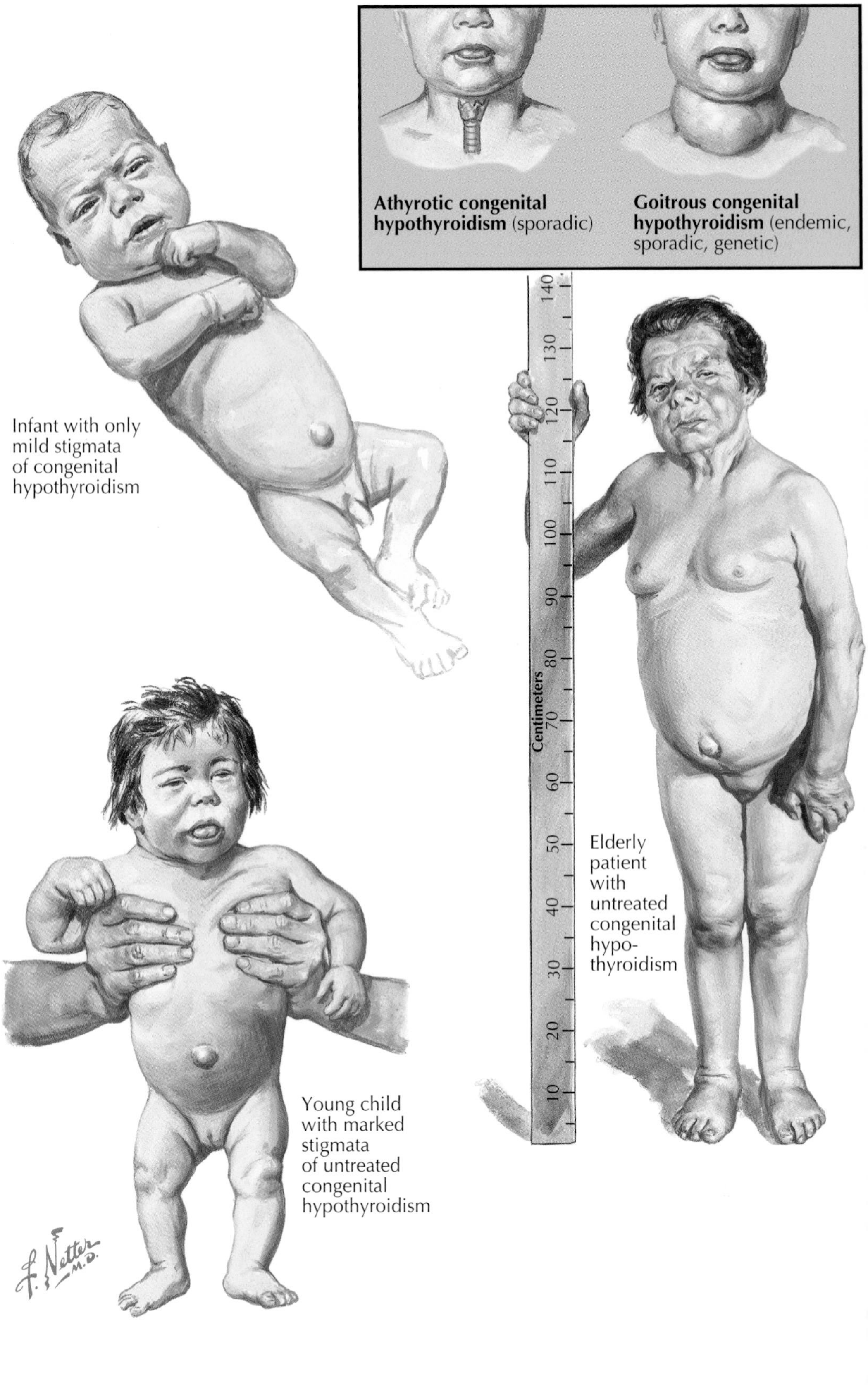

Athyrotic congenital hypothyroidism (sporadic)

Goitrous congenital hypothyroidism (endemic, sporadic, genetic)

Young child with marked stigmata of untreated congenital hypothyroidism

Elderly patient with untreated congenital hypothyroidism

nose is frequently flat and thick; the lips are thick; the mouth remains open, and a large, thick tongue protrudes. The voice is flat and harsh. The neck is usually short and thick. The skin is dry and cool and presents a picture of nonpitting edema. There is usually marked hyperkeratosis in the skin over the anterior abdominal wall. The hair is fine, lifeless, dry, and often quite sparse. Juvenile patients with untreated congenital hypothyroidism may also have a marked growth of fine,

short hair, of a lanugo type, over the shoulders, upper arms, and face.

The physical features of children with congenital hypothyroidism may be confused with the features observed in trisomy 21. Persons with trisomy 21 have finer features, absent coarse skin, slanted eyes, a palmar crease, and excessive extensor flexibility of the fingers arc. On laboratory evaluation, babies with trisomy 21 have normal blood concentrations of TSH and T4.

Plate 2-18

Thyroid

EUTHYROID GOITER

Euthyroid (nontoxic) goiters occur throughout the world, although they is more common in areas where the iodine content in the water and soil is low. In iodine-deficient goiters, there is characteristic enlargement of the thyroid with a moderate-sized, nontoxic, diffuse goiter that occurs in both boys and girls at about the time of puberty. Such goiters are diffuse in the early stage; later, they may become nodular, feeling hard in one area or cystic in another. Nodular goiters may be more or less symmetric or quite asymmetric. Such a goiter, if allowed to progress, may descend beneath the sternum and produce the picture of an intrathoracic goiter. With the increase in goiter size, especially if some of it is lodged beneath the sternum, obstructive symptoms may result from distortion of the trachea, esophagus, nerves, or jugular veins. This may occur because the thoracic inlet is a small area (~5 × 10 cm) that has bony boundaries—first ribs laterally, first thoracic vertebral body posteriorly, and manubrial and sternal bones anteriorly. Typically, these multinodular goiters grow very slowly, and the development of early obstructive symptoms can be quite insidious. Dyspnea on exertion may be the first symptom related to a substernal goiter. With advancing tracheal compression, stridor may become evident. Other thoracic inset compressive symptoms include dysphagia, vocal cord palsy from recurrent laryngeal nerve compression, and Horner syndrome from compression of the cervical sympathetic chain. On physical examination, the Pemberton maneuver may be used to detect thoracic inlet obstruction. The patient is asked to hold the arms straight up vertically for 1 minute; if the patient develops marked facial plethora, cyanosis, or stridor, the result is considered positive for thoracic inlet obstruction.

Occasionally, a nodular goiter may enlarge in one area very suddenly, producing pain that may be referred to the ear, neck structures, or shoulder. This is frequently explained on the basis of a hemorrhage into a follicle or into an adenoma or a large cyst in the thyroid.

In such multinodular goiters, adenomas of various types may be observed, and these may present various kinds of histologic structures. Some may be capable of function and may develop hyperfunction, resulting in a clinical picture of hyperthyroidism in an adenomatous goiter, a so-called "hot nodule" (see Plates 2-12 and 2-13). Cancer is much less common in these multinodular goiters than in thyroids with a single nodule. However, the fact that the goiter is multinodular does not rule out the possibility of cancer's developing or being found in it.

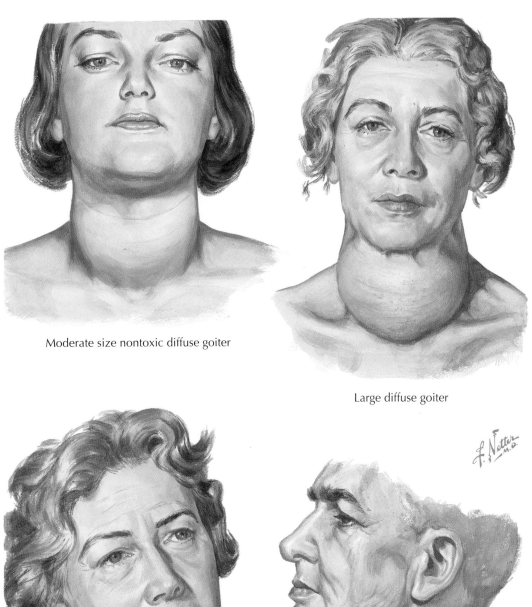

Moderate size nontoxic diffuse goiter

Large diffuse goiter

Nodular goiters

Hyperthyroidism should be excluded by measuring the serum thyrotropin concentration. Thyroid ultrasonography is helpful in assessing the structure of the suprasternal component of a multinodular goiter. If needed, the extent of substernal goiters can be determined with either computed tomography or magnetic resonance imaging. If prominent nodules are present, the underlying pathophysiology can be assessed with ultrasound-guided fine-needle aspiration biopsy.

The indications for surgical removal of such thyroids may fall into several categories: (1) cosmetic reasons that may impel the patient to seek surgical removal of the gland; (2) sudden enlargement of the gland, especially if the site of rapid growth is hard, suggesting a neoplastic change; and (3) most importantly, to correct any obstructive symptoms produced by the impingement of such a large mass on either the trachea or the esophagus.

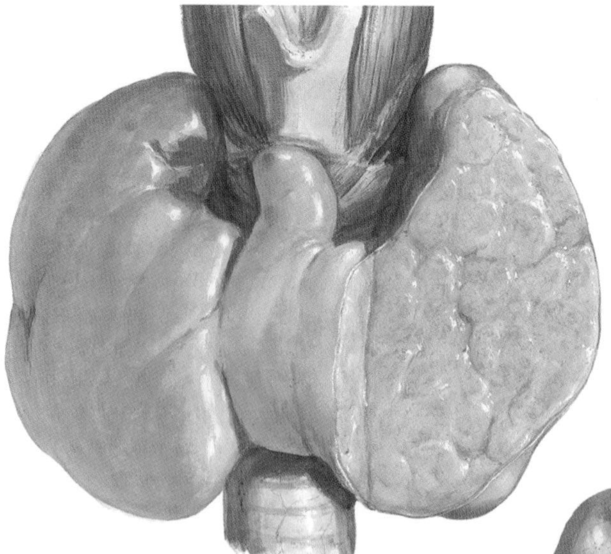

Plate 2-19

Endocrine System

GROSS PATHOLOGY OF GOITER

The term "goiter" refers to an enlargement of the thyroid gland. In general, the prevalence of goiter depends on the dietary iodine intake. Thus, goiters may be endemic in geographic areas of iodine deficiency. Early in the development of a nontoxic goiter, the gland is usually diffusely and uniformly enlarged, with an increase in the size of the pyramidal lobe. This is known as a diffuse nontoxic, or colloid, goiter. Nontoxic goiters are eightfold more common in females and frequently become evident in adolescence or pregnancy. Such glands may be two to three times the normal size or even larger. The patient may become aware of the condition because others have commented on the fullness of the neck, because shirt collars may feel too tight, or because it may become difficult to swallow. Large goiters may compress the trachea and result in stridor. Venous engorgement from narrowing of the thoracic inlet may occur. Most simple and multinodular goiters are associated with a euthyroid state.

On physical examination, the gland feels firm but not hard. As the process progresses, with the advancing age of the patient the thyroid may become asymmetric and multinodular, which is evident on gross examination of the gland. Significant variations in the size and structure of the nodules become apparent. In very long-standing nodular goiters, hemorrhages into various sites in the gland, cyst formation, fibrosis, and even calcification are likely to be observed. On chest radiographs, asymmetric goiters typically cause lateral displacement of the trachea; in addition, any retrosternal extension of such a goiter may, if calcified, initially simulate intrapulmonary calcifications.

The cut surface of a colloid goiter shows a uniform amber color with a translucent appearance. Colloid goiters may weigh anywhere from 40 to 1000 g or more. The thyroid gland is distorted in shape and nodular, with some nodules partially or completely separated from the gland. The gross pathology appearance on cut section typically shows areas of nodularity, fibrosis, hemorrhage, and calcification. Some nodules may show cystic change, and some may have a thickened fibrous connective tissue capsule and have the general appearance of a follicular neoplasm.

Cytologic examination from fine-needle aspiration biopsy of colloid nodules typically shows colloid and mixed cell populations with relatively few cells in the aspirate. The types of cells usually seen on cytologic examination include follicular cells with uniform nuclei, inflammatory cells, and Hürthle cells. Hypercellular foci within a multinodular goiter may simulate a follicular neoplasm.

Microscopic examination of the colloid nodular goiter may reveal every conceivable type of benign adenoma, including a highly undifferentiated trabecular pattern or

Diffuse colloid goiter

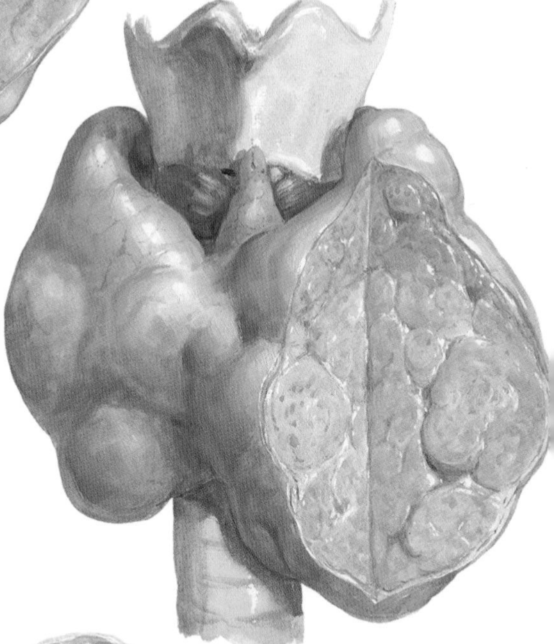

Nodular goiter; variation in size and structure of nodules

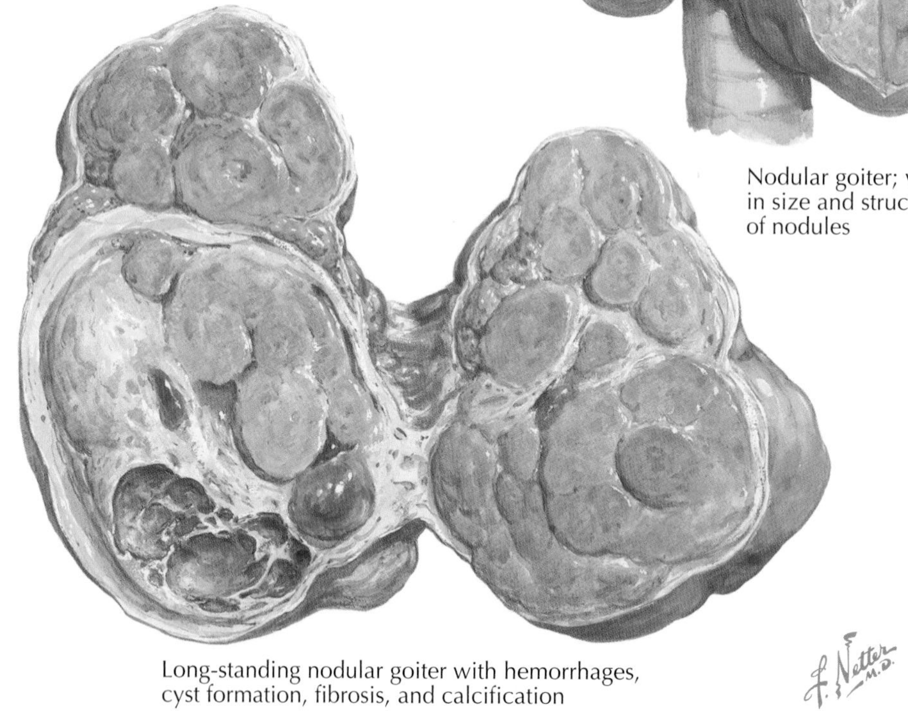

Long-standing nodular goiter with hemorrhages, cyst formation, fibrosis, and calcification

the earliest stage of differentiation of tubular structure, the structure of microfollicles, or the picture of a hyperplastic adenoma. The follicles—usually lined by flattened epithelium with involutional changes—can be of varying size and as large as 2 mm in diameter. Large distended follicles may coalesce to create cystic areas.

Rarely, within these nodules may be seen various types of cancerous growths, such as differentiated thyroid carcinomas (papillary and follicular). However, the cancerous changes in such thyroids are much less common than they are in those of patients presenting with a single nodule in the thyroid. Thoracic inlet obstructive symptoms represent the most important indication for therapeutic intervention, but the rare occurrence of a small malignancy must always be kept in mind.

Plate 2-24

Thyroid

FOLLICULAR THYROID CARCINOMA

Follicular thyroid carcinoma (FTC) is one of the three thyroid epithelial–derived thyroid cancers (papillary thyroid carcinoma [PTC] and anaplastic thyroid carcinoma being the other two). After PTC, FTC is the second most common type of thyroid cancer, accounting for 10% of cases. Compared with PTC, FTC occurs more commonly in older persons; the peak incidence is between 40 and 60 years of age and is threefold more common in women than in men. FTC is more common in iodine-deficient regions of the world.

FTC may present as a small nodule or as a large mass within the thyroid. Unlike PTC, FTC usually has a solitary intrathyroidal focus. Cytologic examination of a thyroid fine-needle aspiration biopsy specimen cannot be used to distinguish between FTC and a benign follicular adenoma. FTC can be diagnosed only on the basis of en bloc thyroid tissue removed at surgery and documentation of tumor capsule or vascular invasion.

Histologically, FTC shows a fairly well-organized follicular pattern, with small but frequently irregular follicles lined by high cuboidal epithelium. The follicles with a more orderly arrangement commonly contain colloid. Findings consistent with PTC (e.g., psammoma bodies) are absent. Although tumor extension through the capsule or vascular invasion is usually present in patients with FTC, minimally invasive FTC is a subtype that is encapsulated and is associated with a good prognosis. Widely invasive FTC, however, extends into blood vessels and adjacent thyroid tissue and is associated with a poor prognosis.

Most FTCs appear to be monoclonal, and approximately 40% are associated with somatic point mutations in the *RAS* oncogenes, a finding associated with a more aggressive tumor.

FTC frequently metastasizes early via hematogenous dissemination; distant metastases are evident at the time of primary tumor detection in 15% of patients with FTC. The most common sites of metastatic disease are bone and lung (less common sites of involvement include the liver, brain, urinary bladder, and skin). Neck lymph node involvement is much less common in FTC than in PTC. Skeletal metastases, when biopsied, may look like normal thyroid tissue.

FTC tends to have a more aggressive clinical course than PTC. A worse prognosis is associated with larger tumor size, distant metastasis, and vascular invasion. Insular carcinoma is a poorly differentiated form of FTC that is associated with a poor prognosis. Hürthle cell carcinoma is an oncocytic variant of FTC (see Plate 2-26).

The treatment of patients with FTC is similar to that for those with PTC. Total thyroidectomy with central

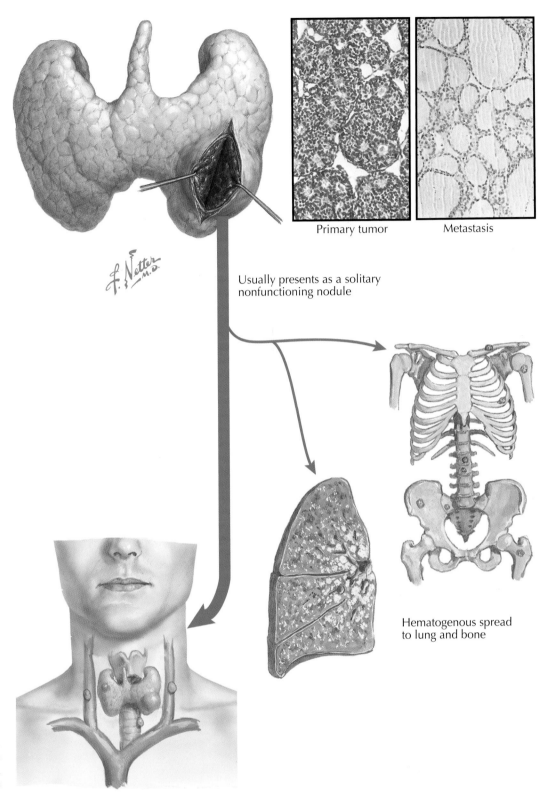

Primary tumor

Metastasis

Usually presents as a solitary nonfunctioning nodule

Hematogenous spread to lung and bone

Rare neck lymph node involvement

compartment lymph node dissection is the treatment of choice. Preoperative neck ultrasonography with lymph node mapping is essential in planning a successful operation. FTC cells are able to retain radioactive iodine 131 (^{131}I) but not as well as normal thyroid follicular cells. Iodine 131 may be administered after surgery to destroy thyroid remnant tissue in the thyroid bed and microscopic metastatic disease. After treatment, levothyroxine replacement therapy is initiated to suppress pituitary thyrotropin, with the intent to prevent thyrotropin-driven growth of any residual FTC cells. External-beam radiation therapy may be used when primary or metastatic disease cannot be resected. Systemic chemotherapy may be needed in the small subset of patients whose disease is refractory to all other treatment options. In addition, molecular pathway–blocking drugs (e.g., tyrosine kinase inhibitors) may be beneficial in patients with refractory disease.

Plate 2-25

Endocrine System

MEDULLARY THYROID CARCINOMA

Medullary thyroid carcinoma (MTC) is a neoplasm of the thyroid parafollicular or "C cells." Approximately 3% of all thyroid malignancies prove to be MTC. The C cells are located in the upper portion of each thyroid lobe and originate from the embryonic neural crest; thus, from the clinical and histologic perspectives, MTC is more of a neuroendocrine tumor than a thyroid neoplasm.

In approximately 80% of patients, MTC is sporadic, but it may be familial either as part of multiple endocrine neoplasia type 2 (MEN 2) syndrome or familial MTC (FMTC). Sporadic MTC typically presents as a solitary thyroid nodule at age 40 to 60 years, with a slight female preponderance. MTC is easily diagnosed by fine-needle aspiration biopsy of a thyroid nodule. At the time of diagnosis, more than half of patients with sporadic MTC have metastatic disease, typically involving regional lymph nodes.

MTC secretes the hormone calcitonin. Markedly elevated levels of calcitonin may be found in patients with MTC and may result in severe diarrhea. Also, because of its neuroendocrine embryology, MTC has the potential to secrete other hormones that may cause additional clinical symptomatology. For example, MTC may hypersecrete corticotropin and cause Cushing syndrome.

On histology, MTC shows a solid trabecular pattern with closely packed cells, with considerable variation in hyperchromatism and the size of the nuclei. The cells usually immunostain for calcitonin, galectin-3, and carcinoembryonic antigen.

Inherited MTC is associated with mutations in the *RET* proto-oncogene and presents as MEN 2A, MEN 2B, or FMTC. The penetrance of MTC in patients with MEN 2 is 100%. Men and women are affected with equal frequency. Patients with MEN 2B have a more aggressive form of MTC, and they should have prophylactic thyroidectomy in the first year of life. Patients with inherited MTC that is not recognized earlier in life typically present between the ages of 20 and 30 years. However, when the risk of familial MTC is known, MTC can be diagnosed before it is palpable or clinically evident. After the specific *RET* proto-oncogene mutation has been identified in the proband, at-risk family members can have genetic testing for the specific mutation to determine their risk for MTC.

Even patients with apparently sporadic MTC should have genetic testing for mutations in the *RET* proto-oncogene because approximately 7% have a mutation. This finding can facilitate genetic testing of at-risk family members to identify individuals with MTC and treat them surgically before metastases develop.

All patients with MTC should have biochemical testing to exclude primary hyperparathyroidism and pheochromocytoma (components of MEN 2). Serum calcitonin concentration should be measured preoperatively in all patients with MTC. The higher the serum calcitonin concentration, the more likely it is that the

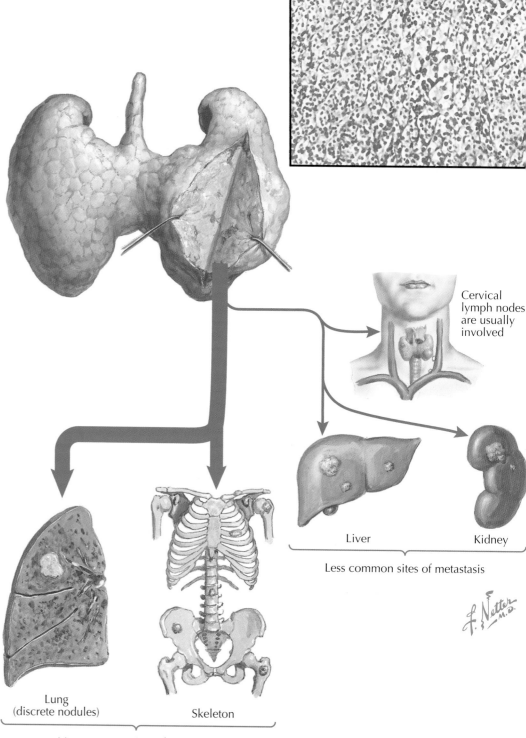

Cervical lymph nodes are usually involved

Liver   Kidney

Less common sites of metastasis

Lung (discrete nodules)   Skeleton

Most common sites of metastasis

patient has metastatic disease and will not be cured with thyroidectomy.

The treatment of choice is total thyroidectomy. Prognosis is determined in part by the age at the time of diagnosis (the older the patient, the poorer the prognosis). For patients with familial disease, the prognosis is determined by the age at which thyroidectomy is performed; cure rates are higher when thyroidectomy

is performed at a younger age. Serum calcitonin concentration should be measured postoperatively to determine if a surgical cure has been achieved. Metastatic disease may involve the neck, mediastinum, lungs, liver, bone, and kidneys. Persistent metastatic disease that cannot be surgically resected may be treated with molecular pathway–blocking drugs (e.g., tyrosine kinase inhibitors).

Plate 3-3

Adrenal

ANATOMY AND BLOOD SUPPLY OF THE ADRENAL GLANDS
(Continued)

SURGICAL APPROACHES TO THE ADRENAL GLANDS

The pathologic process, tumor size, patient size, and previous operations are all factors that help determine the surgical approach to the adrenal glands. No one particular approach can be considered suitable for all cases, and the removal of a diseased gland or an adrenal tumor may, at times, present formidable difficulties.

Open Transabdominal Adrenalectomy

The patient is in the supine position, and the incision is typically in an extended subcostal location. A midline incision may be used if the patient has a narrow costal angle or bilateral adrenal disease is present. The approach to the left adrenal gland is typically through the gastrocolic ligament into the lesser sac. The left adrenal is exposed by lifting the inferior surface of the pancreas upward, Gerota fascia is opened, and the upper pole of the kidney is retracted inferiorly. The approach to the right adrenal gland involves mobilizing the hepatic flexure of the colon inferiorly and retracting the right lobe of the liver upward.

Open Posterior Adrenalectomy

Compared with the open anterior approach, the open posterior approach causes less pain, ileus, and other complications. The patient is in the prone position and the incision is either curvilinear extending from the 10th rib (4 cm from the midvertebral line) to the iliac crest (8 cm from the midvertebral line) or a single straight incision over the 12th rib with a small vertical paravertebral upward extension. The 12th rib is resected, the pleura is reflected upward, and Gerota fascia is incised.

Laparoscopic Transabdominal Adrenalectomy

Since its description in 1992, laparoscopic adrenalectomy has rapidly become the procedure of choice for unilateral adrenalectomy when the adrenal mass is smaller than 8 cm and there are no frank signs of malignancy (e.g., invasion of contiguous structures). The postoperative recovery time and long-term morbidity associated with laparoscopic adrenalectomy are significantly reduced compared with open adrenalectomy. The patient is placed in the lateral decubitus position with the side to be operated facing upward. Four trocars are placed in a straight line, 1 to 2 cm below the subcostal margin. On the right side, the liver with the gallbladder is retracted upward, and the retroperitoneum is incised. On the left side, the left colonic flexure and the descending colon are mobilized inferiorly and medially to expose the upper pole of the left kidney, and the retroperitoneum is incised.

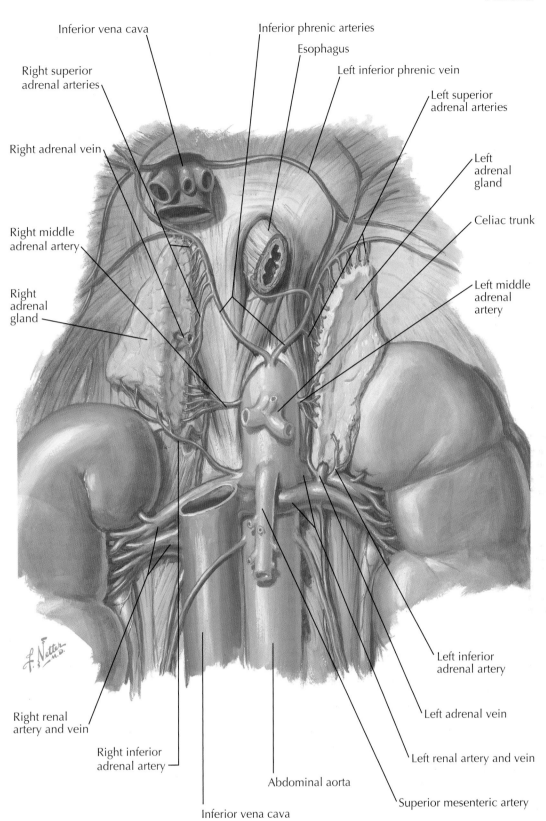

Posterior Retroperitoneoscopic Adrenalectomy

A minimally invasive posterior approach to the adrenal is favored by some endocrine surgeons and is advantageous in patients who have had previous anterior upper abdominal operations. The patient is in the prone position, and three trocars are used. A gas pressure of 20 to 25 mm Hg allows the creation of sufficient space in the retroperitoneum to facilitate the operation.

Keys to Successful Adrenal Surgery

The keys to successful adrenal surgery are appropriate patient selection, knowledge of anatomy, delicate tissue handling, meticulous hemostasis, and experience with the approach used. Familiarity with the vascular anomalies of the blood supply of the adrenal glands is indispensable. Finally, the gland should be handled gently because it fractures easily when traumatized, jeopardizing its complete removal.

Plate 3-4

Endocrine System

INNERVATION OF THE ADRENAL GLANDS

Relative to their size, the adrenal glands have a richer innervation than other viscera. The sympathetic preganglionic fibers for these glands are the axons of cells located in the intermediolateral columns of the lowest two or three thoracic and highest one or two lumbar segments of the spinal cord. They emerge in the anterior rootlets of the corresponding spinal nerves; pass in the white rami communicantes to the homolateral sympathetic trunks; and leave them in the greater, lesser, and least thoracic and first lumbar splanchnic nerves, which run to the celiac, aorticorenal, and renal ganglia. Some fibers end in these ganglia, but most pass through them without relaying and enter numerous small nerves that run outward on each side from the celiac plexus to the adrenal glands. These nerves are joined by direct contributions from the terminal parts of the greater and lesser thoracic splanchnic nerves, and they communicate with the homolateral phrenic nerve and renal plexus. Small ganglia exist on the adrenal nerves and within the actual adrenal medulla; a proportion of sympathetic fibers may relay in these ganglia.

Parasympathetic fibers are conveyed to the celiac plexus in the celiac branch of the posterior vagal trunk, and some of these are involved with adrenal innervation and may relay in ganglia in or near the gland.

On each side, the adrenal nerves form an adrenal plexus along the medial border of the adrenal gland. Filaments associated with occasional ganglion cells spread out over the gland to form a delicate subcapsular plexus, from which fascicles or solitary fibers penetrate the cortex to reach the medulla, apparently without supplying cortical cells en route, although they do supply cortical vessels. Most of the branches of the adrenal plexus, however, enter the gland through or near its hilum as compact bundles, some of which accompany the adrenal arteries. These bundles run through the cortex to the medulla, where they ramify profusely and mostly terminate in synaptic-type endings around the medullary chromaffin cells; some fibers invaginate but do not penetrate the plasma membranes of these cells. The preganglionic sympathetic fibers end directly around the medullary cells because these cells are derived from the sympathetic anlage and are the homologues of sympathetic ganglion cells. Other fibers innervate the adrenal vessels, including the central vein.

Catecholamines are released from the adrenal medullary and sympathoneuronal systems—both are key components of the fight-or-flight reaction. The signs and symptoms of the fight-or-flight reaction include cutaneous and systemic vasoconstriction with cold and clammy skin, anxiety, agitation, piloerection, tachycardia, dilated pupils, hyperventilation, hyperglycemia, decreased gastrointestinal motility, and decreased urinary output. This reaction is triggered by neural signals from several sites in the brain (e.g., the hypothalamus, pons, and medulla), leading to synapses on cell bodies in the intermediolateral cell columns of the thoracolumbar spinal cord. The preganglionic sympathetic nerves leave the spinal cord and synapse in paravertebral and preaortic ganglia of the sympathetic chain. Preganglionic axons from the lower thoracic and lumbar ganglia innervate the adrenal medulla via the splanchnic nerve and ramify about cells of the medulla. Acetylcholine is the neurotransmitter in the ganglia, and the postganglionic fiber releases norepinephrine. The chromaffin cell of the adrenal medulla is a "postganglionic fiber equivalent," and its chemical transmitters are epinephrine and norepinephrine.

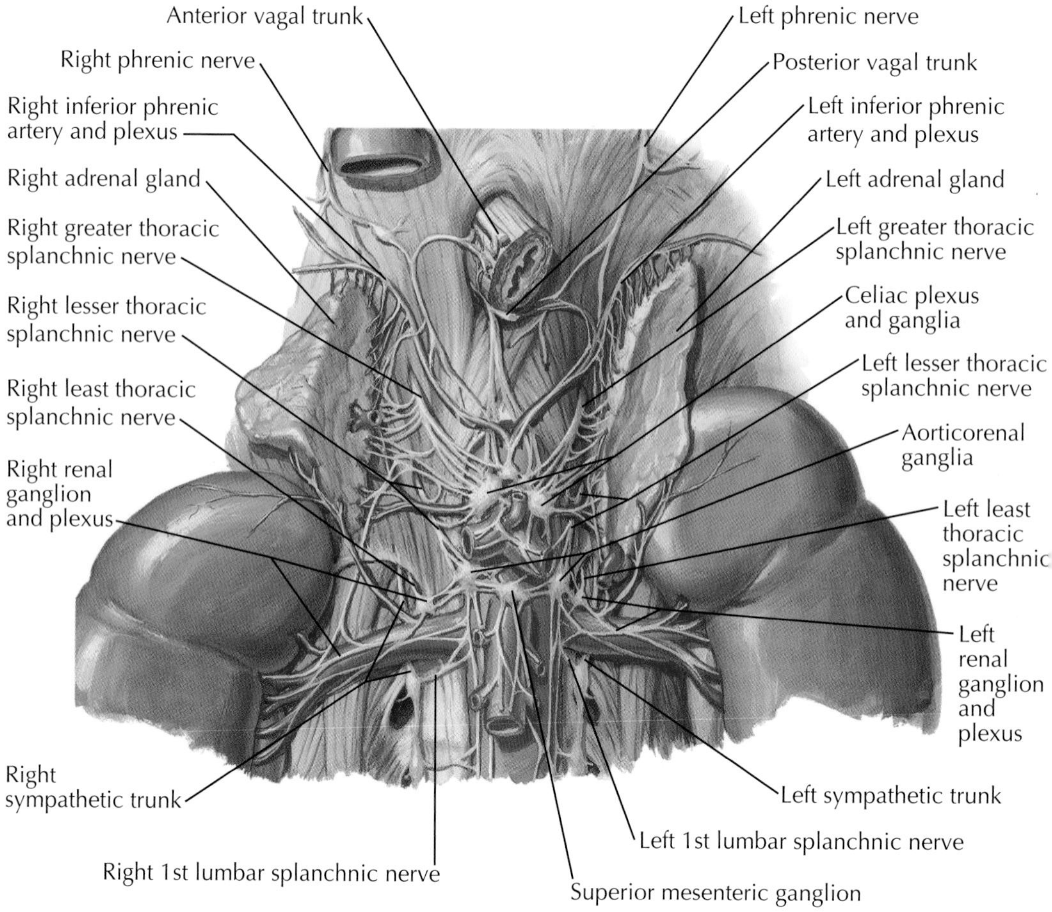

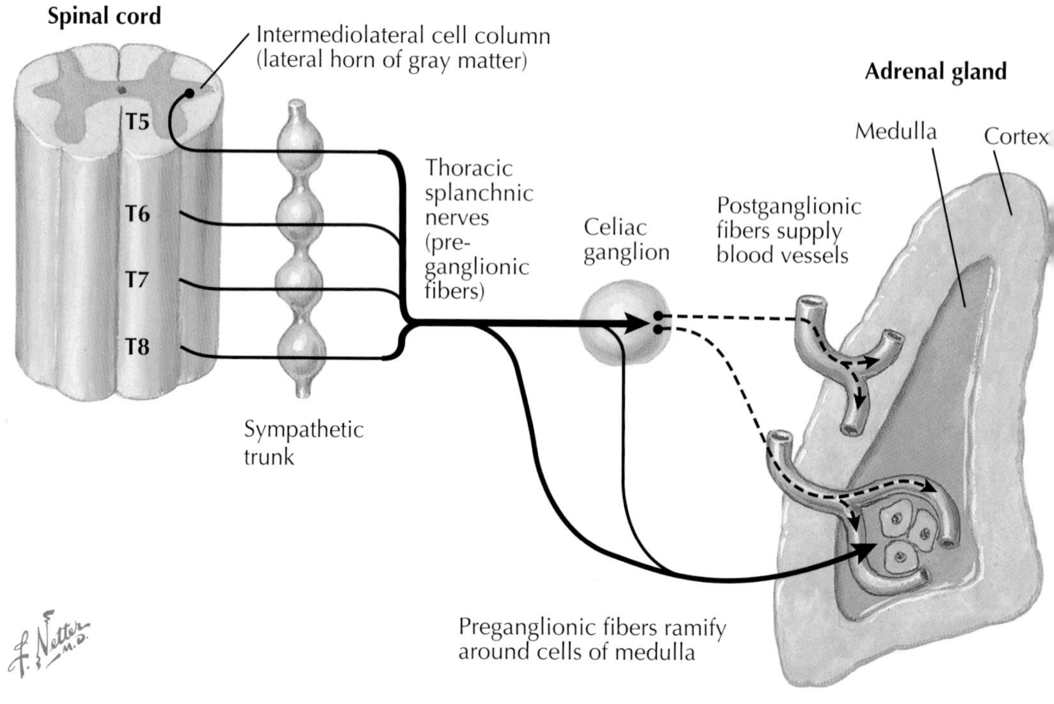

Plate 3-10

Adrenal

TESTS USED IN THE DIAGNOSIS OF CUSHING SYNDROME

The evaluation of Cushing syndrome can be considered in three steps: (1) case-detection testing, (2) confirmatory testing, and (3) subtype testing.

CASE-DETECTION TESTING

Case detection testing should start with measurements of 24-hour urinary free cortisol (UFC), 11 PM salivary cortisol, and serum cortisol concentrations measured at 8 AM and 4 PM. Unfortunately, the diagnosis of the Cushing syndrome is usually not straightforward. For example, a normal 24-hour UFC value does not exclude Cushing syndrome—10% to 15% of patients with Cushing syndrome have normal 24-hour UFC excretion in one of four measurements. In addition, all forms of endogenous Cushing syndrome can produce cortisol in a cyclical fashion that confounds the biochemical documentation and interpretation of suppression testing. If the clinical suspicion for Cushing syndrome is high and the 24-hour UFC excretion results are normal, obtaining multiple 24-hour UFC measurements is indicated (every month for 4 months). The baseline 24-hour UFC measurements may also be increased by alcoholism, depression, severe illness, or high urine volume (>4 L). When measured by tandem mass spectrometry, the upper limit of the reference range for 24-hour UFC is 45 µg (124 nmol).

Salivary cortisol concentrations, obtained at 11 PM, are 92% sensitive for Cushing syndrome. Lack of diurnal variation in serum cortisol concentrations is a finding that is also supportive evidence for glucocorticoid secretory autonomy.

The 1-mg overnight dexamethasone suppression test (DST) is an additional case-detection test. At 11 PM, 1 mg of dexamethasone is administered, and serum cortisol is measured the following morning at 8 AM. The serum cortisol concentration in healthy persons suppresses to below 1.8 µg/dL (50 nmol/L). In addition to Cushing syndrome, causes for cortisol nonsuppression with the overnight 1-mg DST include patient error in taking dexamethasone, increased cortisol-binding globulin (e.g., with estrogen therapy or pregnancy), obesity, ingestion of a drug that accelerates dexamethasone metabolism (e.g., anticonvulsants, phenobarbital, primidone, rifampin), renal failure, alcoholism, psychiatric disorder (e.g., depression), stress, or laboratory error.

CONFIRMATORY TESTING

Additional confirmatory studies are not needed if the baseline 24-hour UFC excretion is more than 200 µg/24 h (>552 nmol/24 h) and the clinical picture is consistent with Cushing syndrome. However, when the clinical findings are "soft" and when the 24-hour UFC excretion is less than 200 µg/24 h (<552 nmol/24 h), autonomous hypercortisolism should be confirmed with the 2-day low-dose DST (dexamethasone, 0.5 mg orally every 6 hours for 48 hours). A 24-hour UFC excretion more than 10 µg/24 h (28 nmol/24 h) confirms the diagnosis. However, the low-dose DST is far from perfect (79% sensitivity, 74% specificity, and 71% accuracy). The low-dose DST works best when the clinician has a low index of suspicion for Cushing syndrome. If clinical suspicion is high, normal suppression with low-dose DST does not exclude corticotropin (adrenocorticotropic hormone [ACTH])–dependent Cushing syndrome; patients with mild pituitary-dependent disease can demonstrate suppression with low-dose DST.

THE EVALUATION OF CUSHING SYNDROME CAN BE CONSIDERED IN 3 STEPS:

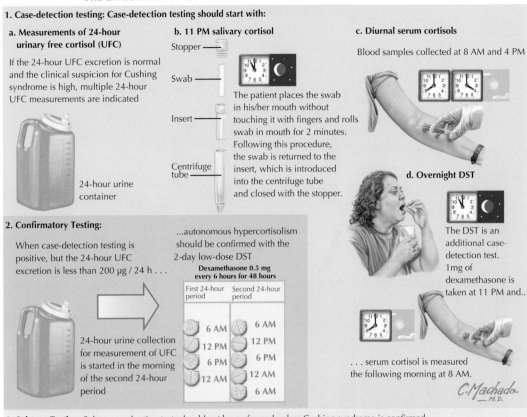

1. Case-detection testing: Case-detection testing should start with:

a. Measurements of 24-hour urinary free cortisol (UFC)

If the 24-hour UFC excretion is normal and the clinical suspicion for Cushing syndrome is high, multiple 24-hour UFC measurements are indicated

24-hour urine container

b. 11 PM salivary cortisol

Stopper

Swab

Insert

Centrifuge tube

The patient places the swab in his/her mouth without touching it with fingers and rolls swab in mouth for 2 minutes. Following this procedure, the swab is returned to the insert, which is introduced into the centrifuge tube and closed with the stopper.

c. Diurnal serum cortisols

Blood samples collected at 8 AM and 4 PM

d. Overnight DST

The DST is an additional case-detection test. 1mg of dexamethasone is taken at 11 PM and...

... serum cortisol is measured the following morning at 8 AM.

2. Confirmatory Testing:

When case-detection testing is positive, but the 24-hour UFC excretion is less than 200 µg/24 h . . .

24-hour urine collection for measurement of UFC is started in the morning of the second 24-hour period

...autonomous hypercortisolism should be confirmed with the 2-day low-dose DST

Dexamethasone 0.5 mg every 6 hours for 48 hours

First 24-hour period	Second 24-hour period
6 AM	6 AM
12 PM	12 PM
6 PM	6 PM
12 AM	12 AM
	6 AM

3. Subtype Testing: Subtype evaluation tests should not be performed unless Cushing syndrome is confirmed.

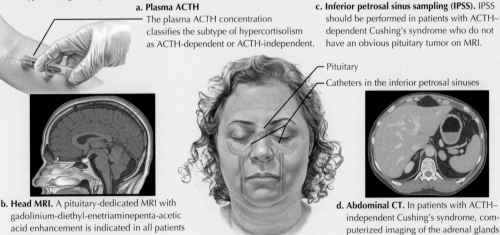

a. Plasma ACTH
The plasma ACTH concentration classifies the subtype of hypercortisolism as ACTH-dependent or ACTH-independent.

c. Inferior petrosal sinus sampling (IPSS). IPSS should be performed in patients with ACTH–dependent Cushing's syndrome who do not have an obvious pituitary tumor on MRI.

Pituitary

Catheters in the inferior petrosal sinuses

b. Head MRI. A pituitary-dedicated MRI with gadolinium-diethyl-enetriaminepenta-acetic acid enhancement is indicated in all patients with ACTH–dependent Cushing syndrome.

d. Abdominal CT. In patients with ACTH–independent Cushing's syndrome, computerized imaging of the adrenal glands usually indicates the type of adrenal disease.

SUBTYPE TESTING

Subtype evaluation tests should not be performed unless Cushing syndrome is confirmed. The application of these tests should be personalized; there is no algorithm that can be applied to all patients with Cushing syndrome. Many of these tests may be superfluous and would delay lifesaving therapy in patients with severe clinical Cushing syndrome.

The plasma ACTH concentration classifies the subtype of hypercortisolism as ACTH dependent (normal to high levels of ACTH) or ACTH independent (undetectable ACTH). A pituitary-dedicated magnetic resonance image (MRI) with gadolinium-diethyl-enetriaminepenta-acetic acid enhancement is indicated in all patients with ACTH-dependent Cushing syndrome. If a definite pituitary tumor is found (≥4 mm or larger) and the clinical scenario is consistent with pituitary disease (e.g., female gender, slow onset of disease, and baseline 24-hour UFC <

fivefold increased above the reference range), then additional studies are usually not required before definitive treatment. Smaller apparent pituitary lesions (<4 mm) are common in healthy persons and should be considered nonspecific; inferior petrosal sinus sampling (IPSS) should be performed. Also, if the pituitary MRI findings are normal (seen in ~50% of patients with pituitary-dependent Cushing syndrome), performing IPSS should be seriously considered.

In patients with ACTH-independent Cushing syndrome, computed tomography (CT) imaging of the adrenal glands usually indicates the type of adrenal disease—adrenal adenoma (usually 3–6 cm in diameter), adrenocortical carcinoma (usually 5–20 cm in diameter), bilateral macronodular hyperplasia (massive nodular bilateral adrenal enlargement), or primary pigmented nodular adrenocortical disease (PPNAD) (on CT, the adrenal glands may appear normal or micronodular).

Plate 3-11   Endocrine System

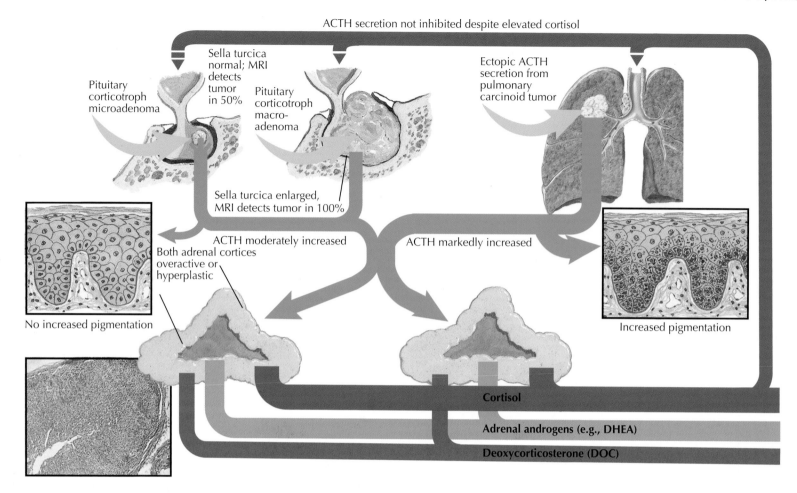

CUSHING SYNDROME:
PATHOPHYSIOLOGY

The underlying pathophysiology of endogenous Cushing syndrome is either corticotropin (adrenocorticotropic hormone [ACTH]) dependent or ACTH independent.

ACTH-dependent Cushing syndrome results in bilateral adrenocortical hyperplasia. An ACTH-secreting pituitary adenoma (Cushing disease) is the most common cause of endogenous hypercortisolism. Tumorous ectopic hypersecretion of ACTH (ectopic ACTH syndrome) or corticotropin-releasing hormone (CRH) are less common causes. Eutopic CRH hypersecretion is a very rare cause.

ACTH-independent Cushing syndrome may be caused by adrenocortical adenoma, adrenocortical carcinoma, ACTH-independent macronodular adrenal hyperplasia (AIMAH), or primary pigmented nodular adrenocortical disease (PPNAD) (see Plate 3-12).

The clinical presentation of Cushing syndrome is determined by the underlying pathophysiology. When there are markedly excessive adrenal androgens (e.g., with ectopic ACTH syndrome or adrenocortical carcinoma), hirsutism, acne, and scalp hair recession may be prominent. When the cortisol levels are markedly increased (e.g., with ectopic ACTH syndrome), severe hypertension and hypokalemia may be prominent. When the hypercortisolism develops slowly over years (e.g., pituitary-dependent Cushing syndrome, AIMAH, or PPNAD), central obesity, osteoporosis, and proximal muscle weakness may be the most prominent features. With markedly increased levels of ACTH (e.g.,

with ectopic ACTH syndrome or pituitary macroadenoma–dependent Cushing syndrome), skin hyperpigmentation may be a prominent feature.

ADRENOCORTICOTROPIC HORMONE–DEPENDENT CUSHING SYNDROME

Most patients with Cushing syndrome have pituitary-dependent disease. Approximately 95% of pituitary corticotroph tumors are microadenomas (≤10 mm), and 50% of the time they are not visible on pituitary-dedicated magnetic resonance imaging. The serum ACTH concentrations in patients with ACTH-secreting microadenomas are typically in the reference range but are inappropriate for the prevailing hypercortisolism. In contrast, the serum ACTH concentrations in patients with ACTH-secreting macroadenomas are usually above the reference range and may result in hyperpigmentation. The increased blood concentrations of ACTH result in bilateral adrenocortical hyperplasia and hypersecretion of cortisol. The adrenal cortices are typically mildly hyperplastic and typically weigh 6 to 12 g each (the normal adrenal gland weight is 4–6 g each). With ectopic ACTH syndrome, the adrenal glands usually weigh more than 12 g each.

The signs and symptoms, as well as the pathology, of Cushing syndrome are primarily caused by excess cortisol, but adrenal androgens may be elevated, and there may be excess mineralocorticoid effect. When a corticotroph adenoma of the pituitary is the source of excess ACTH, histologic sections of the pituitary gland typically demonstrate a pituitary microadenoma that stains for ACTH on immunohistochemistry, and the surrounding nontumorous corticotrophs are hyalinized—known as *Crooke hyaline change*. The latter is also seen

in all forms of hypercortisolism (e.g., ectopic ACTH, adrenal dependent, and exogenous). It is atrophy of the normally ACTH-producing basophilic corticotrophs because of negative feedback by cortisol. The corticotroph adenoma cells are relatively resistant to negative feedback inhibition by cortisol. The blood concentration of dehydroepiandrosterone sulfate (DHEA-S)—an ACTH-dependent adrenal androgen—is mildly increased in patients with pituitary-dependent Cushing syndrome. Selective transnasal endoscopic adenectomy is the treatment of choice for patients with ACTH-secreting pituitary tumors.

The nonpituitary tumor hypersecretion of ACTH in the ectopic ACTH syndrome results in marked bilateral adrenocortical hyperplasia and hypercortisolism. The increased serum cortisol concentrations inhibit hypothalamic CRH and pituitary ACTH secretion. The most common cause of ectopic ACTH syndrome is a bronchial carcinoid tumor. Other tumors that can produce ACTH include small cell lung cancer, medullary thyroid carcinoma, thymic carcinoid, pancreatic neuroendocrine tumors, and pheochromocytoma. The mineralocorticoid excess state caused by ectopic ACTH secretion is related to the high rates of cortisol production that overwhelm 11β-hydroxysteroid dehydrogenase type 2 enzyme activity, allowing free access of cortisol to the mineralocorticoid receptor. Deoxycorticosterone (DOC) levels may also be increased in severe ACTH-dependent Cushing syndrome and contribute to the hypertension and hypokalemia in this disorder. Complete resection of the ectopic ACTH-secreting tumor is the treatment of choice to cure Cushing syndrome. If the tumor cannot be resected, bilateral laparoscopic adrenalectomy should be considered.

Plate 3-11

Adrenal

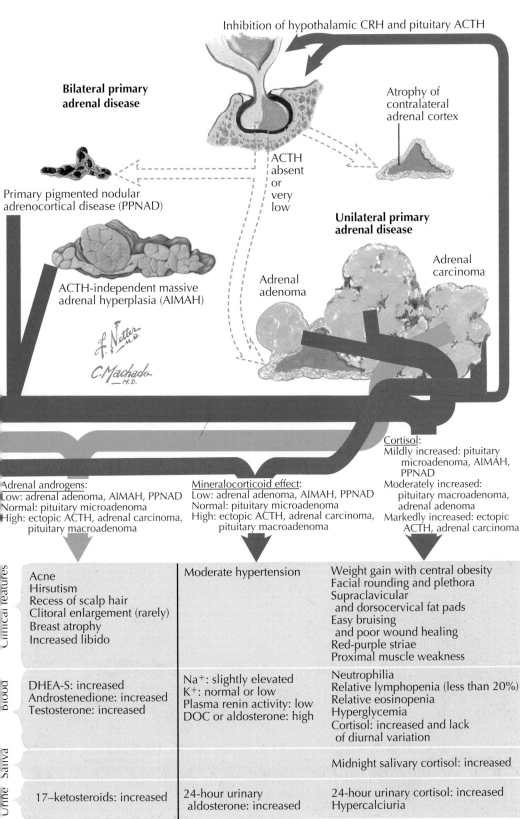

Inhibition of hypothalamic CRH and pituitary ACTH

**Bilateral primary
adrenal disease**

Atrophy of
contralateral
adrenal cortex

Primary pigmented nodular
adrenocortical disease (PPNAD)

ACTH
absent
or
very
low

**Unilateral primary
adrenal disease**

Adrenal
carcinoma

ACTH-independent massive
adrenal hyperplasia (AIMAH)

Adrenal
adenoma

Cortisol:
Mildly increased: pituitary
  microadenoma, AIMAH,
  PPNAD
Moderately increased:
  pituitary macroadenoma,
  adrenal adenoma
Markedly increased: ectopic
  ACTH, adrenal carcinoma

Adrenal androgens:
Low: adrenal adenoma, AIMAH, PPNAD
Normal: pituitary microadenoma
High: ectopic ACTH, adrenal carcinoma,
  pituitary macroadenoma

Mineralocorticoid effect:
Low: adrenal adenoma, AIMAH, PPNAD
Normal: pituitary microadenoma
High: ectopic ACTH, adrenal carcinoma,
  pituitary macroadenoma

Clinical features		
Acne Hirsutism Recess of scalp hair Clitoral enlargement (rarely) Breast atrophy Increased libido	Moderate hypertension	Weight gain with central obesity Facial rounding and plethora Supraclavicular and dorsocervical fat pads Easy bruising and poor wound healing Red-purple striae Proximal muscle weakness
DHEA-S: increased Androstenedione: increased Testosterone: increased	Na+: slightly elevated K+: normal or low Plasma renin activity: low DOC or aldosterone: high	Neutrophilia Relative lymphopenia (less than 20%) Relative eosinopenia Hyperglycemia Cortisol: increased and lack of diurnal variation
		Midnight salivary cortisol: increased
17–ketosteroids: increased	24-hour urinary aldosterone: increased	24-hour urinary cortisol: increased Hypercalciuria

(row labels at left: Clinical features / Blood / Saliva / Urine)

CUSHING SYNDROME:
PATHOPHYSIOLOGY (Continued)

In the rare case of ectopic CRH syndrome, the CRH secretion by the ectopic neoplasm (e.g., bronchial carcinoid tumor, pheochromocytoma) causes pituitary corticotroph hyperplasia and hypersecretion of ACTH.

ADRENOCORTICOTROPIC HORMONE–INDEPENDENT CUSHING SYNDROME

In the presence of a cortisol-secreting benign cortical adenoma of the adrenal cortex, there is a complete inhibition of hypothalamic CRH and pituitary ACTH production through the negative feedback mechanism by excess cortisol. Thus, the adrenal cortex from the contralateral adrenal and the ipsilateral cortex adjacent to a cortisol-secreting adrenal adenoma become atrophic. Adrenal adenomas typical secrete only cortisol, so that the ACTH-dependent adrenal androgens (measured as DHEA-S in the blood and 17-ketosteroids in the urine) are very low (frequently below the assay limit of detection). To generate enough cortisol secretion to cause clinical Cushing syndrome, cortisol-secreting adrenal adenomas are typically at least 2.5 cm in diameter. Unilateral laparoscopic adrenalectomy is the treatment of choice to cure Cushing syndrome associated with solitary adrenocortical adenoma.

A carcinoma of the adrenal cortex may be limited to the adrenal gland or may be metastatic (regional lymph nodes or distant to liver and lungs). Here, too, the adjacent cortex and the contralateral adrenal gland cortex become atrophic. Approximately half of adrenocortical carcinomas are hormone producing; they may hypersecrete a single hormone or multiple hormones (e.g., glucocorticoids, mineralocorticoids, adrenal androgens). With hormonally active adrenocortical carcinomas, the blood concentration of DHEA-S is typically increased. In addition, DOC and aldosterone may be hypersecreted, resulting in hypokalemic hypertension. Open laparotomy with en bloc tumor resection, if possible, is the treatment of choice for adrenocortical carcinomas. However, even with apparent curative surgery, the recurrence rate is high, and the overall 5-year survival is 30%.

AIMAH is bilateral massive macronodular cortical hyperplasia (the adrenal glands typically weigh 100–500 g each). In some cases, the pathogenesis of AIMAH involves inappropriate expression of ectopic receptors (e.g., gastric inhibitory polypeptide, β-adrenergic, vasopressin, serotonin, or luteinizing hormone) or overexpression of eutopic receptors. The mechanism underlying the promiscuous expression of the ectopic receptors is unknown. These patients typically have mild and slowly progressive Cushing syndrome. If feasible, bilateral laparoscopic adrenalectomy is the treatment of choice to cure Cushing syndrome associated with AIMAH.

PPNAD may occur in sporadic or familial forms (as part of the Carney complex) (see Plate 3-12). The hypercortisolism in individuals with PPNAD is caused by multiple, pigmented, autonomously functioning adrenocortical nodules. Patients with PPNAD tend to be young and have mild signs and symptoms related to hypercortisolism, have marked osteoporosis (presumably because of long-standing mild hypercortisolism before clinical detection), and may have cyclic disease. Baseline hormonal evaluation documents increased levels of cortisol in the blood and urine, suppressed ACTH, suppressed serum DHEA-S, and a paradoxical increase in urinary free cortisol with dexamethasone-suppression testing. In patients with PPNAD, the adrenal glands are usually of normal size, and most are studded with black, brown, or red nodules ranging in size from 1 mm to 3 cm. Most of the pigmented nodules are smaller than 4 mm in diameter and are interspersed in the adjacent atrophic cortex. PPNAD may occur as part of the Carney complex, which is characterized by spotty skin pigmentation (pigmented lentigines and blue nevi on the face—including the eyelids, vermilion borders of the lips, the conjunctivae, the sclera—and the labia and scrotum); myxomas (cardiac atrium, cutaneous, and mammary); testicular large-cell calcifying Sertoli cell tumors; growth hormone–secreting pituitary adenomas; and psammomatous melanotic schwannomas. Bilateral laparoscopic adrenalectomy is the treatment of choice to cure Cushing syndrome associated with PPNAD.

Plate 3-12

Endocrine System

CUSHING'S SYNDROME IN A PATIENT WITH THE CARNEY COMPLEX

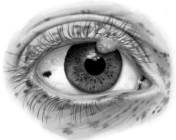

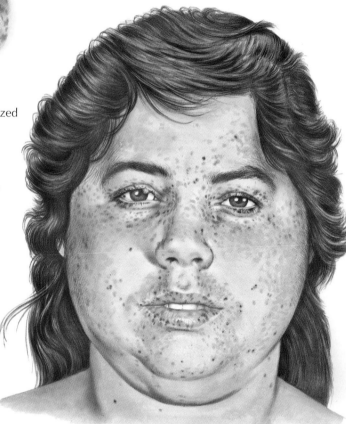

The Carney complex is characterized by spotty skin pigmentation. Pigmented lentigines and blue nevi can be seen on the face—including the eyelids, vermilion borders of the lips, the conjunctivae, the sclera—and the labia and scrotum.

CUSHING SYNDROME CAUSED BY PRIMARY PIGMENTED NODULAR ADRENOCORTICAL DISEASE

A rare form of Cushing syndrome is corticotropin (adrenocorticotropic hormone [ACTH])-independent primary pigmented nodular adrenocortical disease (PPNAD), which may be sporadic or familial (as part of the Carney complex). The hypercortisolism in individuals with PPNAD is caused by multiple, pigmented, autonomously functioning adrenocortical nodules. Patients with PPNAD may present with the typical signs and symptoms of hypercortisolism, including central weight gain, hyperglycemia, proximal muscle weakness, purple-red abdominal striae, hypertension, and menstrual cycle disturbance. However, patients with PPNAD tend to be young (i.e., younger than 30 years), have mild signs and symptoms related to hypercortisolism, have marked osteoporosis (presumably because of long-standing mild hypercortisolism before clinical detection), and may have cyclic disease. Baseline hormonal evaluation documents increased levels of cortisol in the blood and urine, suppressed ACTH, suppressed serum dehydroepiandrosterone sulfate, and a paradoxical increase in urinary free cortisol with dexamethasone suppression testing.

In patients with this disease, the adrenal glands are usually of normal size, and most are studded with black, brown, or red nodules ranging in size from 1 mm to 3 cm. Most of the pigmented nodules are smaller than 4 mm in diameter and are interspersed in the adjacent atrophic cortex. The weight of a PPNAD adrenal gland is either normal (e.g., 4 g) or mildly enlarged (e.g., 5–15 g). The cells in the PPNAD nodules contain granular brown pigment (lipofuscin) and are globular with clear or eosinophilic cytoplasm. PPNAD may occur as part of the Carney complex, which is characterized by spotty skin pigmentation (pigmented lentigines and blue nevi on the face—including the eyelids, vermilion borders of the lips, the conjunctivae, and the sclera—and the labia and scrotum); myxomas (cardiac atrium, cutaneous, and mammary); testicular large-cell calcifying Sertoli cell tumors; growth hormone–secreting pituitary adenomas; and psammomatous melanotic schwannomas.

Additional features of the Carney complex can include:

▶ Myxomas: cardiac atrium, cutaneous (e.g., eyelid), and mammary

▶ Testicular large-cell calcifying Sertoli cell tumors

▶ Growth hormone–secreting pituitary adenomas

▶ Psammomatous melanotic schwannomas

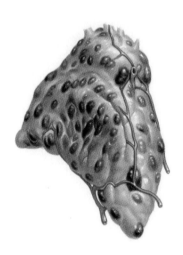

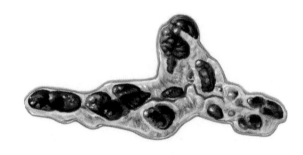

PPNAD adrenal glands are usually of normal size, and most are studded with black, brown, or red nodules. Most of the pigmented nodules are less than 4 mm in diameter and interspersed in the adjacent atrophic cortex.

Approximately half of the patients diagnosed with PPNAD prove to have the Carney complex. Approximately 60% of the cases of the Carney complex are familial. Thus far, mutations in three genes have been associated with PPNAD: *PRKAR1A*, *PDE11A*, and *MYH8*. However, because there are families with Carney complex that do not have mutations in one of these three genes, studies are ongoing to identify additional loci. Heterozygous inactivating mutations in *PRKAR1A*—an apparent tumor suppressor gene that encodes the protein kinase A regulatory 1α subunit—are found in approximately 70% of patients with the Carney complex. In most familial cases, the Carney complex appears to be autosomal dominant in inheritance. Germline mutations in *PRKAR1A* may also be present in patients with isolated PPNAD.

Bilateral laparoscopic adrenalectomy is the treatment of choice to cure Cushing syndrome associated with PPNAD.

MAJOR BLOCKS IN ABNORMAL STEROIDOGENESIS

Genetically determined deficiencies in the enzymes responsible for the biosynthesis of cortisol are referred to as *blocks in adrenal steroidogenesis*. Congenital adrenal hyperplasia (CAH) refers to clinical disorders associated with the decreased production of cortisol and the secondary corticotropin (adrenocorticotropic hormone [ACTH])–driven increased production of precursor steroids that have precursor-specific activity at the mineralocorticoid or androgen receptors.

CONGENITAL LIPOID HYPERPLASIA

The steroidogenic acute regulatory protein (StAR) mobilizes cholesterol from the outer mitochondrial membrane to the inner mitochondrial membrane, where the rate-limiting steroid side-chain cleavage enzyme (P450scc) cleaves cholesterol to pregnenolone. Mutations in the genes encoding either StAR or P450scc result in congenital lipoid adrenal hyperplasia, the most severe form of CAH. This disorder is characterized by a deficiency in all adrenal and gonadal steroid hormones and an ACTH-driven buildup of cholesterol esters in the adrenal cortex. Congenital lipoid adrenal hyperplasia is an autosomal recessive disorder usually caused by mutations in the gene that encodes StAR. The steroidogenic defect progresses with age, suggesting that the cholesterol ester accumulation causes further dysfunction of the adrenocortical cells.

3β-HYDROXYSTEROID DEHYDROGENASE DEFICIENCY

Pregnenolone is converted to progesterone by 3β-hydroxysteroid dehydrogenase (3β-HSD) by a reaction involving dehydrogenation of the 3-hydroxyl group to a keto group and isomerization of the double bond at C5. The type I isoenzyme of 3β-HSD (3β-HSD1) is present in the placenta, liver, and brain, and the type II isoenzyme of 3β-HSD (3β-HSD2) is present in the adrenal cortex and gonads. Mutations in the β-HSD2 gene (*HSD3B2*) cause a rare form of CAH associated with deficiencies in cortisol, aldosterone, and gonadal steroids. Because of the block at 3β-HSD2, there is an accumulation of Δ⁵-pregnenolone, 17α-hydroxypregnenolone, dehydroepiandrosterone (DHEA), and DHEA sulfate (DHEA-S).

17α-HYDROXYLASE DEFICIENCY

Progesterone is hydroxylated to 17-hydroxyprogesterone through the activity of 17α-hydroxylase (P450c17). 17-Hydroxylation is a prerequisite for glucocorticoid synthesis (the zona glomerulosa does not express P450c17). P450c17 also possesses 17,20-lyase activity, which results in the production of the C19 adrenal androgens (DHEA and androstenedione). Deficiency of P450c17 is another rare form of CAH caused by mutations in *CYP17A1*. It is inherited in an autosomal recessive fashion and causes an ACTH-driven increased production of 11-deoxycorticosterone and corticosterone—both of which have some activity at the mineralocorticoid receptor—leading to hypokalemia and hypertension. The deficiency in 17,20-lyase activity results in decreased androgen and estrogen production because the androgen substrate is not present to be aromatized to estrogens.

IV. 21-HYDROXYLASE DEFICIENCY

21-Hydroxylation of either progesterone in the zona glomerulosa or 17-hydroxyprogesterone in the zona fasciculata is performed by 21-hydroxylase (P450c21) to yield 11-deoxycorticosterone or 11-deoxycortisol, respectively. Deficiency of P450c21 is the most common form of CAH, accounting for more than 90% of cases. 21-Hydroxylase deficiency is inherited in an autosomal recessive fashion and leads to an ACTH-driven increased production of progesterone, 17-hydroxyprogesterone, and adrenal androgens.

V. 11β-HYDROXYLASE DEFICIENCY

The final step in cortisol biosynthesis is the conversion of 11-deoxycortisol to cortisol by 11β-hydroxylase (P450c11β). Deficiency of P450c11β is the second most common form of CAH. 11β-Hydroxylase deficiency is inherited in an autosomal recessive fashion and leads to an ACTH-driven buildup of 11-deoxycortisol, 11-deoxycorticosterone, and adrenal androgens. This disorder is caused by mutations in the *CYP11B1* gene.

Additional Enzymatic Steps

In the zona glomerulosa, aldosterone synthase (P450c11AS) converts corticosterone to aldosterone via the intermediate 18-hydroxycorticosterone. Whereas aldosterone secretion is confined to the zona glomerulosa through the restricted expression of aldosterone synthase, the zona glomerulosa cannot synthesize cortisol because it does not express 17α-hydroxylase. In the zona reticularis, high levels of cytochrome b5 facilitate 17,20-lyase activity on P450c17 and the production of DHEA. DHEA is either converted to androstenedione by 3β-HSD or sulfated in the zona reticularis by the DHEA sulfotransferase to form DHEA-S. Androstenedione may be converted to testosterone by 17β-ketosteroid reductase (17β-HSD3) in the adrenal glands or gonads. The interconversion of cortisol and cortisone via 11β-hydroxysteroid dehydrogenase (11β-HSD) regulates local corticosteroid hormone action. There are two distinct 11β-HSD isozymes. Type 1 (11β-HSD1) is expressed primarily in the liver and converts cortisone to cortisol; type 2 (11β-HSD2) is found in the mineralocorticoid receptor in the kidney, colon, and salivary glands and inactivates cortisol to cortisone.

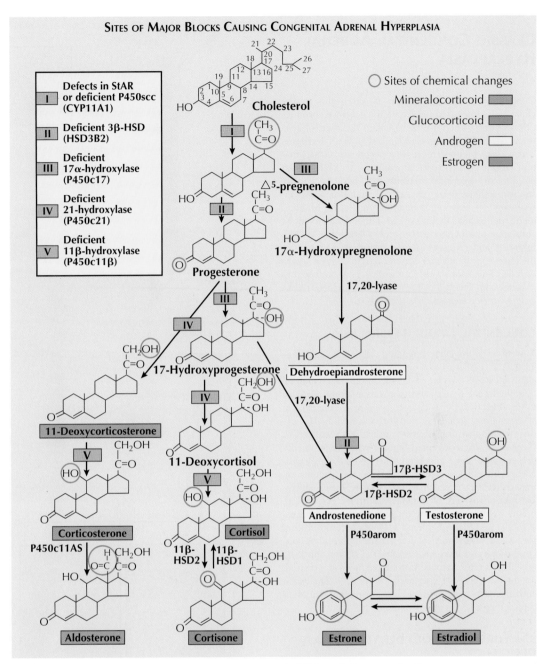

SITES OF MAJOR BLOCKS CAUSING CONGENITAL ADRENAL HYPERPLASIA

I	Defects in StAR or deficient P450scc (CYP11A1)
II	Deficient 3β-HSD (HSD3B2)
III	Deficient 17α-hydroxylase (P450c17)
IV	Deficient 21-hydroxylase (P450c21)
V	Deficient 11β-hydroxylase (P450c11β)

Sites of chemical changes
Mineralocorticoid
Glucocorticoid
Androgen
Estrogen

Plate 3-14

Endocrine System

CLASSIC CONGENITAL ADRENAL HYPERPLASIA

Congenital adrenal hyperplasia (CAH) refers to the clinical disorders associated with the decreased production of cortisol because of blocks in the cortisol synthetic enzyme pathway (see Plate 3-13). With decreased cortisol production, there is a secondary corticotropin (adrenocorticotropic hormone [ACTH])–driven buildup of precursor steroids that have precursor-specific activity at the mineralocorticoid or androgen receptors. In addition, depending on the site of enzymatic deficiency, deficiency of mineralocorticoid or androgen production may occur. Depending on the mutation and resultant degree of protein dysfunction, the deficiency in adrenal enzyme activity may be severe or mild. The most severe forms of CAH are referred to as *classic*, and the milder forms of CAH are referred to as *late-onset* or *nonclassic* (see Plate 3-16).

CONGENITAL LIPOID HYPERPLASIA

Mutations in the genes encoding either the steroidogenic acute regulatory protein (StAR) or the steroid side-chain cleavage enzyme (P450scc) result in congenital lipoid adrenal hyperplasia, the most severe form of CAH. This disorder is characterized by a deficiency in all adrenal and gonadal steroid hormones and an ACTH-driven buildup of cholesterol esters in the adrenal cortex. Neonates with congenital lipoid hyperplasia usually present with signs and symptoms of marked adrenocortical insufficiency (e.g., hyperemesis, hypotension, hyperkalemia, hyponatremia) shortly after birth. Because of the lack of testicular androgen production, infants with a 46,XY karyotype have female external genitalia (see Plates 4-13 and 4-15). Laboratory testing shows low serum cortisol and plasma aldosterone concentrations and increased serum ACTH concentration and plasma renin activity. If not recognized and treated, congenital lipoid hyperplasia is lethal. Treatment consists of glucocorticoid and mineralocorticoid replacement.

3β-HYDROXYSTEROID DEHYDROGENASE DEFICIENCY

Pregnenolone is converted to progesterone by 3β-hydroxysteroid dehydrogenase (3β-HSD). Mutations in the 3β-HSD2 gene (*HSD3B2*) cause a rare form of CAH associated with deficiency in cortisol, aldosterone, and gonadal steroids. The clinical presentation of CAH caused by 3β-HSD deficiency is similar to that of StAR deficiency—infants present with signs and symptoms of both cortisol and aldosterone deficiencies. The excess dehydroepiandrosterone (DHEA) may cause mild virilization in infants with a 46,XX karyotype. The phenotype in infants with a 46,XY karyotype varies from normal to hypospadias to female external genitalia. Late-onset forms of 3β-HSD also exist (see Plate 3-16). In addition to hyperkalemia, hyponatremia, cortisol deficiency, and aldosterone deficiency, laboratory studies show increased baseline blood concentrations of DHEA and DHEA sulfate (DHEA-S). Because most of the adrenal androstenedione production is dependent on the conversion of DHEA to androstenedione by 3β-HSD, androstenedione levels are not increased in this form of CAH. Exaggerated increases in the blood concentrations of Δ⁵-pregnenolone and DHEA are observed with the cosyntropin-stimulation test.

Affected patients are treated with glucocorticoid and mineralocorticoid replacement and, at puberty, with gonadal steroid replacement.

17α-HYDROXYLASE DEFICIENCY

Progesterone is hydroxylated to 17-hydroxyprogesterone through the activity of 17α-hydroxylase (P450c17). 17α-Hydroxylase deficiency is a rare form of CAH caused by mutations in *CYP17A1*. It is inherited in an autosomal recessive fashion and causes ACTH-driven increased production of 11-deoxycorticosterone and corticosterone—both of which have some activity at the mineralocorticoid receptor—leading to hypokalemia and hypertension. The deficiency in 17,20-lyase activity results in decreased androgen and estrogen production because the androgen substrate is not present to be aromatized to estrogens. The clinical presentation may not occur until puberty when individuals with a 46,XX karyotype are found to have primary amenorrhea, absent secondary sexual development, hypertension, and hypokalemia. Individuals with a 46,XY karyotype who are phenotypically female, are usually not evaluated until the lack of pubertal development; they have female external genitalia, intraabdominal testes, short vagina, absent uterus and fallopian tubes, hypertension, and hypokalemia (see Plate 4-15). Laboratory studies show hypokalemia, low plasma renin activity, and low plasma aldosterone concentration. Blood concentrations of ACTH, progesterone, 11-deoxycorticosterone, luteinizing hormone, and follicle-stimulating hormone are increased. Decreased blood concentrations of 17-hydroxyprogesterone, 11-deoxycortisol, cortisol, DHEA, DHEA-S, androstenedione, testosterone, and estradiol are observed. Treatment includes replacement of glucocorticoid and gonadal steroids.

Little or no inhibition of hypothalamic CRH or pituitary ACTH production because of deficient cortisol

Pigmentation caused by increased ACTH

Hypothalamus

Adeno-hypophysis

ACTH greatly increased

Hyperplasia of adrenal cortex

Cortisol

11-Deoxycortisol

11-Deoxycorticosterone

17α-Hydroxyprogesterone

Progesterone

Cholesterol

Block 20

Δ⁵-Pregnenolone

17-Hydroxypregnenolone

Corticosterone

Aldosterone

Adrenal androgens (greatly increased because of lack of cortisol inhibition of ACTH and 21 block)

Lipoid hyperplasia of adrenal cortex

H & E stain

Fat stain

Plate 3-14

Adrenal

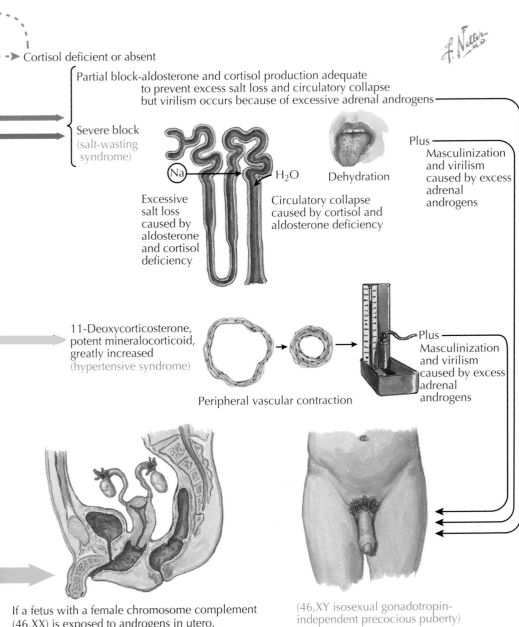

Cortisol deficient or absent

Partial block-aldosterone and cortisol production adequate to prevent excess salt loss and circulatory collapse but virilism occurs because of excessive adrenal androgens

Severe block (salt-wasting syndrome)

Na   H₂O   Dehydration

Excessive salt loss caused by aldosterone and cortisol deficiency

Circulatory collapse caused by cortisol and aldosterone deficiency

Plus Masculinization and virilism caused by excess adrenal androgens

11-Deoxycorticosterone, potent mineralocorticoid, greatly increased (hypertensive syndrome)

Peripheral vascular contraction

Plus Masculinization and virilism caused by excess adrenal androgens

If a fetus with a female chromosome complement (46,XX) is exposed to androgens in utero, androgenization of the external genitalia occurs (46,XX disorder of sex development)

(46,XY isosexual gonadotropin-independent precocious puberty)

Deficiency in all adrenal and gonadal steroid hormones

Because of the lack of testicular androgen production, neonates with a 46,XY karyotype have female external genitalia (46,XY disorder of sex development)

CLASSIC CONGENITAL ADRENAL HYPERPLASIA (Continued)

21-HYDROXYLASE DEFICIENCY

21-Hydroxylation of either progesterone in the zona glomerulosa or 17-hydroxyprogesterone in the zona fasciculata is performed by 21-hydroxylase (P450c21) to yield deoxycorticosterone or 11-deoxycortisol, respectively. Deficiency of P450c21 is the most common form of CAH, accounting for more than 90% of all cases. Classic 21-hydroxylase deficiency presents in infancy with typical signs and symptoms of adrenal insufficiency and androgen excess. Ambiguous genitalia are found in infants with a 46,XX karyotype (see Plate 4-12). Depending on the severity of the enzymatic defect and its effect on the mineralocorticoid synthetic pathway, classic 21-hydroxylase deficiency may be referred to as *salt wasting* or *simple virilizing*. In both forms of classic 21-hydroxylase deficiency, a markedly increased (greater than sixfold above the upper limit of the reference range) blood concentration of 17-hydroxyprogresterone is diagnostic. In borderline cases, a cosyntropin-stimulation test may be needed to demonstrate the enzymatic block. Additional blood tests usually show low blood concentrations of 11-deoxycortisol, cortisol, 11-deoxycorticosterone, and aldosterone (the latter two in the salt-wasting form). Increased blood concentrations of the following are usually observed: progesterone, 17-hydroxyprogesterone, androstenedione, and ACTH. Plasma renin activity is usually increased. Newborn screening for 21-hydroxylase deficiency by measuring 17-hydroxyprogesterone in a dried blood sample is routinely performed in the United States and in many other countries.

11β-HYDROXYLASE DEFICIENCY

Deficiency of 11β-hydroxylase (P450c11β) is the second most common form of CAH. With more severe defects in 11β-hydroxylase function, neonates with a 46,XX karyotype are born with ambiguous genitalia, and neonates with a 46,XY karyotype are born with penile enlargement. With *CYP11B1* mutations that result in decreased, but not absent, 11β-hydroxylase activity, affected individuals may present later in childhood with hypertension and precocious puberty or in young adulthood with hypertension, acne, hirsutism, and oligomenorrhea or amenorrhea. Although 11-deoxycortisol has no glucocorticoid activity, 11-deoxycorticosterone has mineralocorticoid activity, and when produced in excess, it can cause hypertension, hypokalemia, low plasma renin activity, and low plasma aldosterone concentration. Additional findings on laboratory testing in patients with 11β-hydroxylase deficiency include increased blood concentrations of 11-deoxycortisol, 11-deoxycorticosterone, DHEA, DHEA-S, androstenedione, and testosterone.

APPARENT MINERALOCORTICOID EXCESS

The interconversion of cortisol and cortisone via 11β-hydroxysteroid dehydrogenase (11β-HSD) regulates local corticosteroid hormone action. There are two distinct 11β-HSD isozymes. Type 1 (11β-HSD1) converts cortisone to cortisol; type 2 (11β-HSD2) inactivates cortisol to cortisone. Apparent mineralocorticoid excess is the result of impaired 11β-HSD2 activity. Cortisol can be a potent mineralocorticoid, and as a result of the enzyme deficiency, high levels of cortisol accumulate in the kidneys. Thus, 11β-HSD2 normally excludes physiologic glucocorticoids from the nonselective mineralocorticoid receptor by converting them to the inactive 11-keto compound, cortisone. Decreased 11β-HSD2 activity may be hereditary or secondary to pharmacologic inhibition of enzyme activity by glycyrrhizic acid, the active component of licorice root (*Glycyrrhiza glabra*). The clinical phenotype of patients with apparent mineralocorticoid excess includes hypertension, hypokalemia, metabolic alkalosis, low plasma renin activity, low plasma aldosterone concentration, and normal plasma cortisol levels. The diagnosis is confirmed by demonstrating an abnormal ratio of cortisol to cortisone (e.g., >10:1) in a 24-hour urine collection. The apparent mineralocorticoid excess state caused by ectopic ACTH secretion, seen in patients with Cushing syndrome, is related to the high rates of cortisol production that overwhelm 11β-HSD2 activity.

Plate 3-15

Endocrine System

THE BIOLOGIC ACTIONS OF ADRENAL ANDROGENS

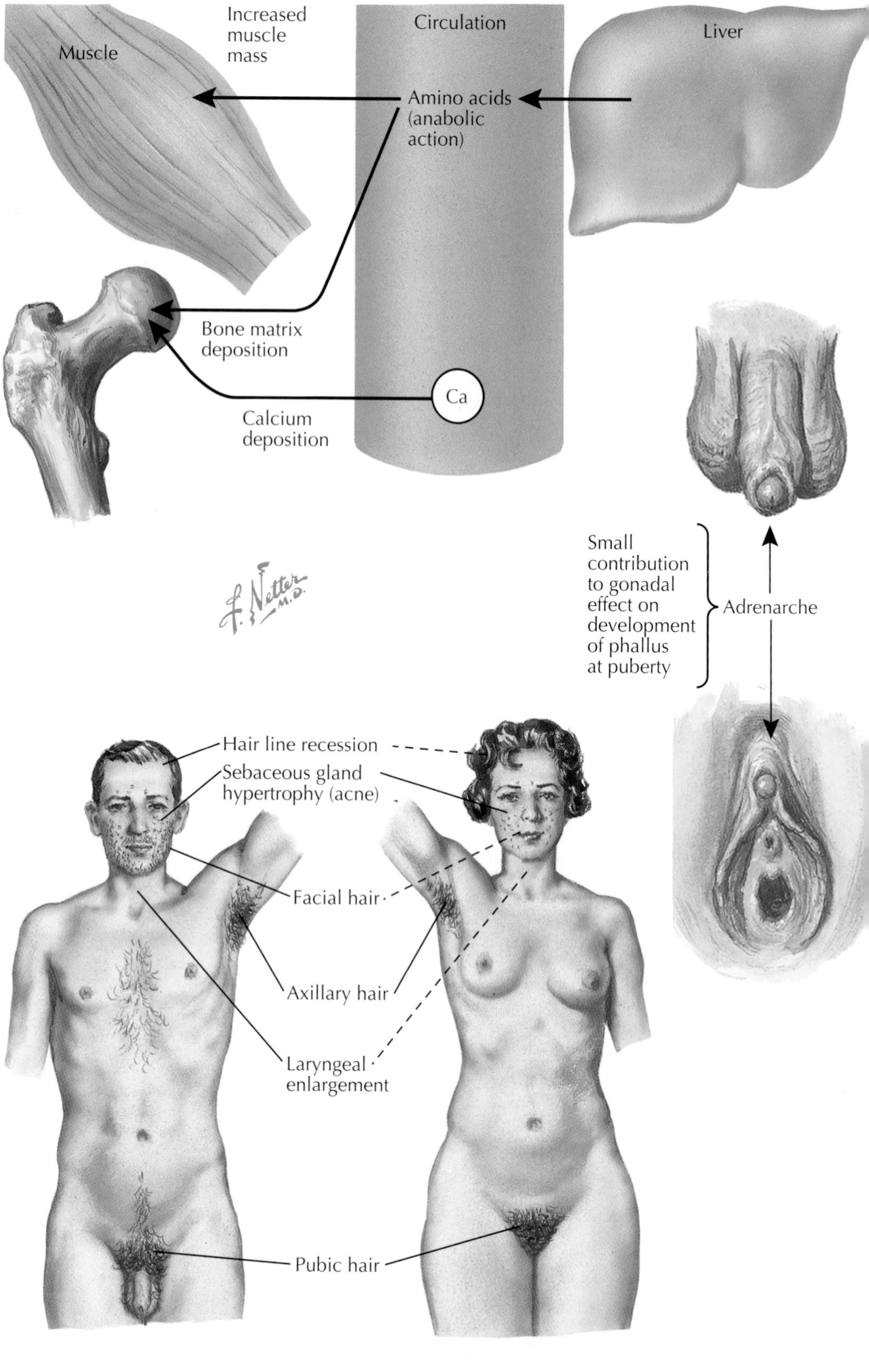

Androgens produced by the adrenal cortex in both sexes include dehydroepiandrosterone (DHEA), DHEA sulfate (DHEA-S), androstenedione, and testosterone. In varying degrees, adrenal androgens have an anabolic effect leading to increased muscle mass. They stimulate male sex characteristics, including an increase in facial hair, recession of the scalp hairline, hypertrophy of sebaceous glands and acne, enlargement of larynx resulting in the deep male voice, secondary sex hair growth in axillary and pubic regions, hair growth over the chest and around the nipples, and development of the phallus in puberty. Although the main source of androgens in men is gonadal, in most women, the adrenal glands are the primary source of androgens. Indeed, a key sign of primary adrenal failure in women is loss of axillary and pubic hair.

Adrenarche is a biochemical event, defined as the increase in adrenal androgens that occurs between 6 and 8 years of age. Pubarche is a phenotypic event, defined as the growth of sexual hair in the suprapubic area and the axillae. Adrenal androgens are the primary factors that facilitate pubic and axillary hair growth in girls; labial hair usually precedes axillary hair growth. In boys, the role of adrenal androgens is not as clear because of the dominant role of testicular testosterone production. Adrenal androgens appear to be an important factor in the onset of puberty and the maturation of the hypothalamic–pituitary–gonadal complex. Adrenarche and pubarche are considered premature when pubic hair growth appears before age 8 years in girls and before age 9 years in boys. Premature adrenarche, which is more common in girls, is associated with taller height, increased body odor and acne, and a bone age that is advanced by 1 to 2 years.

Adrenal androgens may have additional physiologic roles yet to be delineated. DHEA-S may serve as a large sex steroid depot. DHEA-S is converted to testosterone and estradiol in peripheral tissues; a sulfatase converts DHEA-S to DHEA, which is then converted to androstenedione by 3β-hydroxysteroid dehydrogenase. Androstenedione is metabolized to either testosterone or estradiol by 17β-hydroxysteroid dehydrogenase and P450 aromatase, respectively. DHEA may also act as a neurosteroid in the central nervous system; however, a DHEA-specific receptor has not yet been identified.

Androgenic (anabolic) steroids have been used surreptitiously by athletes to increase muscle mass and to enhance physical performance. The prevalence of their use is difficult to determine, but approximately 6% of high school boys and 2% of high school girls have reported using androgenic steroids at least once. Anabolic steroids are prohibited by the International Olympic Committee and the National Collegiate Athletic Association for use in competition. Athletes often take several performance-enhancing drugs in various patterns (e.g., simultaneously, consecutively, escalating doses, or intermittently) in an attempt to increase the overall effect on performance. Adverse effects include suppression of endogenous testicular function (resulting in transient infertility and decreased testicular size), gynecomastia (because testosterone is aromatized to estradiol), erythrocytosis, increased liver enzymes and peliosis hepatitis (only with oral 17-α-alkylated androgens), mood disorders and aggressive behavior, decreased serum high-density lipoprotein cholesterol concentrations, increased low-density lipoprotein cholesterol concentrations, virilization in women (e.g., hirsutism, temporal hair recession, acne, deepening of the voice, and clitoral enlargement), premature epiphyseal fusion, and stunting of growth in adolescents. Athletes may take additional agents to mask the visible side effects of high-dose anabolic steroids; for example, athletes may take human chorionic gonadotropin to counteract the decrease in testicular size, an aromatase inhibitor or estrogen receptor antagonist to counteract the gynecomastia, and a 5α-reductase inhibitor to prevent balding and acne.

Plate 3-16   Adrenal

ADULT ANDROGENITAL SYNDROMES

Adult adrenogenital syndromes are disorders associated with excess adrenal androgen effects in adults. The causes of adrenal androgen excess in adults include late-onset (nonclassic) congenital adrenal hyperplasia (CAH), familial glucocorticoid resistance, Cushing syndrome, and androgen-secreting adrenal neoplasms. Because of the presence of more potent testicular androgens, adrenal androgen excess in men may go undetected because of lack of symptomatology. However, women with adrenal androgen excess usually present with varying degrees of masculinization and menstrual dysfunction (see Plates 4-14 and 4-15).

Hirsutism is defined as excessive male-pattern coarse hair growth in women (e.g., cheeks, upper lip, chin, midline chest, male escutcheon, inner thighs, and midline lower back). Virilization, reflecting a more severe form of androgen excess, is defined as the development of signs and symptoms of masculinization in women. The signs and symptoms of masculinization include increased muscle bulk, loss of female body contours, deepening of the voice, breast atrophy, clitoromegaly, temporal balding, and androgenic flush (plethora of the face, neck, and upper chest). The normal size of the clitoris is smaller than 10 mm in length and smaller than 7 mm in width.

LATE-ONSET (NONCLASSIC) CONGENITAL ADRENAL HYPERPLASIA

Partial enzymatic blocks in 3β-hydroxysteroid dehydrogenase, 21-hydroxylase, and 11β-hydroxylase may all present in late-onset or nonclassic forms (also referred to as adult-onset, attenuated, incomplete, and cryptic adrenal hyperplasia) and be responsible for hirsutism, menstrual irregularities, and varying degrees of virilization. Late-onset 3β-hydroxysteroid dehydrogenase deficiency should be suspected in symptomatic women who have markedly increased blood concentrations of dehydroepiandrosterone sulfate (DHEA-S) and low levels of androstenedione. The diagnosis can be confirmed with cosyntropin-stimulation testing and demonstration of a marked increase in 17-hydroxypregnenolone and DHEA but no increase in 17-hydroxyprogesterone and androstenedione. Late-onset 11-hydroxylase deficiency may have an identical presentation to that of 3β-hydroxysteroid dehydrogenase deficiency, but the laboratory profile is different. With 11-hydroxylase deficiency, the baseline levels of progesterone, 17-hydroxyprogesterone, and androstenedione are increased above the reference range, and all three increase dramatically after cosyntropin stimulation. A partial block at 11β-hydroxylase is associated with increased blood concentrations of 11-deoxycortisol, 11-deoxycorticosterone, DHEA, and androstenedione. In addition to symptoms related to androgen excess, individuals with partial 11β-hydroxylase deficiency may have hypertension and hypokalemia. Cosyntropin-stimulation testing may be needed to confirm the block at 11β-hydroxylase. Treatment for late-onset CAH includes glucocorticoid replacement to suppress the excess corticotropin (adrenocorticotropic hormone [ACTH]) secretion, with the goal of avoiding overtreatment and resultant Cushing syndrome.

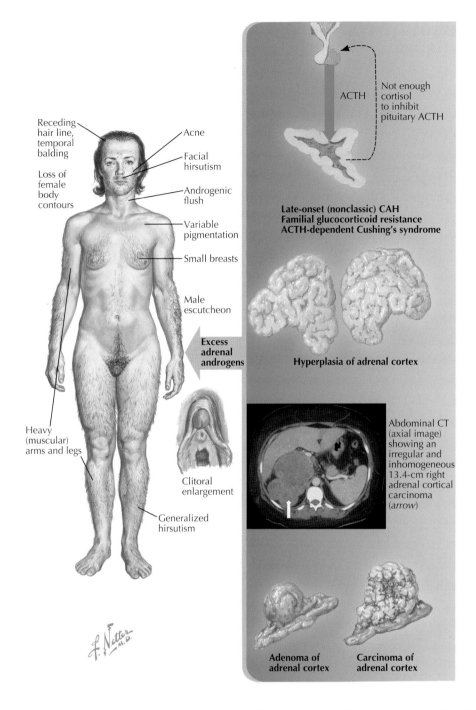

Receding hair line, temporal balding

Loss of female body contours

Acne

Facial hirsutism

Androgenic flush

Variable pigmentation

Small breasts

Male escutcheon

Excess adrenal androgens

Heavy (muscular) arms and legs

Clitoral enlargement

Generalized hirsutism

Not enough cortisol to inhibit pituitary ACTH

ACTH

Late-onset (nonclassic) CAH
Familial glucocorticoid resistance
ACTH-dependent Cushing's syndrome

Hyperplasia of adrenal cortex

Abdominal CT (axial image) showing an irregular and inhomogeneous 13.4-cm right adrenal cortical carcinoma (*arrow*)

Adenoma of adrenal cortex

Carcinoma of adrenal cortex

FAMILIAL GLUCOCORTICOID RESISTANCE

Familial glucocorticoid resistance is caused by mutations in the glucocorticoid receptor gene. These mutations inhibit the action of cortisol, leading to increased ACTH secretion and adrenocortical hyperplasia. With the increased mass action of cortisol production, there is increased production of adrenal androgens (e.g., DHEA) and mineralocorticoids (e.g., 11-deoxycorticosterone). Thus, individuals with familial glucocorticoid resistance present clinically in a very similar way to those with late-onset 11β-hydroxylase deficiency with signs and symptoms of androgen excess, hypertension, and hypokalemia.

ADRENOCORTICOTROPIC HORMONE–DEPENDENT CUSHING SYNDROME

The hypersecretion of ACTH in patients with ACTH-dependent Cushing syndrome leads to the production

of excess adrenal androgens and weak mineralocorticoids (see Plate 3-9).

ANDROGEN-SECRETING ADRENAL NEOPLASMS

Androgen-secreting adrenal neoplasms are rare. Androgen hypersecretion occurs more often with adrenocortical carcinoma than with adrenal adenomas. The most common hypersecreted androgen is DHEA, followed by androstenedione and testosterone. The distinction between adenoma and carcinoma can usually be made before surgery on the basis of the imaging phenotype on computed tomography (CT). Whereas testosterone-secreting adenomas are usually small (e.g., 1 cm in diameter), homogeneous, and low in density on CT, androgen-secreting adrenocortical carcinomas are almost always more than 4 cm in diameter (average diameter, 10 cm), are inhomogeneous, and have a higher density on CT.

Plate 3-17

Endocrine Syster

THE BIOLOGIC ACTIONS OF ALDOSTERONE

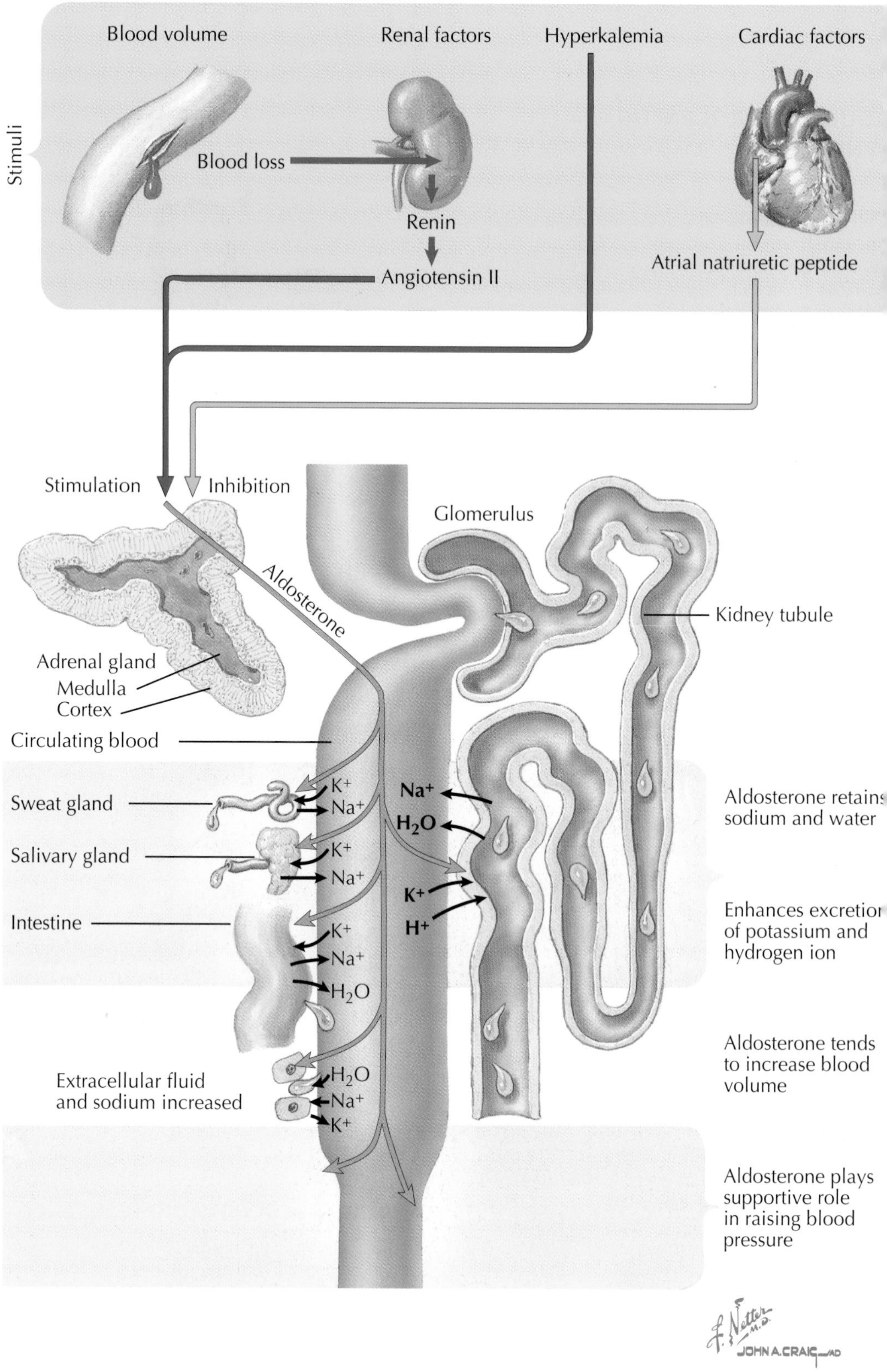

Aldosterone secretion is stimulated by angiotensin II, hyperkalemia, and (to a lesser extent) corticotropin; aldosterone secretion is inhibited by atrial natriuretic factor and hypokalemia. Approximately 50% to 70% of aldosterone circulates bound to either albumin or weakly to corticosteroid-binding globulin; 30% to 50% of total plasma aldosterone is free. Thus, aldosterone has a relatively short half-life of 15 to 20 minutes. In the liver, aldosterone is rapidly inactivated to tetrahydroaldosterone. The normal peripheral blood concentration of aldosterone ranges between 0 and 21 ng/dL.

The classic functions of aldosterone are regulation of extracellular volume and control of potassium homeostasis. These effects are mediated by binding of free aldosterone to the mineralocorticoid receptor in the cytosol of epithelial cells, principally the distal tubules in the kidney, where it facilitates the exchange of sodium for potassium and hydrogen ions. The action of angiotensin II on aldosterone involves a negative feedback loop that also includes extracellular fluid volume. The main function of this feedback loop is to modify sodium homeostasis and, secondarily, to regulate blood pressure. Thus, sodium restriction activates the renin–angiotensin–aldosterone axis. The effects of angiotensin II on both the adrenal cortex and the renal vasculature promote renal sodium conservation. Conversely, with suppression of renin release and suppression of the level of circulating angiotensin, aldosterone secretion is reduced and renal blood flow is increased, thereby promoting sodium loss. The renin–angiotensin–aldosterone loop is very sensitive to dietary sodium intake. Sodium excess enhances the renal and peripheral vasculature responsiveness and reduces the adrenal responsiveness to angiotensin II. Sodium restriction has the opposite effect. Thus, sodium intake modifies target tissue responsiveness to angiotensin II, a fine tuning that appears to be critical to maintaining normal sodium homeostasis without a chronic effect on blood pressure.

Mineralocorticoid receptors have tissue-specific expression. For example, the tissues with the highest concentrations of these receptors are the distal nephron, colon, and hippocampus. Lower levels of mineralocorticoid receptors are found in the rest of the gastrointestinal tract, sweat glands, salivary glands, and heart. Transport to the nucleus and binding to specific binding domains on targeted genes lead to their increased expression. Aldosterone-regulated kinase appears to be a key intermediary, and its increased expression leads to modification of the apical sodium channel, resulting in increased sodium ion transport across the cell membrane. The increased luminal negativity augments tubular secretion of potassium by the tubular cells and hydrogen ion by the interstitial cells. Glucocorticoids and mineralocorticoids bind equally to the mineralocorticoid receptor. Specificity of action is provided in many tissues by the presence of a glucocorticoid-degrading enzyme, 11β-hydroxysteroid dehydrogenase, which prevents glucocorticoids from interacting with the receptor. Mineralocorticoid "escape" refers to the counterregulatory mechanisms that are manifested after 3 to 5 days of excessive mineralocorticoid administration. Several mechanisms contribute to this escape, including renal hemodynamic factors and an increased level of atrial natriuretic peptide.

In addition to the classic genomic actions mediated by aldosterone binding to cytosolic receptors,

mineralocorticoids have acute, nongenomic actions caused by activation of an unidentified cell surface receptor. This action involves a G protein signaling pathway and probably modification of the sodium–hydrogen exchange activity. This effect has been demonstrated in both epithelial and nonepithelial cells.

Aldosterone has additional, nonclassic effects primarily on nonepithelial cells. These actions, although probably genomic and therefore mediated by activation of the cytosolic mineralocorticoid receptor, do not include modification of sodium–potassium balance.

Aldosterone-mediated actions include the expression o several collagen genes; genes controlling tissue growt factors, such as transforming growth factor β and plas minogen activator inhibitor type 1; or genes mediatin inflammation. The resultant actions lead to microan giopathy; acute necrosis; and fibrosis in various tissue such as the heart, vasculature, and kidney. Increase levels of aldosterone are not necessary to cause thi damage; an imbalance between the volume or sodiur balance state and the level of aldosterone appears to b the critical factor.

Plate 3-18

Adrenal

PRIMARY ALDOSTERONISM

Hypertension, suppressed renin, and increased aldosterone secretion characterize the syndrome of primary aldosteronism (PA), which was first described in 1955 by Jerome Conn. Bilateral idiopathic hyperaldosteronism (IHA) and aldosterone-producing adenoma (APA) are the most common subtypes of PA. A much less common form, unilateral adrenal hyperplasia (UAH), is caused by zona glomerulosa hyperplasia of predominantly one adrenal gland. Two forms of familial hyperaldosteronism (FH) have been described: FH type I and FH type II. FH type I, or glucocorticoid-remediable aldosteronism (GRA), is autosomal dominant in inheritance and is associated with variable degrees of hyperaldosteronism, and aldosterone hypersecretion suppresses with exogenous glucocorticoids. FH type II refers to the familial occurrence of APA, IHA, or both. Very rarely, excessive aldosterone may be secreted by a neoplasm outside of the adrenal gland (e.g., ovary).

PA is the most common form of identifiable secondary hypertension, affecting 5% of all patients with hypertension. Most patients with PA do not have hypokalemia and present with asymptomatic hypertension, which may be mild or severe. Aldosterone excess results in the renal loss of potassium and hydrogen ions. When hypokalemia does occur, it is usually associated with alkalosis, and patients may present with nocturia and polyuria (caused by hypokalemia-induced failure in renal concentrating ability), palpitations, muscle cramps, or positive Chvostek and Trousseau signs. Patients with hypertension and hypokalemia, treatment-resistant hypertension, hypertension and adrenal incidentaloma, onset of hypertension younger than 20 years, or severe hypertension should undergo testing for PA, as should patients for whom a diagnosis of secondary hypertension is being considered. Case finding can be completed with a simple morning (8–10 AM) blood test (ratio of plasma aldosterone concentration [PAC] to plasma renin activity [PRA]) in a seated, ambulatory patient. The patient may take any antihypertensive drugs except mineralocorticoid receptor (MR) antagonists or high-dose amiloride. Hypokalemia is associated with false-negative ratios, and any potassium deficit should be corrected before testing. The PAC:PRA ratio is a case-finding test with sensitivity and specificity of approximately 75%. All patients with an increased PAC:PRA ratio should undergo confirmatory testing, a step completed with aldosterone-suppression testing (e.g., oral sodium loading, saline-suppression testing, captopril-stimulation testing, or fludrocortisone-suppression testing).

Unilateral adrenalectomy in patients with APA or UAH results in normalization of hypokalemia in all; hypertension is improved in all and is cured in approximately 30% to 60% of these patients. In IHA, unilateral or bilateral adrenalectomy seldom corrects the hypertension. IHA and GRA should be treated medically. Therefore, for patients who want to pursue a surgical cure, the accurate distinction between the subtypes of PA is a critical step. The subtype evaluation may require one or more tests, the first of which is imaging the adrenal glands with computed tomography (CT). When a small, solitary, hypodense macroadenoma (>1 cm and <2 cm) and normal contralateral adrenal morphology are found on CT in a patient younger than 40 years with PA, unilateral adrenalectomy is a reasonable therapeutic option. However, in many cases, CT may show

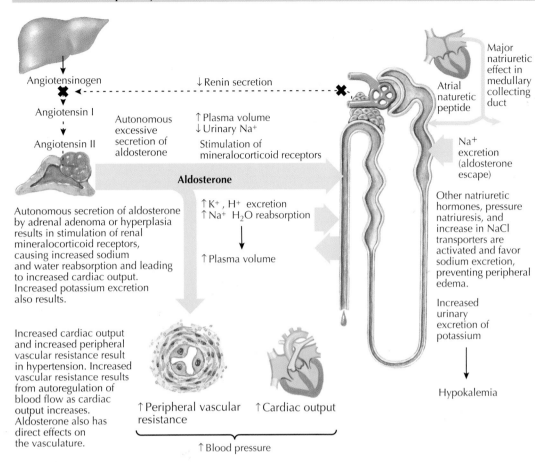

Mechanisms in primary aldosteronism

Angiotensinogen

↓ Renin secretion

Angiotensin I

Angiotensin II

Autonomous excessive secretion of aldosterone

↑Plasma volume
↓Urinary Na+

Stimulation of mineralocorticoid receptors

Aldosterone

Atrial naturetic peptide

Major natriuretic effect in medullary collecting duct

Na+ excretion (aldosterone escape)

Autonomous secretion of aldosterone by adrenal adenoma or hyperplasia results in stimulation of renal mineralocorticoid receptors, causing increased sodium and water reabsorption and leading to increased cardiac output. Increased potassium excretion also results.

↑K+, H+ excretion
↑Na+ H2O reabsorption

↑Plasma volume

Other natriuretic hormones, pressure natriuresis, and increase in NaCl transporters are activated and favor sodium excretion, preventing peripheral edema.

Increased urinary excretion of potassium

Increased cardiac output and increased peripheral vascular resistance result in hypertension. Increased vascular resistance results from autoregulation of blood flow as cardiac output increases. Aldosterone also has direct effects on the vasculature.

↑Peripheral vascular resistance

↑Cardiac output

Hypokalemia

↑Blood pressure

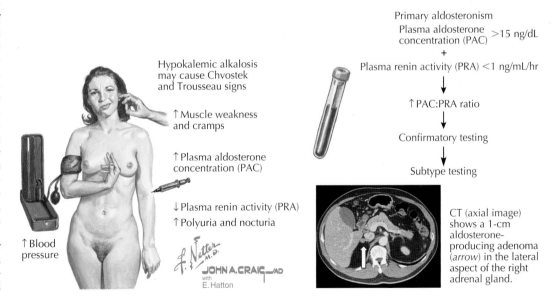

Clinical features

Hypokalemic alkalosis may cause Chvostek and Trousseau signs

↑Muscle weakness and cramps

↑Plasma aldosterone concentration (PAC)

↓Plasma renin activity (PRA)
↑Polyuria and nocturia

↑Blood pressure

J. Netter M.D.
JOHN A. CRAIG—AD
with E. Hatton

Primary aldosteronism
Plasma aldosterone concentration (PAC) >15 ng/dL
+
Plasma renin activity (PRA) <1 ng/mL/hr

↑PAC:PRA ratio

Confirmatory testing

Subtype testing

CT (axial image) shows a 1-cm aldosterone-producing adenoma (arrow) in the lateral aspect of the right adrenal gland.

normal-appearing adrenal glands, minimal unilateral adrenal limb thickening, unilateral microadenomas (≤1 cm), or bilateral macroadenomas. Thus, adrenal venous sampling (AVS) is usually essential to direct appropriate therapy in patients with PA who want to pursue a surgical treatment option (see Plate 3-19).

The treatment goal is to prevent the morbidity and mortality associated with hypertension, hypokalemia, and cardiovascular damage. The cause of the PA helps to determine the appropriate treatment. Normalization of blood pressure should not be the only goal in managing patients with PA. In addition to the kidney and colon, MRs are present in the heart, brain, and blood vessels. Excessive secretion of aldosterone is associated with increased cardiovascular morbidity. Therefore, normalization of circulating aldosterone concentrations or MR blockade should be part of the management plan for all patients with PA. Unilateral laparoscopic adrenalectomy is an excellent treatment option for patients with APA or UAH. Patients with IHA and GRA should be treated medically with an MR antagonist.

Plate 3-19

Endocrine Syste█

ADRENAL VENOUS SAMPLING FOR PRIMARY ALDOSTERONISM

Most patients with primary aldosteronism have either bilateral idiopathic hyperaldosteronism, which is optimally treated medically with mineralocorticoid receptor blockade, or a unilateral aldosterone-producing adenoma, which may be treated surgically with unilateral laparoscopic adrenalectomy (see Plate 3-18). Multiple studies have shown that the accuracy of adrenal computed tomography in localizing the source of aldosterone excess is poor (~50%) and that in patients with primary aldosteronism who wish to pursue the surgical option for hypertension management, adrenal venous sampling (AVS) is a key step.

The keys to successful AVS include appropriate patient selection, careful patient preparation, focused technical expertise, a defined protocol, and accurate data interpretation. A center-specific, written protocol is mandatory. Most centers use a continuous cosyntropin infusion (50 μg/h started 30 minutes before sampling and continued throughout the procedure) during AVS for the following reasons: (1) to minimize stress-induced fluctuations in aldosterone secretion during nonsimultaneous AVS, (2) to maximize the gradient in cortisol from adrenal vein to inferior vena cava (IVC) and thus confirm successful sampling of the adrenal veins, and (3) to maximize the secretion of aldosterone from an aldosterone-producing adenoma.

The adrenal veins are sequentially catheterized through the percutaneous femoral vein approach under fluoroscopic guidance Correct catheter tip location is confirmed with injection of a small amount of contrast medium. Blood is obtained by gentle aspiration from both adrenal veins. Successful catheterization may require an array of catheter configurations; intraprocedural steam-shaping of the catheter tip may be helpful to facilitate access to the adrenal veins. In addition, the placement of side holes very close to the catheter tip may facilitate the blood draw.

The right adrenal vein enters the IVC posteriorly several centimeters above the right renal vein. It is more difficult to catheterize than the left one for a variety of reasons—it is short, small in caliber, and often has an angulated path causing the catheter tip to impact the intima, making blood aspiration problematic. Because of its short length, sometimes it does not support a stable catheter position during respiratory motion. Rarely, it arises in conjunction with a hepatic vein branch and needs to be separately engaged using a specific catheter shape to match the anatomy. Additionally, some physicians confuse the right adrenal vein with adjacent small hepatic vein branches, which are frequently encountered entering the IVC near the adrenal vein region. However, contrast injections clearly distinguish hepatic vein anatomy from that of the adrenal gland.

The left adrenal vein is a tributary of the inferior phrenic vein, which enters the roof of the left renal vein near the lateral margin of the vertebral column in almost all patients. The venous sample from the left side is typically obtained from the common inferior phrenic vein close to the junction of the adrenal vein. Usually, it is rapidly catheterized, and the blood aspiration is easy to achieve.

The final sample needs to be from a pure background source isolated from any possible contamination from the adrenal venous drainage. Traditionally, it is stated

to be the "IVC" sample, although it should be from the external iliac vein; it is free of contamination from collateral left adrenal venous effluent, which on rare occasions drains through a large left gonadal vein caudally into the internal iliac veins.

To minimize the time lag between the sampling of the adrenal veins, the right adrenal vein is sampled first because it is usually more time consuming and will be quickly followed by the left sample in almost all cases. The final sample is from the external iliac vein. This

approach allows all three samples to be close in phys█ ologic time frame. Aldosterone and cortisol concentra█ tions are measured in the blood from all three sites (i.e█ right adrenal vein, left adrenal vein, and IVC). All █ the blood samples should be assayed at 1:1, 1:10, an█ 1:50 dilutions; absolute values are mandatory.

At centers with experience with AVS, the complica█ tion rate is 2.5% or less. Complications can includ█ symptomatic groin hematoma, adrenal hemorrhag█ and dissection of an adrenal vein.

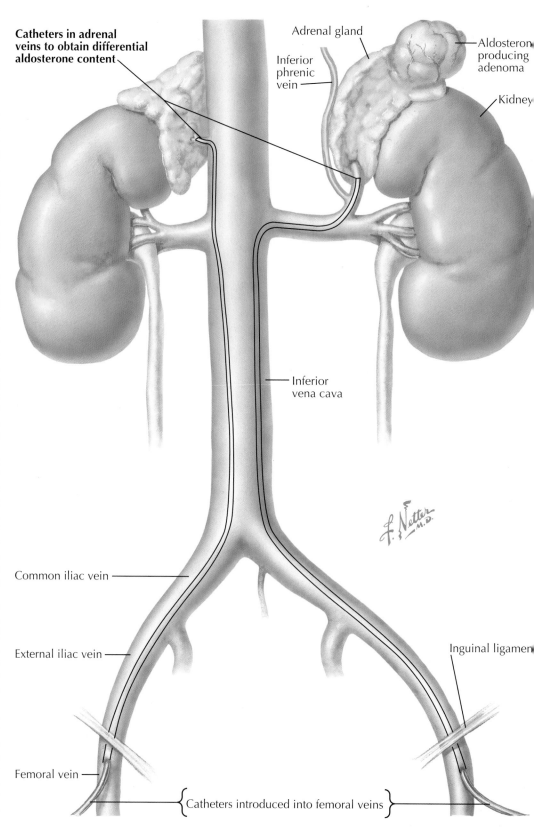

Catheters in adrenal veins to obtain differential aldosterone content

Adrenal gland

Aldosteron█ producing adenoma

Inferior phrenic vein

Kidney

Inferior vena cava

Common iliac vein

External iliac vein

Inguinal ligamen█

Femoral vein

Catheters introduced into femoral veins

REPRODUCTION

Plate 4-1

Endocrine System

DIFFERENTIATION OF GONADS

FACTORS INFLUENCING NORMAL AND ABNORMAL GONADAL DIFFERENTIATION

Whether the primordial gonad differentiates as a testis or as an ovary is determined by genetic information coded on the X and Y chromosomes. The differentiation of all the other anatomic and functional features that distinguish male from female stem secondarily from the effect of testicular or ovarian secretions on their respective primordial structures. The Y chromosome possesses male-determining genes that direct the primitive gonad to develop as a testis, even in the presence of more than one X chromosome. Two X chromosomes are essential for the formation of normal ovaries; individuals with a single X chromosome (karyotype, 45,XO; Turner syndrome) develop gonads that usually display only the most rudimentary form of differentiation.

Although many patients with congenitally defective gonads have an abnormal karyotype caused by meiotic nondisjunction, similar patients may have normal-appearing sex chromosomes or chromosomal abnormalities not explainable on this basis. In individuals with chromosomal mosaicism, the various tissues may have multiple cell lines of differing chromosomal makeup. Mosaicism arises from mitotic nondisjunction or chromosomal loss occurring after fertilization. Other patients may have deletions or translocations of small chromosomal fragments. If these rearrangements disrupt the sex-determining genes, the effect on gonadal structure may be as devastating as in instances where a total chromosome is lost. In other individuals, mutations in sex-determining genes may cause a specific enzymatic error, leading to defective gonadal structure or hormonal secretion.

STAGES IN GONADAL DIFFERENTIATION

Undifferentiated Stage

At the sixth week of gestation, the primitive gonad is represented by a well-demarcated genital ridge running along the dorsal root of the mesentery. The cortical portion of the ridge consists of a cloak of coelomic epithelial cells. The mature ovary is derived principally from these cortical cells. Large primordial germ cells are also found in these superficial layers that are capable of differentiating as either oogonia or spermatogonia.

The medullary, or interior, portion of the primitive gonad is composed of a mesenchyme, in which sheets of epithelial cells are condensed to form the primary sex cords. This medullary portion has the potential to further differentiate as a testis.

Testicular Differentiation

Testicular differentiation is determined by the Y chromosome *SRY* gene and a related homeobox gene, *SOX9* (an autosomal gene). *SRY* regulates *SOX9* expression. *SOX9* in turn directly regulates transcription of antimüllerian hormone (AMH) by Sertoli cell precursors. AMH causes müllerian duct regression. As the primitive gonad becomes a testis, the inner portion of the primary sex cords becomes a collecting system connecting the seminiferous tubules with the mesonephric, or wolffian, duct. The peripheral portions of the sex cords join with ingrowths of coelomic epithelium (containing primordial germ cells) to form seminiferous tubules. Most of the cortex, however, becomes isolated by the tunica albuginea and the tunica vaginalis, which are the only cortical vestiges in the mature testis. Interstitial

cells of Leydig become abundant at about 8 weeks and secrete androgenic hormone necessary for the development of male external genitalia. Leydig cells disappear shortly after birth and are not seen again until the onset of adolescence.

Ovarian Differentiation

Ovarian development occurs several weeks later than testicular differentiation. Ovarian differentiation is determined by the lack of expression of *SRY*, *SOX9*, and AMH. There is likely a mechanism to repress autosomal testis-inducing genes (e.g., *SOX9*) and to activate

ovary-inducing genes (e.g., *WNT4* and *NR0B1* [*DAX1*]). At this time, the cortex undergoes intense proliferation, and strands of epithelial cells (called secondary sex cords) push into the interior of the gonad. Primordial germ cells are carried along in this inward migration. Clumps from the secondary sex cords fragment off to form primordial follicles. While the ovary is thus forming, the primary sex cords recede to the hilum, leaving stromal and connective tissue cells behind. Leydig cells and the rete ovarii persist as medullary remnants in the ovary. Proliferation of the cortex ceases at about 6 months.

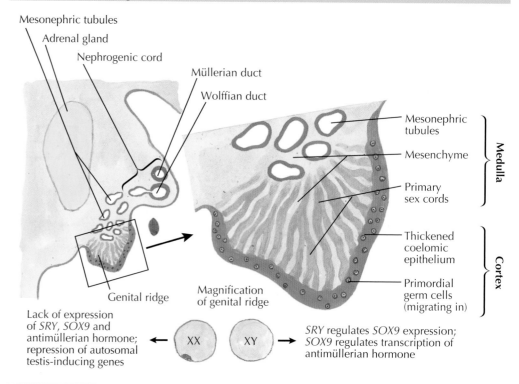

Undifferentiated stage

Mesonephric tubules
Adrenal gland
Nephrogenic cord
Müllerian duct
Wolffian duct

Mesonephric tubules — Medulla
Mesenchyme
Primary sex cords

Thickened coelomic epithelium — Cortex
Primordial germ cells (migrating in)

Genital ridge
Magnification of genital ridge

Lack of expression of *SRY*, *SOX9* and antimüllerian hormone; repression of autosomal testis-inducing genes ← XX XY → *SRY* regulates *SOX9* expression; *SOX9* regulates transcription of antimüllerian hormone

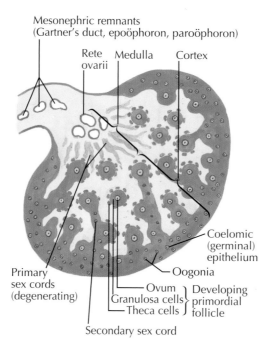

Female (primitive ovary)

Mesonephric remnants (Gartner's duct, epoöphoron, paroöphoron)
Rete ovarii
Medulla
Cortex

Primary sex cords (degenerating)
Coelomic (germinal) epithelium
Oogonia
Ovum
Granulosa cells } Developing primordial follicle
Theca cells
Secondary sex cord

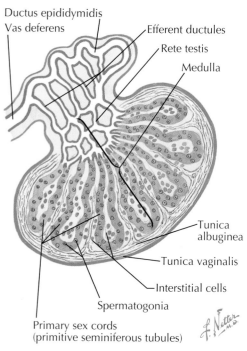

Male (primitive testis)

Ductus epididymidis
Vas deferens
Efferent ductules
Rete testis
Medulla

Tunica albuginea
Tunica vaginalis
Interstitial cells
Spermatogonia
Primary sex cords (primitive seminiferous tubules)

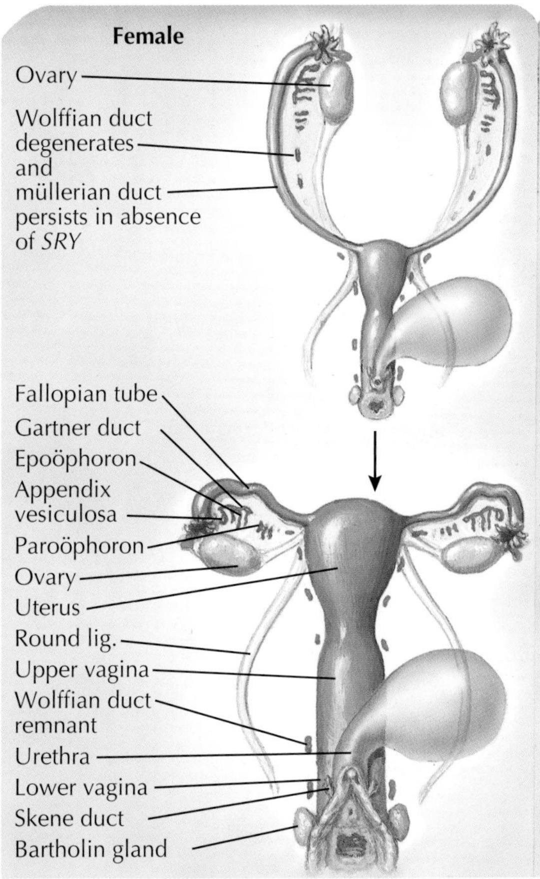

Plate 4-2   Reproduction

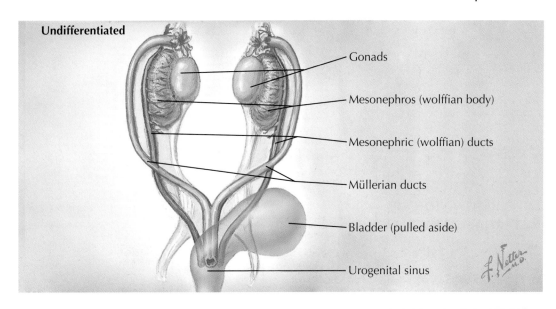

Undifferentiated

- Gonads
- Mesonephros (wolffian body)
- Mesonephric (wolffian) ducts
- Müllerian ducts
- Bladder (pulled aside)
- Urogenital sinus

Female

- Ovary
- Wolffian duct degenerates and müllerian duct persists in absence of SRY

Male

- Testis
- Degenerating müllerian duct
- Persistent wolffian duct (vas deferens)

Female labels:
- Fallopian tube
- Gartner duct
- Epoöphoron
- Appendix vesiculosa
- Paroöphoron
- Ovary
- Uterus
- Round lig.
- Upper vagina
- Wolffian duct remnant
- Urethra
- Lower vagina
- Skene duct
- Bartholin gland

Male labels:
- Vas deferens
- Seminal vesicle
- Prostatic utricle
- Prostate gland
- Bulbourethral gland
- Vas deferens
- Appendix epidymidis
- Appendix testis
- Epididymis
- Vasa efferentia
- Testis
- Gubernaculum

DIFFERENTIATION OF GENITAL DUCTS

The early embryo of either sex is equipped with identical primitive gonads that have the capacity to develop into either testes or ovaries. In the case of the internal genital ducts, however, the early embryo has both a male and a female set of primordial structures. The müllerian ducts have the potential to develop into fallopian tubes, a uterus, and the upper portion of the vagina. The mesonephric, or wolffian, ducts have the capacity to develop into the vas deferens and the seminal vesicles. The large wolffian body, containing the proximal mesonephric ducts, becomes the epididymis.

During the third fetal month, either the müllerian or the wolffian structures normally complete their development, and involution occurs simultaneously in the other set. Vestigial remnants of the other duct system, however, persist into adult life. In females, the mesonephric structures are represented by the epoöphoron, paroöphoron, and the ducts of Gartner. In males, the only müllerian remnant normally present is the appendix testis.

The direction in which these genital ducts develop is a direct consequence of the gonadal differentiation that occurred somewhat earlier. Testicular differentiation is determined by the Y chromosome *SRY* gene and a related homeobox gene, *SOX9* (an autosomal gene). *SRY* regulates *SOX9* expression. *SOX9* in turn directly regulates transcription of antimüllerian hormone (AMH) by Sertoli cell precursors. AMH causes müllerian duct regression through apoptosis and mesenchymal-epithelial cell remodeling. Müllerian ducts are nearly completely absent by 10 weeks; then the derivatives of the mesonephric system complete their normal male development.

Ovarian differentiation is determined by the lack of expression of SRY, *SOX9*, and AMH. There is likely a

mechanism to repress autosomal testis-inducing genes (e.g., *SOX9*) and to activate ovary-inducing genes (e.g., *WNT4* and *NR0B1* [*DAX1*]). In this setting, the müllerian structures proceed to become the uterus and fallopian tubes, and the mesonephric structures become vestigial. It should be emphasized that female development is not dependent on any ovarian secretion because in the absence of any gonads at all, the uterus and fallopian tubes develop normally.

In the female, ovarian differentiation is determined by the lack of expression of *SRY*, *SOX9*, and antimüllerian hormone. Müllerian structures proceed to become the uterus and fallopian tubes, and the wolffian ducts become vestigial.

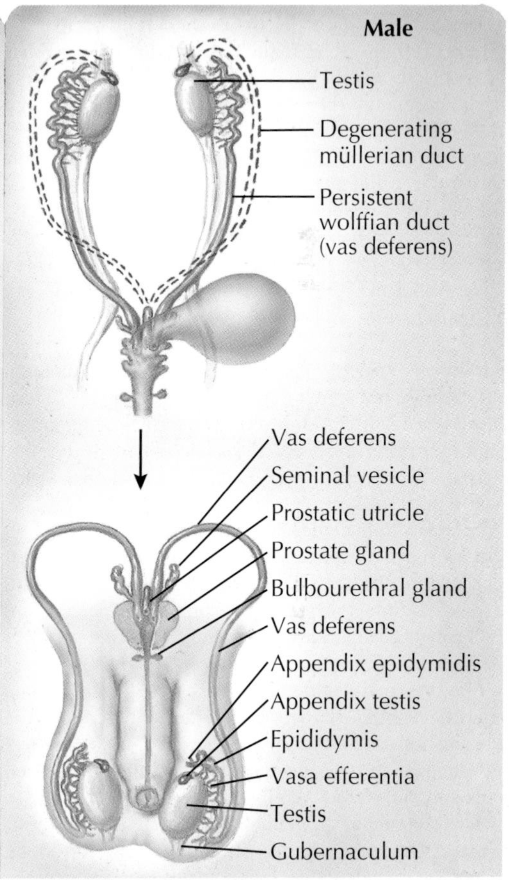

In the male, the Y chromosome–encoded *SRY* regulates *SOX9* expression. *SOX9* regulates transcription of antimüllerian hormone, causing the müllerian ducts to degenerate and wolffian ducts to persist and differentiate.

It is clear that *SRY* is the key factor in testis determination. However, multiple other factors must be repressed or activated for normal testicular development. This concept is evidenced by the findings of 46,XX males with testes who do not have a Y chromosome and by 46,XY females with gonadal dysgenesis who have an intact *SRY* gene. Thus, non–Y chromosomal factors must contribute in a clinically important way to testis determination.

Plate 4-3   Endocrine System

DIFFERENTIATION OF EXTERNAL GENITALIA

Before the ninth week of gestation, both sexes have a urogenital sinus and an identical external appearance. At this undifferentiated stage, the external genitalia consist of a genital tubercle beneath which is a urethral groove, bounded laterally by urethral folds and labioscrotal swellings. The male and female derivatives of these structures are shown in Plate 4-3.

The urogenital slit is formed at an even earlier stage when the perineal membrane partitions it from a single cloacal opening. Thereafter, the bladder and both genital ducts find a common outlet in this sinus.

The vagina develops as a diverticulum of the urogenital sinus in the region of the müllerian tubercle and becomes contiguous with the distal end of the müllerian ducts. About two-thirds of the vagina originates in the urogenital sinus, and about one-third is of müllerian origin.

In normal male development, the vaginal remnant is tiny because the müllerian structures atrophy before this diverticulum develops very far. In male pseudohermaphroditism, however, a sizable remnant of this vaginal diverticulum may persist as a blind vaginal pouch.

In normal female development, the vagina is pushed posteriorly by a downgrowth of connective tissue, so that by the 12th fetal week, it has acquired a separate external opening. In female pseudohermaphroditism, the growth of this septum is inhibited, leading to persistence of the urogenital sinus.

The principal distinctions between male and female external genitalia at this stage of development are the location and size of the vaginal diverticulum, the size of the phallus, and the degree of fusion of the urethral folds and labioscrotal swellings.

As in the case of the genital ducts, there is an inherent tendency for the external genitalia to develop along feminine lines. Masculinization of the external genitalia is brought about by exposure to androgenic hormones during the process of differentiation. Normally, the androgenic hormone is testosterone, derived from the Leydig cells of the fetal testis. The critical factor in determining whether masculinization will occur, however, is not the source of the androgen but rather its timing and its amount. In female pseudohermaphroditism caused by congenital adrenal hyperplasia, the fetal adrenal glands secrete sufficient androgen to bring about some masculinization of the external genitalia. In other instances, androgenic hormone may be derived from the maternal circulation.

By the 12th fetal week, the vagina has migrated posteriorly, and androgens will no longer cause fusion of the urethral and labioscrotal folds. Clitoral hypertrophy, however, may occur at any time in fetal life or even after birth.

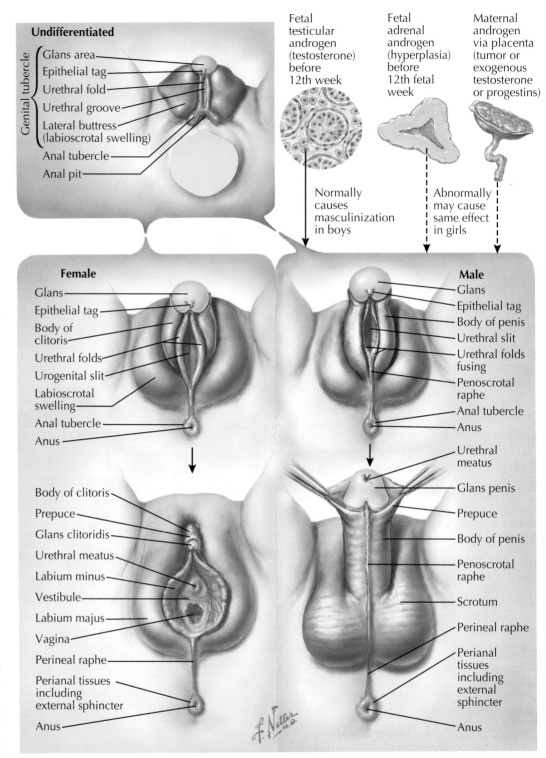

Female and male derivatives of urogenital sinus and external genitalia

Female derivative	Primordial structure	Male derivative
Vagina (lower two-thirds) Paraurethral glands (of Skene) Bartholin glands	Urogenital sinus	Prostatic utricle (vagina masculina) Prostate Bulbourethral glands (of Cowper)
Clitoris Corpora cavernosa Glands clitoridis	External genitalia *Genital tubercle*	Penis Corpora cavernosa Glans penis
Labia minora	*Urethral folds*	Corpus spongiosum (enclosing penile urethra)
Labia majora	*Labioscrotal swellings*	Scrotum

Plate 4-4

Reproduction

TESTOSTERONE AND ESTROGEN SYNTHESIS

Three glands that originate in the coelomic cavity—the adrenal cortex, the ovary, and the testis—produce steroids under the influence of tropic hormones of the anterior pituitary, corticotropin (adrenocorticotropic hormone [ACTH]) and gonadotropins. Cleaving cholesterol into pregnenolone (the C_{21} precursor of all active steroid hormones) and isocaproaldehyde is the critical first step, and it occurs in a limited number of sites in the body (adrenal cortex, testicular Leydig cells, ovarian theca cells, trophoblast cells of the placenta, and certain glial and neuronal cells of the brain). The roles of different steroidogenic tissues are determined by how this process is regulated and how pregnenolone is subsequently metabolized. Androgens have 19 carbon atoms (C19 steroids), and estrogens have 18 carbon atoms (C18 steroids).

Pregnenolone is converted to 17α-hydroxypregnenolone by 17α-hydroxylase (P450c17). P450c17 also possesses 17,20-lyase activity, which results in the production of the C19 adrenal androgens (dehydroepiandrosterone [DHEA] and androstenedione). Most of the adrenal androstenedione production is dependent on the conversion of DHEA to androstenedione by 3β-hydroxysteroid dehydrogenase. Androstenedione may be converted to testosterone by 17β-ketosteroid reductase (17β-HSD3) in the adrenal glands or gonads.

Androstenedione and testosterone are secretory products of the Leydig cells, which are found in abundance in the testis but are present in only small numbers in the hilar region of the ovary. In men, 95% of testosterone (7 mg/d) is produced by the testicles under the control of luteinizing hormone. The local effect of testosterone can be amplified by conversion via type 2 5α-reductase to the more potent dihydrotestosterone. This local amplification system occurs at the hair follicle and the prostate gland. Testosterone is bound to sex hormone–binding globulin in the blood. Conjugation with glucuronic acid takes place in the liver. Much of the conjugated testosterone is excreted in its water-soluble form by the kidney with a little free, unconjugated testosterone.

DHEA, a precursor of androstenedione and testosterone, is found mostly in the 17-ketosteroid fraction in the urine and is derived largely from the adrenal cortex. It is a weak androgen that makes up more than 60% of the 17-ketosteroids. The normal excretion value for 17-ketosteroids is higher in men than in women, presumably because of the contribution by the testis of some DHEA and a variety of other 17-ketosteroids.

The ovary contains at least three differential secretory zones: the granulosa cells of the follicle, engaged in estrogen formation; the theca cells, having a tendency to produce somewhat more androgens; and the

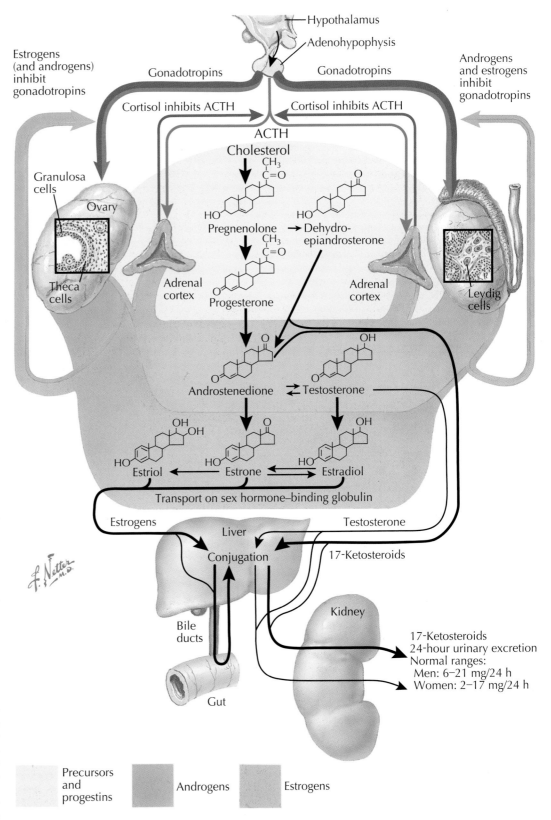

hilar cells, predominantly involved in androgen formation. The balance of these cellular elements ensures a normal degree of femininity; conversely, an imbalance leads to androgenicity. Within the ovary there are also the cells of the corpus luteum, which produce the bulk of progesterone.

Testosterone and androstenedione, respectively, are precursors of estradiol and estrone. Hydroxylation of the 19-carbon initiates a series of reactions that aromatize the A ring of the steroid nucleus, and this aromatization

is, in fact, characteristic of estrogens. Estradiol is more potent than estrone; estriol is purely an excretory product, which is extremely weak biologically.

The estrogens are bound in blood by sex hormone–binding globulin and albumin. Inactivation of estrogen occurs in the liver through conversion to less active estrogens (i.e., estradiol to estrone to estriol), oxidation to totally inert compounds, or conjugation to glucuronic acid. There is considerable enterohepatic circulation because estrogens are excreted in the bile.

Plate 4-5

Endocrine System

TANNER STAGES OF BREAST DEVELOPMENT

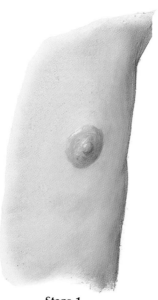

Stage 1
Elevation of papilla only

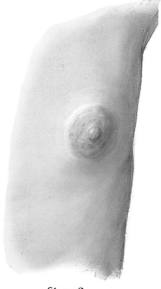

Stage 2
Breast bud: elevation of breast and papilla as a small mound and enlargement of areolar diameter

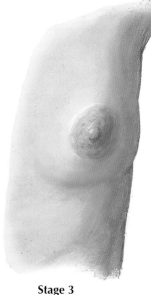

Stage 3
Additional enlargement of breast and areola with no separation of their contours

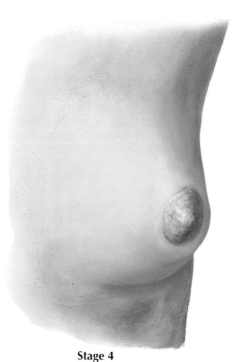

Stage 4
Areola and papilla project from surface of breast to form secondary mound

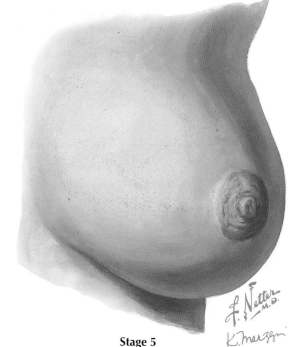

Stage 5
Mature stage with projection of papilla only with recession of the areola to the general contour of the breast

NORMAL PUBERTY

TIMING OF PUBERTY

Although it is often thought of as a distinct event, puberty is part of a lifelong process of hypothalamic–pituitary–gonadal development. Puberty is a biologic transition during which secondary sex characteristics develop, a linear growth spurt occurs, fertility is realized, and psychosocial changes occur. *Adrenarche* refers to the adrenal component of pubertal maturation and usually occurs earlier than gonadarche (the maturation of the hypothalamic–pituitary–gonadal system). *Thelarche* refers to pubertal breast development.

Before the onset of puberty, conspicuous physical differences between boys and girls are largely confined to the anatomy of their genital organs. The mean age of puberty onset is 10.6 years (range, 7–13 years) in white girls and 8.9 years (range, 6–13 years) in African American girls. The mean age of puberty onset in boys is 11 years (range, 9–14 years); some African American boys start puberty between 8 to 9 years.

The factors that lead to the maturation of the gonadotropin-releasing hormone pulse generator and thus trigger the onset of puberty are multiple and not yet fully understood. For example, body weight is one factor that triggers puberty, and the mechanism may involve leptin, a hormone produced in adipocytes. Puberty does not occur in animal models that are deficient in leptin but can be induced by leptin administration.

Most of the physical changes that begin at puberty are attributable to an increase in androgens and estrogens from the gonads and reticular zone of the adrenal cortex. The gonads are activated by pituitary luteinizing hormone (LH) and follicle-stimulating hormone (FSH), which, until this time, are not secreted in clinically important amounts in normally developing children. Corticotropin (adrenocorticotropic hormone [ACTH]) and a yet to be identified adrenal androgen–stimulating factor (perhaps of pituitary origin) appear to be responsible for adrenarche.

The capacity to secrete both androgens and estrogens is inherent in the adrenal glands, as well as in the gonads of both sexes. Enlargement of the reticular zone of the adrenal cortex and increased secretion of adrenal androgens occur at about the same time that the ovaries exhibit heightened activity. Androgenic hormones from both the adrenals and ovaries increase the growth rate and the development of pubic hair, later axillary hair, and seborrhea and acne. Both androgens and estrogens have a stimulatory effect on epiphysial maturation, and as fusion occurs, the rate of linear growth rapidly decelerates.

Approximately 18% of total adult height accrues during the pubertal growth spurt. Although the pubertal growth velocity is slightly lower in girls, they reach their peak height velocity about 2 years earlier than boys. In boys, the peak height velocity is approximately 9.5 cm per year at an average age of 13.5 years, whereas, in girls, the peak height velocity is approximately 8.3 cm per year at an average age of 11.5 years. Because of a longer duration of pubertal growth, boys on average gain 10 more centimeters of increased height than girls through the pubertal growth spurt, thus accounting for the general difference in sex-dependent adult height. Normal growth spurt in girls is dependent on growth hormone, insulinlike growth factor 1 (IGF-1), and estrogen. In boys, growth is dependent on growth hormone, IGF-1, estrogen, and testosterone. Increased pubertal blood estradiol concentrations appear to trigger hypothalamic–pituitary activity that results in increased growth hormone pulse amplitude and frequency. Serum IGF-1 concentrations peak during puberty and remain increased for approximately 2 years after the pubertal growth spurt before falling into the adult reference ranges.

Plate 4-6

Reproduction

TANNER STAGES OF FEMALE PUBIC HAIR DEVELOPMENT

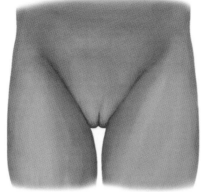

Stage 1
The vellus over the pubes is the same
as that over the anterior abdominal wall

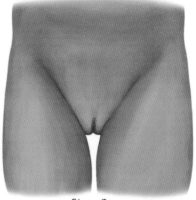

Stage 2
Sparse slightly pigmented, downy hair along
the labia that is straight or only slightly curled

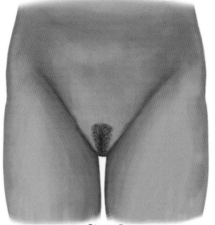

Stage 3
Hair spreads sparsely over the pubic
region and is darker, coarser, and curlier

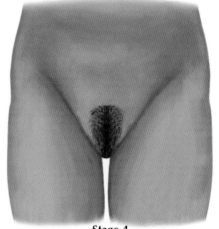

Stage 4
Hair is adult type, but the area covered is
smaller than in most adults, and there is no
spread to the medial surface of the thighs

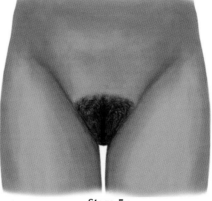

Stage 5
Hair is adult in quantity and type, distributed as an inverse
triangle, and spreads to the medial surface of the thighs but
not up the midline anterior abdominal wall

NORMAL PUBERTY (Continued)

The upper body to lower body segment ratio (U:L ratio) is defined as the distance from the top of the head to the top of the pubic ramus, divided by the length from the bottom of the feet to the top of the pubic ramus. The U:L ratio is approximately 1.7 at birth, 1.4 at 1 year of age, 1.0 at 10 years of age, 0.92 in white adults, and 0.85 in African American adults. The U:L ratios are the same in females and males. Eunuchoid proportions (decreased U:L ratio) develop in patients with hypogonadism, in whom epiphyseal fusion is delayed and the extremities grow for a prolonged period of time. Eunuchoid proportions are also seen patients with estrogen receptor deficiency or defects in estrogen synthesis. Patients who produce excess estrogen (aromatase excess), however, have advanced skeletal maturation, an increased U:L ratio, and short adult height.

Almost 50% of total body calcium in girls and slightly more than 50% in boys is laid down in bone mineral during puberty. After puberty, boys have 50% more total body calcium than girls. During puberty, the hips enlarge more in girls, and the shoulders become wider in boys. The pelvic inset widens in girls because of the growth of the os acetabuli. Men have 50% more lean body mass and skeletal mass than women, and women generally have twice the amount of body adipose tissue (distributed in the upper arms, thighs, and upper back) than men. Cardiovascular changes that occur during puberty include a greater aerobic reserve.

Marshall and Tanner developed a staging system to document the sequence of changes of secondary sexual characteristics. The Tanner stages are based on visual criteria to document five stages of pubertal development with regard to breast and pubic hair development in girls and genital and pubic hair development in boys. Stage 1 is the prepubertal state, and stage 5 is the adult state.

FEMALE PUBERTY

The three main phenotypic pubertal events in girls are increased height velocity, breast development (thelarche, under the control of ovarian estrogen secretion), and growth of axillary and pubic hair (under the control of androgens secreted by the ovaries and adrenal glands). An increase in height velocity is usually the first sign of puberty in girls. Most girls grow only approximately 2.5 cm in height after menarche. The stages of breast and pubic hair development usually progress in concert, but discordance may occur, and they are best classified separately The mean age of puberty onset is 10.6 years (range, 7–13 years) in white girls and 8.9 years (range, 6–13 years) in African American girls.

Pubertal breast enlargement (thelarche) is associated with increased amounts of glandular and connective tissue. The size and shape of breasts are determined by genetic factors, nutritional factors, and exposure to estrogen. Initially, breast development may be unilateral and then asynchronous. In the prepubertal girl (Tanner stage 1), there is elevation of papilla (see Plate 4-5). Tanner stage 2 is the breast bud stage, with enlargement of the areolar diameter and elevation of breast and papilla as a small mound. The mean age of onset of Tanner stage 2 breast development is 10.3 years in white girls and 9.5 years in African American girls. In Tanner stage 3, there is further enlargement of breast and areola, but with no separation of their contours. In Tanner stage 4, the areola and papilla project above the level of the breast to form a secondary mound. In Tanner stage 5, the mature breast has formed, there is recession of the areola, and only the papilla projects from the surface of the breast. The diameter of the papilla increases from 3 to 4 mm (in Tanner breast stages 1 through 3) to an average diameter of 9 mm in Tanner stage 5.

Plate 4-7

Endocrine System

TANNER STAGES OF MALE PUBIC HAIR AND GENITAL DEVELOPMENT

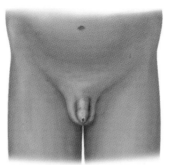

Stage 1

Penis, testes, and scrotum are the same size and proportion as in early childhood

The vellus hair over the pubic region is the same as that on the abdominal wall

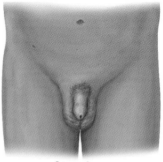

Stage 2

Testes and scrotum enlarge, and scrotal skin shows a change in texture and reddening

Sparse growth of straight or slightly curled pigmented hair appearing at the base of the penis

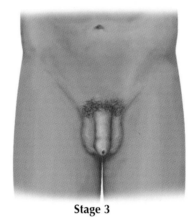

Stage 3

Penile growth in length more than width; further growth of the testes and scrotum

Hair is coarser, curlier, and darker, spread sparsely over the junction of the pubes

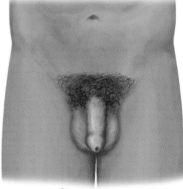

Stage 4

Further penile growth and development of the glans; further enlargement of testes and scrotum

Adult-type hair, but area covered less than in most adults; no spread to the medial surface of the thighs

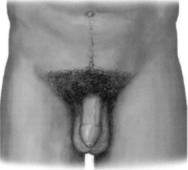

Stage 5

Genitalia are adult in size and shape

Adult in quantity and type of hair, distributed as an inverse triangle; spread is to the medial surface of the thighs

NORMAL PUBERTY (Continued)

In the prepubertal girl (Tanner pubic hair stage 1), there is vellus-type hair over the pubic region, but it is not different from that over the anterior abdominal wall (see Plate 4-6). In Tanner stage 2, early pubic hair becomes evident; it is slightly pigmented and straight or slightly curled, appearing along the labia. The mean age of onset of Tanner stage 2 pubic hair development is 10.4 years in white girls and 9.4 years in African American girls. During Tanner stage 3, the hair spreads sparsely over the pubic region, and it becomes coarser, darker, and curlier. In Tanner stage 4, the hair is adult in type, but it covers a smaller area than in most adults and it does not appear on the medial surface of the thighs. In Tanner stage 5, the appearance is that of an adult in distribution (including the medial surface of the thighs), quantity, and type.

During the progression through the pubic hair stages, the vaginal mucosa undergoes changes because of estrogen effects. The vaginal mucosa loses its prepubertal reddish glistening form and becomes thickened and dull because of cornification of the vaginal epithelium. Several months before menarche, there is vaginal secretion of clear or whitish discharge. The length of the vagina increases, and the labia minor and majora become thickened and rugated. There is a rounding of body contours, a fat pad develops in the mons pubis, and the clitoris increases in size. The uterus enlarges from a prepubertal length of 3 cm to a postpubertal length of 8 cm. The endometrium begins to proliferate during the first stages of puberty.

In white girls in the United States, the average age of menstruation (menarche) onset is 12.8 years; it is 6 months earlier in African American girls. Menarche occurs 1 to 3 years after the onset of puberty, typically during Tanner stage 4. Ovulation does not occur until some additional months have elapsed. Until then, the menses are often erratic, and even then, anovulatory cycles are common for the first 2 years after menarche. Progesterone is secreted only as corpora lutea are formed after ovulation. When this occurs, the proliferative endometrium is transformed into a secretory type. The peak in ovarian primordial follicles is reached at 20 weeks of fetal life, and no additional germ cells develop after this time point. Under gonadotropin stimulation during puberty, the ovaries become microcystic with the development of follicles more than 4 mm in diameter. The ovarian volume increases from a prepubertal size of 0.2 to 1.6 mL to 2.8 to 15 mL during puberty.

Axillary hair development is evident by age 12 years in more than 90% of African American girls and 70% of white girls. The development of acne—sometimes the most obvious initial sign of puberty in a girl—is caused by adrenal and ovarian androgen secretion. Acne represents a dysfunction of the pilosebaceous unit, where there is follicular occlusion and inflammation as a result of androgenic stimulation. Facial changes occur during puberty in both boys and girls with enlargement of the nose, mandible, maxilla, and frontal sinuses. In girls, the pituitary gland increases in height from an average of 6 mm before puberty to an average of 10 mm by Tanner stage 5.

MALE PUBERTY

The three main phenotypic pubertal events in boys are increased height velocity, genitalia development (under the control of pituitary gonadotropins and testicular testosterone secretion), and growth of axillary and pubic hair (under the control of androgens secreted by the testicles and adrenal glands). The first sign of puberty in boys is usually testicular growth; in the United States, this occurs approximately 6 months after the onset of breast development in girls.

Plate 4-8

Reproduction

HORMONAL EVENTS IN FEMALE AND MALE PUBERTY

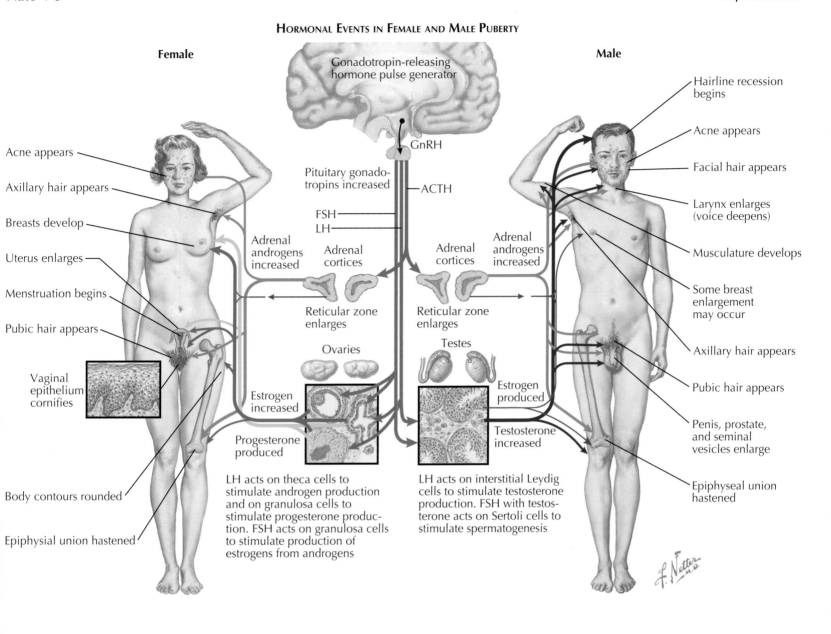

Female

Acne appears

Axillary hair appears

Breasts develop

Uterus enlarges

Menstruation begins

Pubic hair appears

Vaginal epithelium cornifies

Body contours rounded

Epiphysial union hastened

Gonadotropin-releasing hormone pulse generator

GnRH

Pituitary gonado-tropins increased

ACTH

FSH

LH

Adrenal androgens increased

Adrenal cortices

Adrenal cortices

Adrenal androgens increased

Reticular zone enlarges

Reticular zone enlarges

Ovaries

Testes

Estrogen increased

Estrogen produced

Progesterone produced

Testosterone increased

LH acts on theca cells to stimulate androgen production and on granulosa cells to stimulate progesterone produc-tion. FSH acts on granulosa cells to stimulate production of estrogens from androgens

LH acts on interstitial Leydig cells to stimulate testosterone production. FSH with testos-terone acts on Sertoli cells to stimulate spermatogenesis

Male

Hairline recession begins

Acne appears

Facial hair appears

Larynx enlarges (voice deepens)

Musculature develops

Some breast enlargement may occur

Axillary hair appears

Pubic hair appears

Penis, prostate, and seminal vesicles enlarge

Epiphyseal union hastened

NORMAL PUBERTY (Continued)

Testicular volume, which correlates with the stages of puberty, can be measured by comparing the testes with model ellipsoids (orchidometer) that have volumes ranging from 1 to 35 mL. The increase in size is pri-marily caused by seminiferous tubule growth. The main cell type in the seminiferous cords before puberty is the Sertoli cell, whereas in mature men, germ cells are the predominant cell type. With the increased LH levels with puberty, adult-type Leydig cells appear. Sperma-togenesis starts between ages 11 and 15 years. Onset of puberty is predicted when a testis is more than 4 mL in volume. In adults, the average testicle has a volume of 29 mL; the right testis is usually slightly larger than the left, and the left testis is usually located lower in the scrotum than the right testis. When the phallus is meas-ured, it should be flaccid and stretched. The phallus length is approximately 6 cm prepubertally and 12 cm in white men. The male areolar diameter also increases during puberty. The normal age range for onset of puberty in boys is 9 to 14 years.

In Tanner genital development stage 1 (prepubertal), the penis, testes, and scrotum are the same as in early childhood (see Plate 4-7). In Tanner stage 2, the testes and scrotum start to enlarge, and the scrotal skin starts to redden and change in texture. The average age at Tanner genital stage 2 is 11.2 years. In Tanner stage 3, penile growth has started, more evident in length than width, and there is also further enlargement of the testes and scrotum. In Tanner stage 4, the penis increases in size (both length and width), and the glans of the penis starts to develop; the testicles and scrotum continue to enlarge, and the scrotal skin becomes darker. In Tanner stage 5, the genitalia are adult in size and shape, and no further enlargement occurs.

In Tanner pubic hair development stage 1 in boys, the hair over the pubic region is vellus in type and is the same as that on the abdominal wall (see Plate 4-7). In Tanner stage 2, there is sparse, straight or slightly cured, lightly pigmented hair that appears at the base of the penis. In Tanner stage 3, the hair is spread sparsely over the pubic area, and it is curlier, darker, and coarser. In Tanner stage 4, the hair, although adult in type, covers a smaller area than in most adults, and it

has not yet spread to the medial surface of the thighs. In Tanner stage 5, the hair is adult in type and quantity and is distributed to the medial surface of the thighs.

The vocal cords lengthen during puberty, and the larynx, cricothyroid cartilage, and laryngeal muscles enlarge. The pitch of the voice changes dramatically between Tanner genital stages 3 and 4. The average age when the adult voice is reached is 15 years. During Tanner pubic hair stage 3, facial hair starts to appear, initially at the corners of the upper lip and cheeks, then spreading to below the lower lip and eventually (after achieving Tanner pubic and genital stages 5) extending to the sides of the cheeks and chin. Axillary hair devel-opment is evident at age 14 years in boys. Acne, caused by testicular and adrenal androgen secretion, appears at an average age of 12 years (range, 9–15 years) and progresses through puberty. Pubertal gynecomastia occurs in about 50% of normally developing boys at an average age of 13 years, and it usually resolves sponta-neously over 1 to 2 years (see Plate 4-25).

Facial changes occur during puberty in both boys and girls with enlargement of the nose, mandible, maxilla, and frontal sinuses.

Plate 4-9

Endocrine System

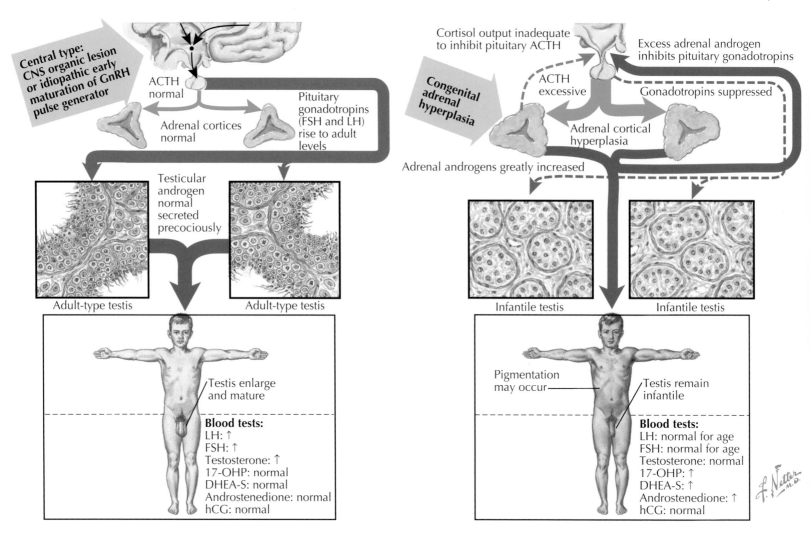

Central type: CNS organic lesion or idiopathic early maturation of GnRH pulse generator

ACTH normal

Adrenal cortices normal

Pituitary gonadotropins (FSH and LH) rise to adult levels

Testicular androgen normal secreted precociously

Adult-type testis

Adult-type testis

Testis enlarge and mature

Blood tests:
LH: ↑
FSH: ↑
Testosterone: ↑
17-OHP: normal
DHEA-S: normal
Androstenedione: normal
hCG: normal

Cortisol output inadequate to inhibit pituitary ACTH

Excess adrenal androgen inhibits pituitary gonadotropins

Congenital adrenal hyperplasia

ACTH excessive

Gonadotropins suppressed

Adrenal cortical hyperplasia

Adrenal androgens greatly increased

Infantile testis

Infantile testis

Pigmentation may occur

Testis remain infantile

Blood tests:
LH: normal for age
FSH: normal for age
Testosterone: normal
17-OHP: ↑
DHEA-S: ↑
Androstenedione: ↑
hCG: normal

PRECOCIOUS PUBERTY

Precocious puberty is the initiation of puberty before the age of 8 years in girls and 9 years in boys. The cause may be benign (normal variant early adrenarche) or more serious (malignant germinoma). When the sexual characteristics are appropriate for the child's sex, it is termed *isosexual precocious puberty*. Inappropriate virilization in girls or feminization in boys is termed *contrasexual precocious puberty*. Precocious puberty is 10-fold more common in girls, in whom the cause is usually central in nature.

GONADOTROPIN-DEPENDENT PRECOCIOUS PUBERTY

Central or true precocious puberty is gonadotropin-dependent and attributable to early maturation of the gonadotropin-releasing hormone (GnRH) pulse generator, a finding that is 20-fold more common in girls than in boys. Although this form of precocious puberty may be triggered by a central nervous system (CNS) process, the cause cannot be identified in 90% of affected girls. This development leads to premature breast (thelarche) and pubic hair (pubarche) changes in girls and premature pubarche and testicular enlargement (gonadarche) in boys. When pubertal changes start, they progress at a pace and in an order found in puberty that starts at a normal age. The blood concentrations of luteinizing hormone (LH), follicle-stimulating hormone (FSH), testosterone, and estradiol are characteristic of those seen in normal puberty. These patients have an advanced bone age and accelerated growth for their age.

Although the etiology is usually idiopathic in girls, head magnetic resonance imaging (MRI) is indicated to exclude a CNS disorder. In boys with central precocious puberty, the etiology is idiopathic in half and a CNS abnormality in the other half. Some considerations in this setting include the following: hamartomas of the tuber cinereum that contain GnRH neurosecretory neurons and function as an ectopic GnRH pulse generator; astrocytoma; ependymoma; hypothalamic or optic gliomas in patients with neurofibromatosis type 1; any neoplasm in the hypothalamic region (e.g., craniopharyngioma) that impinges on the posterior hypothalamus; an adverse effect of CNS radiotherapy (e.g., for tumors or leukemia); hydrocephalus; CNS inflammatory disorder (e.g., sarcoidosis); congenital midline defects; and pineal neoplasms. Hamartomas of the tuber cinereum are not actually tumors but rather congenital malformations that appear on MRI as an isodense fullness of the prepontine, interpeduncular, and posterior suprasellar cisterns. When the diameter of the hamartoma exceeds 1 cm, there is a high risk for seizures, which may be gelastic (laughing), petit mal, or generalized tonic-clonic. A rare cause is a gonadotropin-secreting pituitary tumor. Exposure to androgens (exogenous or endogenous) can trigger maturation of the GnRH pulse generator and central precocious puberty.

GONADOTROPIN-INDEPENDENT PRECOCIOUS PUBERTY

Peripheral or gonadotropin-independent precocious puberty (also referred to as *pseudoprecocious puberty*) is caused by excess secretion of estrogen or testosterone from gonadal or adrenal sources. These patients usually do not follow the normal sequence and pace of puberty (e.g., menstrual bleeding may be the first sign). Depending on the type of sex hormone excess, gonadotropin-independent precocious puberty may be isosexual or contrasexual. Blood concentrations of LH and FSH are suppressed in these patients.

Plate 4-10

Reproduction

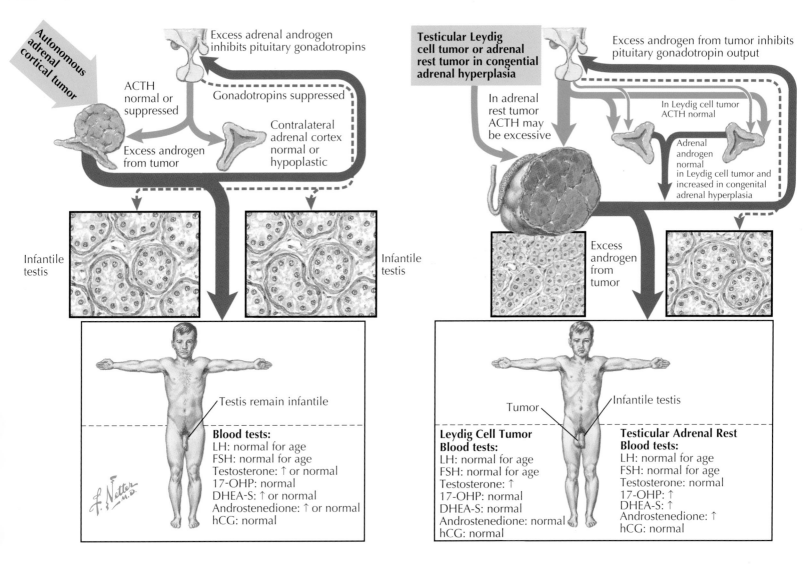

Testis remain infantile

Blood tests:
LH: normal for age
FSH: normal for age
Testosterone: ↑ or normal
17-OHP: normal
DHEA-S: ↑ or normal
Androstenedione: ↑ or normal
hCG: normal

Tumor — Infantile testis

Leydig Cell Tumor Blood tests:
LH: normal for age
FSH: normal for age
Testosterone: ↑
17-OHP: normal
DHEA-S: normal
Androstenedione: normal
hCG: normal

Testicular Adrenal Rest Blood tests:
LH: normal for age
FSH: normal for age
Testosterone: normal
17-OHP: ↑
DHEA-S: ↑
Androstenedione: ↑
hCG: normal

PRECOCIOUS PUBERTY (Continued)

The possible causes of isosexual gonadotropin-independent precocious puberty in girls include the following: exogenous estrogen (e.g., estrogen-containing creams and ointments), follicular ovarian cysts, ovarian neoplasms (e.g., granulosa-cell tumors, gonadoblastoma, and Leydig cell tumors), estrogen-secreting adrenal neoplasms, and McCune-Albright syndrome. McCune-Albright syndrome is associated with mutations in the *GNAS* gene that encodes the α-subunit of the guanosine triphosphate (GTP)–binding protein (Gs) that is involved in adenylate cyclase activation. The disorder is caused by a postzygotic somatic mutation; thus, the extent of tissue involvement depends on how early in development the mutation occurs. The clinical presentation of McCune-Albright syndrome is the triad of gonadotropin-independent precocious puberty, irregularly edged café au lait spots that usually do not cross the midline, and bony fibrous dysplasia (e.g., hyperostosis of the skull base and facial asymmetry) (see Plate 4-11). Based on the tissue distribution of the somatic mutation, other endocrine hyperfunction disorders may be seen in patients with McCune-Albright syndrome, including Cushing syndrome (bilateral adrenal hyperplasia), thyrotoxicosis, hyperparathyroidism (adenoma or hyperplasia), hypophosphatemic vitamin D–resistant rickets, and gigantism (mammosomatotroph hyperplasia). McCune-Albright syndrome–related sexual precocity usually begins in the first 2 years of life with menstrual bleeding caused by autonomously functioning ovarian luteinized follicular cysts.

In boys with isosexual peripheral precocious puberty, the diagnostic considerations include the following: testicular Leydig cell tumors (usually benign); human chorionic gonadotropin (hCG)–secreting germ cell tumors (hCG is an LH receptor agonist) that arise from sites of embryonic germ cells (pineal region of the brain, posterior mediastinum, liver [malignant hepatoma and hepatoblastoma], retroperitoneum, and testicles). Germ cell tumors are malignant but may be indolent (e.g., dysgerminoma) or more aggressive (e.g., choriocarcinoma, embryonal cell carcinoma). Androgen-secreting adrenal tumors and congenital adrenal hyperplasia (e.g., 21-hydroxylase deficiency or, less commonly, 11β-hydroxylase deficiency) are additional considerations of isosexual gonadotropin-independent precocious puberty. Boys can also have a germline autosomal dominant activating mutation in the LH receptor gene that predisposes to early Leydig cell development and testosterone secretion (testotoxicosis). McCune-Albright syndrome does occur in boys, although its occurrence is 50% less common than in girls.

Causes of contrasexual gonadotropin-independent precocious puberty in girls include exogenous androgens (e.g., testosterone gel), androgen-secreting adrenal neoplasms, and congenital adrenal hyperplasia. Causes of contrasexual gonadotropin-independent precocious puberty in boys include exogenous estrogen (e.g., estrogen-containing creams and ointments) and adrenal estrogen-secreting neoplasms.

INCOMPLETE PRECOCIOUS PUBERTY

Incomplete precocious puberty is the descriptor used for premature thelarche or premature adrenarche, both of which may be variants of normal puberty. Usually bone age is not advanced in these settings. Thus, premature thelarche may occur in isolation in normally developing girls, with no other signs of puberty. However, a subset of girls with premature thelarche or premature adrenarche may progress to gonadotropin-dependent precocious puberty. In addition, incomplete precocious puberty may be caused by long-standing, untreated primary hypothyroidism.

Plate 4-11

Endocrine System

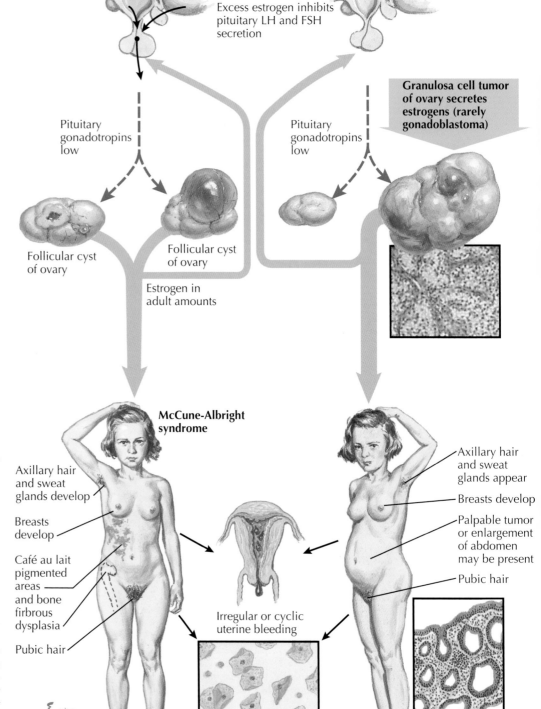

Excess estrogen inhibits pituitary LH and FSH secretion

Granulosa cell tumor of ovary secretes estrogens (rarely gonadoblastoma)

Pituitary gonadotropins low

Pituitary gonadotropins low

Follicular cyst of ovary

Follicular cyst of ovary

Estrogen in adult amounts

McCune-Albright syndrome

Axillary hair and sweat glands develop

Breasts develop

Café au lait pigmented areas and bone firbrous dysplasia

Pubic hair

Irregular or cyclic uterine bleeding

Estrogenic vaginal smear

Axillary hair and sweat glands appear

Breasts develop

Palpable tumor or enlargement of abdomen may be present

Pubic hair

Hyperplastic endometrium

Precocious Puberty
(Continued)

DIAGNOSTIC EVALUATION AND TREATMENT

A focused history and physical examination usually provide clues as to the cause of precocious puberty. For example, headaches, visual changes, or symptoms of diabetes insipidus should increase the suspicion for a mass in the hypothalamic region. All previous height measurements should be plotted on a growth chart. On physical examination, a detailed description of secondary sexual characteristics on the basis of the Tanner staging should be documented (see Plates 4-5 to 4-7). Measurements should be made of testicular volume and penile length in boys and of diameter of breast tissue in girls. The patient should be examined for the presence of multiple café au lait spots; in neurofibromatosis type 1, they are smoother in outline ("coast of California" appearance) than those associated with McCune-Albright syndrome ("coast of Maine" appearance). Complete neurologic examination may provide clues to an underlying CNS process. The abdominal and pelvic examination may detect a hepatic or ovarian mass. Testicular examination may show symmetric testicular enlargement in patients with central precocious puberty or a unilateral nodular enlargement in boys with Leydig cell tumors. Bone age should be evaluated to see if it is advanced compared with chronologic age. Basal blood concentrations of LH, FSH, estradiol, testosterone, 17-hydroxyprogesterone (17-OHP), dehydroepiandrosterone sulfate (DHEA-S), and androstenedione distinguish between central and peripheral precocious puberty. Serum thyrotropin should be measured in all patients with precocious puberty. Blood concentrations of β-hCG and α-fetoprotein may be measured in select cases. Performing a GnRH stimulation test for LH may be necessary to confirm central precocious puberty, in which LH is expected to increase after GnRH administration.

Head MRI is indicated in patients with gonadotropin-dependent precocious puberty. Abdominal and gonadal imaging are indicated in patients with gonadotropin-independent precocious puberty.

Treatment is determined by the cause and pace of precocious puberty. If a CNS lesion is discovered in patients with gonadotropin-dependent precocious puberty, treatment options are usually clear. For example, a dysgerminoma is usually confirmed by biopsy and then treated with radiation therapy, chemotherapy, or both. In patients with idiopathic gonadotropin-dependent precocious puberty (a diagnosis of exclusion), treatment with a GnRH agonist is an effective option to arrest pubertal development, and it improves final adult height compared with final height of patients who are not treated.

The treatment of patients with gonadotropin-independent precocious puberty is directed at the source of sex hormone excess. For example, androgen excess associated with congenital adrenal hyperplasia caused by 21-hydroxylase deficiency is very effectively treated with glucocorticoid replacement.

Plate 4-20

Reproduction

TURNER SYNDROME AND MIXED GONADAL DYSGENESIS: 45,X/46,XY KARYOTYPE

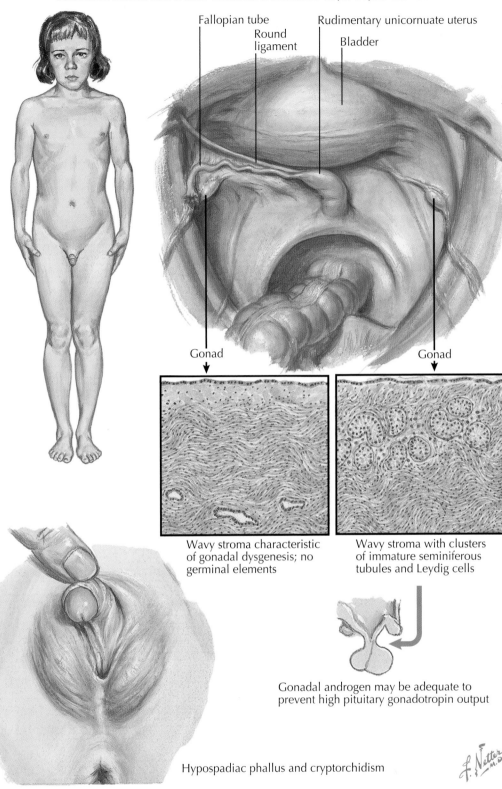

Fallopian tube

Round ligament

Rudimentary unicornuate uterus

Bladder

Gonad

Gonad

Wavy stroma characteristic of gonadal dysgenesis; no germinal elements

Wavy stroma with clusters of immature seminiferous tubules and Leydig cells

Gonadal androgen may be adequate to prevent high pituitary gonadotropin output

Hypospadiac phallus and cryptorchidism

TURNER SYNDROME (GONADAL DYSGENESIS) (Continued)

In the most primitive of such rudimentary testes, only rete tubules and nests of Leydig cells can be identified. In other instances, solid cords of cells resembling the primary sex cords are enmeshed within an abundant mesenchymal matrix. The spectra of testicular development in these cases find their counterparts in all the stages through which a normal testis passes in its embryonic differentiation. The hormonal pattern that emerges at adolescence is frequently a recapitulation of the performance of the Leydig cells in utero. Thus, if these cells were sufficiently abundant to produce virilization of the external genitalia in utero, at adolescence they may be expected to produce androgenic hormones and bring about male secondary sex characteristics. Likewise, gonads in which the cortical elements have differentiated beyond the primitive stage may be expected to bring about some degree of feminization at adolescence.

The time in life when Turner syndrome becomes clinically evident is variable. For example, Turner syndrome may be evident at birth with the typical physical anomalies and lymphedema of the extremities and cutis laxa. It may be diagnosed in childhood because of growth failure, in adolescence with pubertal failure and primary amenorrhea, or later in life with secondary amenorrhea. Turner syndrome should be suspected in all prepubertal girls who are of short stature (<2 standard deviations below the mean height for age) and have at least two of the physical stigmata. In the past, a buccal smear for assessment of Barr bodies (nuclear heterochromatin) was performed in this setting. However, because this technique lacks sensitivity and specificity, it is no longer performed. If Turner syndrome is suspected, a peripheral blood karyotype analysis is indicated. A 46,X karyotype is documented in approximately 75% of patients with Turner syndrome, and the remainder proves to have mosaic forms (e.g., 45,X/46,XX). Blood concentrations of luteinizing hormone and follicle-stimulating hormone are increased above normal in most of these patients throughout all age groups.

Treatment depends in part on the age at diagnosis and the presence of congenital anomalies. Although the short stature is not caused by growth hormone deficiency, the administration of recombinant human growth hormone in childhood—typically initiated when height falls below the fifth percentile for age—enhances growth and final adult height (the typical height gain is between 2 and 6 inches). The reasons for estrogen replacement therapy include inducing sexual development, optimizing adolescent bone development, and optimizing cognitive function. Typically, low-dose estrogen replacement is started around age 13 to 14 years. A progestin is given with the estrogenic agent to prevent endometrial hyperplasia. Treatment of the adult patient with Turner syndrome includes surveillance for potential cardiovascular anomalies with periodic echocardiography. Because of the high risk for hypothyroidism, annual measurement of serum thyrotropin concentration is indicated.

HIRSUTISM AND VIRILIZATION

Hirsutism is defined as excessive male-pattern hair growth in women. The causes of hirsutism are many and diverse—from an ethnic or hereditary disposition toward superfluous hair growth to hyperplasia or neoplasia of the adrenal gland or ovaries. Virilization, reflecting a more severe form of androgen excess, is defined as the development of signs and symptoms of masculinization in a woman (increased muscle bulk, loss of female body contours, deepening of the voice, breast atrophy, clitoromegaly, temporal balding) (see Plate 3-16). Hypertrichosis is not true hirsutism but rather a diffuse increase in total body hair in women or men that may be drug induced (e.g., minoxidil) or associated with other conditions (e.g., anorexia nervosa, malnutrition).

Hair growth has three phases: growth phase (anagen), involution phase (catagen), and rest phase (telogen). Although hair follicle number does not change over time, the size and shape of the hair follicles can change. Hair is either vellus (not pigmented, fine, soft) or terminal (pigmented, thick, coarse). Vellus hair is present on most of the skin. Androgens, in addition to increasing hair follicle size and hair diameter, increase the proportion of time that terminal hairs remain in growth phase at androgen-sensitive body sites. Thus, hirsutism is the development of terminal hair in areas where it does not usually occur in women (e.g., face, midline chest, abdomen, and back). At the scalp, androgens reduce the time that hair is in the growth phase and can result in hair thinning.

The degree of male-pattern terminal hair growth in a woman can be assessed with a modified scale originally developed by Ferriman and Gallwey (see Plate 4-21). The degree of terminal hair growth is graded at nine body areas: upper lip, chin, chest, upper back, lower back, upper abdomen, lower abdomen, upper arms, and thighs. Each area is scored 0 to 4 (0 = no growth of terminal hair and 4 = complete and heavy cover). The sum of these numbers is the modified Ferriman Gallwey hirsutism score. Most women have a modified Ferriman Gallwey hirsutism score of less than 8 (maximum score, 36), but 5% to 10% of women have scores above 8, a level consistent with the diagnosis of hirsutism. Ethnicity has a major influence on body hair in women. For example, despite equivalent circulating androgen levels, most American Indian and Asian women have little body hair, and women of Mediterranean descent have much more.

Hirsutism is usually caused by increased androgen effect, associated with either increased circulating androgen levels or increased local conversion of testosterone to the more potent dihydrotestosterone (DHT) at the hair follicle. The conversion of testosterone to DHT is catalyzed by 5α-reductase and amplifies the androgenic effect. DHT is produced primarily by target tissues. Thus, androgen action is determined in part by the target tissue androgen receptors and 5α-reductase activity. The adrenal glands produce dehydroepiandrosterone (DHEA) and androstenedione. DHEA has no direct androgenic effects but rather serves as a substrate for conversion to androstenedione (which is also androgenically inactive) and then to testosterone. In the ovary, much of the testosterone is aromatized to estradiol. Blood testosterone concentrations in

premenopausal women are determined by direct ovarian secretion (one-third of total) and by the peripheral conversion of androstenedione to testosterone in adipose tissue and skin (two-thirds of total). Increased blood testosterone concentrations usually originate from the ovaries, and increased DHEA sulfate (DHEA-S) concentrations usually originate from the adrenal glands. Excess androstenedione secretion can come from either the adrenal glands or the ovaries.

Polycystic ovary syndrome (PCOS) is the most common cause of clinically evident androgen excess. Hirsutism is often concomitant with obesity, amenorrhea, and infertility. These women typically have anovulatory, irregular menstrual cycles; signs of excess androgen effect (e.g., hirsutism, acne); or increased blood concentrations of androgens. PCOS usually becomes evident shortly after the onset of puberty, and the signs and symptoms gradually progress with age.

Plate 5-3   Pancreas

Relative density of distribution of islets in various parts of pancreas

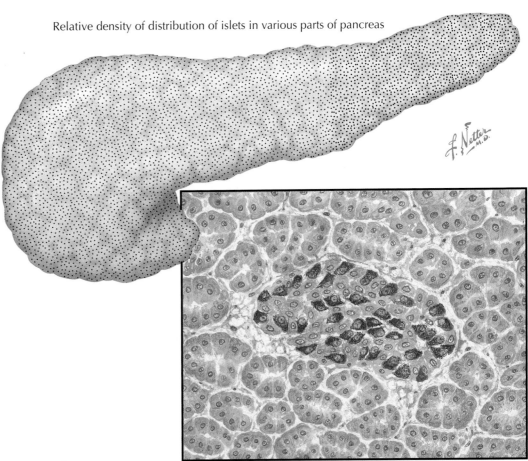

NORMAL HISTOLOGY OF PANCREATIC ISLETS

The pancreas is the union of an endocrine gland (pancreatic islets) and an exocrine gland (acinar and ductal cells). Approximately 85% of pancreatic mass is exocrine, 2% endocrine, 10% extracellular matrix, and 3% blood vessels and ducts. The exocrine (acinar) cells are clustered in acini, divided by connective tissue, and connected to a duct that drains into the pancreatic duct and into the duodenum. Small clusters of endocrine cells—islets of Langerhans—are embedded within the acini of the pancreas. The three main types of endocrine cells are β-cells (75% of endocrine cell mass) that produce insulin, α-cells (20% of endocrine cell mass) that produce glucagon, and δ-cells (5% of endocrine cell mass) that secrete somatostatin. The δ$_2$-cells secrete vasoactive intestinal polypeptide. The pancreatic polypeptide–producing (PP) cells secrete pancreatic polypeptide. Within the islet, the β-cells are in the center and surrounded by the α-cells, δ-cells, and PP cells.

The adult pancreas contains about 1 million islets (varying in size from 40–300 μm) that are more densely distributed in the tail of the gland. The entire mass of islets in a single pancreas weighs only approximately 1 g. Each islet contains approximately 3000 cells. The β-cells are polyhedral in shape and are distributed equally in islets across the pancreas. The α-cells are columnar in shape and are located primarily in islets in the body and tail of the pancreas. The δ-cells are smaller than the α- and β-cells and are frequently dendritic. The PP cells are located primarily in islets in the head and uncinate process of the pancreas. The Gomori aldehyde fuchsin and Ponceau techniques stain the insulin-containing granules in β-cells a deep bluish-purple; the α-cells appear pink or red.

Insulin, discovered in 1920 by Banting and Best, is a 56–amino acid peptide with two chains (α and β chains) joined by two disulfide bridges. β-Cell synthesis of insulin is regulated by plasma glucose concentrations, neural signals, and paracrine effects. The enteric hormones gastric inhibitory peptide, glucagon-like peptide-1 (GLP-1), and cholecystokinin also augment insulin secretion. Somatostatin, amylin, and pancreastatin inhibit insulin release. Cholinergic and β-adrenergic sympathetic innervation stimulate insulin release, and α-adrenergic sympathetic innervation inhibits insulin secretion. Insulin acts by inhibiting hepatic glucose production, glycogenolysis, fatty acid breakdown, and ketone formation. Insulin also facilitates glucose transport into cells and stimulates protein synthesis.

Glucagon is a 29–amino acid single-chain peptide hormone that counteracts the effects of insulin by promoting hepatic glycogenolysis and gluconeogenesis. Glucagon release is inhibited by increased levels of plasma glucose and by GLP-1, insulin, and somatostatin. Glucagon secretion is stimulated by the amino acids arginine and alanine. As with insulin, cholinergic and β-adrenergic sympathetic innervation stimulate glucagon release, and α-adrenergic sympathetic innervation inhibits glucagon secretion.

Somatostatin is a peptide that has two bioactive forms—14–amino acid and 28–acid forms. In general, somatostatin inhibits pancreatic endocrine and exocrine secretions.

Pancreatic polypeptide is a 36–amino acid hormone that inhibits bile secretion, gallbladder contraction, and exocrine pancreatic secretion. Pancreatic polypeptide also regulates hepatic insulin receptor expression. Enteral protein and fat stimulate pancreatic polypeptide secretion.

Amylin (also referred to as islet amyloid polypeptide) is a 37–amino acid hormone secreted by β-cells in concert with insulin. Amylin is synergistic with insulin by slowing gastric emptying, inhibiting digestive secretions, and inhibiting glucagon release. The effects of amylin are centrally mediated.

Section of an islet surrounded by acini (× 220); Gomori aldehyde fuchsin and Ponceau stain: β-granules stain deep purple; α-cells, orange–pink

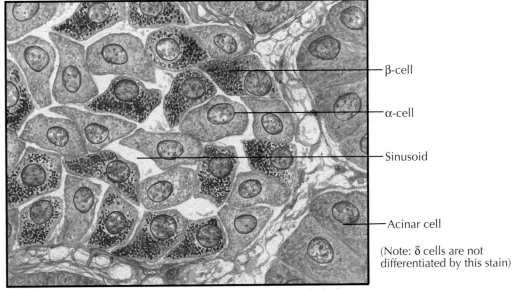

- β-cell
- α-cell
- Sinusoid
- Acinar cell

(Note: δ cells are not differentiated by this stain)

Portion of islet greatly magnified (× 1200); Gomori aldehyde fuchsin and Ponceau stain

Plate 5-4

Endocrine System

INSULIN SECRETION

Pancreatic β-cell production of insulin is regulated by plasma glucose concentration, neural inputs, and the effects of other hormones by paracrine and endocrine actions. Proinsulin consists of an amino-terminal β-chain, a carboxy-terminal α-chain, and a connecting peptide (C-peptide) in the middle. C-peptide functions by allowing folding of the molecule and the formation of disulfide bonds between the α- and β-chains. C-peptide is cleaved from proinsulin by endopeptidases in the β-cell endoplasmic reticulum (ER) to form insulin. Insulin and C-peptide are packaged into secretory granules in the Golgi apparatus. The secretory granules are released into the portal circulation by exocytosis. Insulin is degraded in the liver, kidney, and target tissues; it has a circulating half-life of 3 to 8 minutes. C-peptide does not act at the insulin receptor and is not degraded by the liver; it has a circulating half-life of 35 minutes. Thus, measurement of serum C-peptide concentration serves as a measure of β-cell secretory capacity. Defects in the synthesis and cleavage of insulin can lead to rare forms of diabetes mellitus (e.g., Wakayama syndrome, proinsulin syndromes).

Insulin is released in a pulsatile and rhythmic background pattern throughout the day and serves to suppress hepatic glucose production and mediates glucose disposal by adipose tissue. Superimposed on the background secretion of insulin is the meal-induced insulin release. There are two phases of caloric intake–induced insulin secretion. In the first phase, prestored insulin is released over 4 to 6 minutes. The second phase is a slower onset and longer sustained release because of the production of new insulin.

The regulators of insulin release include nutrients (e.g., glucose and amino acids), hormones (e.g., glucagon-like peptide 1 [GLP-1], somatostatin, insulin, and epinephrine), and neurotransmitters (e.g., acetylcholine, norepinephrine). The β-cells are exquisitely sensitive to small changes in glucose concentration; maximal stimulation of insulin secretion occurs at plasma glucose concentrations more than 400 mg/dL. Glucose enters the β-cells by a membrane-bound glucose transporter (GLUT 2). Glucose is then phosphorylated by glucokinase as the first step in glycolysis (leading to the generation of acetyl-coenzyme A and adenosine triphosphate (ATP) through the Krebs cycle (see Plate 5-6). The rise in intracellular ATP closes (inhibits) the ATP-sensitive potassium (K^+) channels and reduces the efflux of K^+, which causes membrane depolarization and opening (activation) of the voltage-dependent calcium (Ca^{2+}) channels. The resultant Ca^{2+} influx increases the concentration of intracellular Ca^{2+}, which triggers the exocytosis of insulin secretory granules into the circulation. The β-cell Ca^{2+} concentrations can also be increased by the ATP generated from amino acid metabolism.

Insulin release from β-cells can be amplified by cholecystokinin, acetylcholine, gastric inhibitory polypeptide (GIP), glucagon, and GLP-1. Orally administered glucose stimulates a greater insulin response than an equivalent amount of glucose administered intravenously because of the release of enteric hormones (e.g., GLP-1, GIP) that potentiate insulin secretion. This phenomenon is referred to as the *incretin effect*, a finding that has led to new pharmacotherapeutic options in the treatment of patients with type 2 diabetes mellitus (see Plate 5-20). Acetylcholine and cholecystokinin bind to cell surface receptors and activate adenylate cyclase and phospholipase C, which leads to inositol triphosphate (IP₃) breakdown and

mobilization of Ca^{2+} from intracellular stores; activation of protein kinase C also triggers insulin secretion. GLP-1 receptor activation leads to increased cyclic adenosine monophosphate (cAMP) and activation of the cAMP-dependent protein kinase A; the Ca^{2+} signal is amplified by decreasing Ca^{2+} uptake by cellular stores and by activation of proteins that trigger exocytosis of insulin. Somatostatin and catecholamines inhibit insulin secretion through G-protein–coupled receptors and inhibition of adenylate cyclase.

Normal insulin secretion is dependent on the maintenance of an adequate number of functional β-cells (referred to as *β-cell mass*). The β-cells must be able to sense the key regulators of insulin secretion (e.g., blood glucose concentration). In addition, the rates of proinsulin synthesis and processing must be sufficient to maintain adequate insulin secretion. Defects in any of these steps in insulin secretion can lead to hyperglycemia and diabetes mellitus.

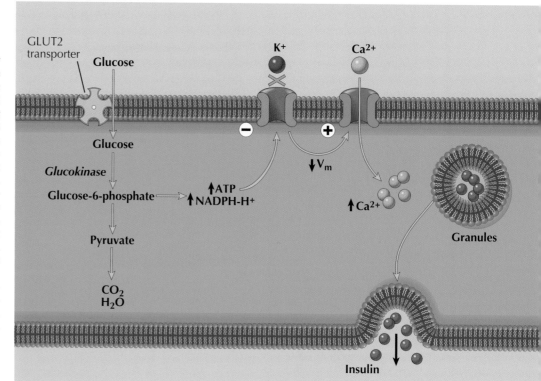

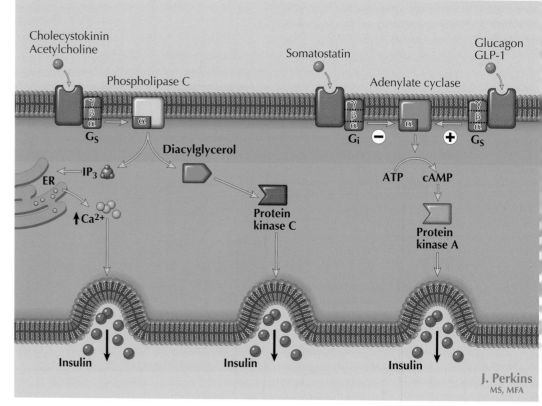

Plate 5-5

Pancreas

ACTIONS OF INSULIN

Insulin is a 56–amino acid polypeptide that consists of two peptide chains (α and β) that are joined by two disulfide bridges. Insulin is secreted into the portal vein and delivered directly to the liver. Approximately 80% of insulin is cleared by the hepatic cell surface insulin receptors with the first pass through the liver. Insulin acts through the insulin receptor and has anabolic effects at target organs to promote synthesis of carbohydrate, fat, and protein.

The insulin receptor, a member of the growth factor receptor family, is a heterotetrameric glycoprotein membrane receptor that has two α- and two β-subunits that are linked by disulfide bonds. The α-subunits form the extracellular portion where insulin binds. The β-subunits form the transmembrane and intracellular portions of the receptor and contain an intrinsic tyrosine kinase activity. Insulin binding to the receptor triggers autophosphorylation on the intracellular tyrosine residues and leads to phosphorylation of insulin receptor substrates (IRS-1, IRS-2, IRS-3, and IRS-4). The phosphorylation of the IRS proteins activates the phophatidylinositol-3-kinase (PI₃ kinase) and mitogen-activated protein kinase (MAPK) pathways. The PI₃ kinase pathway mediates the metabolic (e.g., glucose transport, glycolysis, glycogen synthesis, and protein synthesis) and antiapoptotic effects of insulin. The MAPK pathway has primarily proliferative and differentiation effects. The number of insulin receptors expressed on the cell membrane can be modulated by diet, body type, exercise, insulin, and other hormones. Obesity and high serum insulin concentrations downregulate the number of insulin receptors. Exercise and starvation upregulate the number of insulin receptors.

Glucose oxidation is the major energy source for many tissue types. Cell membranes are impermeable to hydrophilic molecules such as glucose and require a carrier system to transport glucose across the lipid bilayer cell membrane. Glucose transporter 1 (GLUT 1) is present in all tissues and has a high affinity for glucose to mediate a basal glucose uptake in the fasting state. GLUT 2 has a low affinity for glucose and functions primarily at high plasma glucose concentrations (e.g., after a meal). GLUT 3 is a high-affinity glucose transporter for neuronal tissues. GLUT 4 is localized primarily to muscle and adipose tissues.

In muscle, activation of the insulin receptor and the PI₃ kinase pathway leads to recruitment of the glucose transporter GLUT 4 from the cytosol to the plasma membrane. Increased expression of GLUT 4 leads to active transport of glucose across the myocyte cell membrane. Insulin promotes myocyte glycogen synthesis by increasing the activity of glycogen synthase and inhibiting the activity of glycogen phosphorylase. Insulin also enhances protein synthesis by increasing amino acid transport and by phosphorylation of a serine/threonine protein kinase.

In adipose tissue, insulin inhibits lipolysis by promoting dephosphorylation of hormone-sensitive (intracellular) lipase. The decreased breakdown of adipocyte triglycerides to fatty acids and glycerol leads to decreased substrate for ketogenesis. Insulin also induces the production of the endothelial cell–bound lipoprotein lipase, which hydrolyzes triglycerides from circulating lipoproteins to provide free fatty acids for adipocyte uptake. Insulin stimulates lipogenesis by activating acetyl-coenzyme A carboxylase. Increased glucose transport into adipocytes increases the availability of α-glycerol phosphate that is used in the esterification of free fatty acids into triglycerides. The decreased fatty acid delivery to the liver is a key factor in the net impact of insulin to decrease hepatic gluconeogenesis and ketogenesis.

In the liver, insulin stimulates the synthesis of enzymes that are involved in glucose utilization (e.g., pyruvate kinase, glucokinase) and inhibits the synthesis of enzymes involved in glucose production (e.g., glucose 6-phospatase, phosphoenolpyruvate carboxykinase). Insulin enhances glycogen synthesis by increasing phosphatase activity, causing dephosphorylation of glycogen synthase and glycogen phosphorylase. Insulin also promotes hepatic synthesis of triglycerides, very low-density lipoprotein, and proteins.

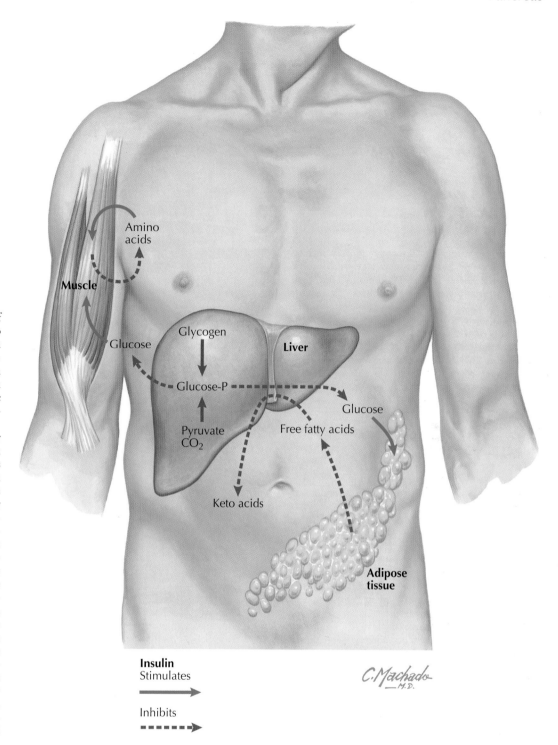

Insulin
Stimulates

Inhibits

Plate 5-6

Endocrine System

GLYCOLYSIS

Glycolysis is the major pathway for glucose metabolism, and it occurs in the cytosol of all cells. Glycolysis breaks down glucose (a 6-carbon molecule) into pyruvate (a 3-carbon molecule). Glycolysis can function either aerobically or anaerobically, depending on the availability of oxygen and the electron transport chain. The ability of glycolysis to provide energy in the form of adenosine triphosphate (ATP) from adenosine diphosphate (ADP) in the absence of oxygen allows tissues to survive anoxia.

Glycolysis occurs when a molecule of glucose 6-phosphate is transformed to pyruvate:

Glucose + 2 ADP + 2 NAD$^+$
+ 2 Inorganic phosphate (P$_i$)
→ 2 Pyruvate + 2 ATP
+ 2 NADH + 2 H$^+$ + 2H$_2$O

Glucose enters glycolysis by phosphorylation to glucose 6-phosophate, an irreversible reaction catalyzed by hexokinase, and ATP serves as the phosphate donor. Glucose 6-phosphate is converted to fructose-6-phosphate by phosphohexose isomerase. This intermediate is then phosphorylated to yield fructose-1,6-diphosphate. At this stage, the hexose molecule is cleaved by aldolase into two 3-carbon compounds: glyceraldehyde 3-phosphate and dihydroxyacetone phosphate. Dihydroxyacetone phosphate is quickly converted to glyceraldehyde 3-phosphate. The aldehyde group (CHO) of glyceraldehyde 3-phosphate is oxidized by a nicotinamide adenine dinucleotide (NAD)–dependent enzyme, and a phosphate group is attached, yielding 1, 3-bisphosphoglycerate. The energy of this oxidative step now rests in the phosphate bond at position 1. This energy is transferred to a molecule of ADP, forming ATP.

Glyceraldehyde 3-phosphate + P$_i$ + NAD + ADP
→ 3-Phosphoglycerate + NADH + ATP

The above reaction yields energy that is not immediately given off as heat but is stored in the form of ATP. Because two molecules of glyceraldehyde 3-phosphate are produced for every molecule of glucose, two molecules of ATP are formed at this step per molecule of glucose undergoing glycolysis. An ensuing transformation of phosphoenolpyruvate to pyruvate (catalyzed by pyruvate kinase) gives rise to another ATP (2 molecules of ATP per molecule of glucose oxidized).

When a tissue possesses the systems for further oxidation of pyruvate, provided oxygen is present, pyruvate is cleaved to acetyl coenzyme A (CoA), and it enters the tricarboxylic acid cycle (see Plate 5-7). However, when the oxidative systems are absent (e.g., in erythrocytes that lack mitochondria) or if oxygen is excluded or is present in insufficient amounts (e.g., under

anaerobic conditions), pyruvate is reduced to lactic acid by the enzyme lactate dehydrogenase. This system provides for the reoxidation of NADH and thus enables its participation again in oxidizing glyceraldehyde 3-phosphate; otherwise, the latter reaction would stop as soon as all the molecules of NAD were reduced.

(A) Glyceraldehyde 3-phosphate + NAD
→ 1,3-Diphosphoglycerate + NADH
(B) Pyruvate + NADH → Lactate + NAD

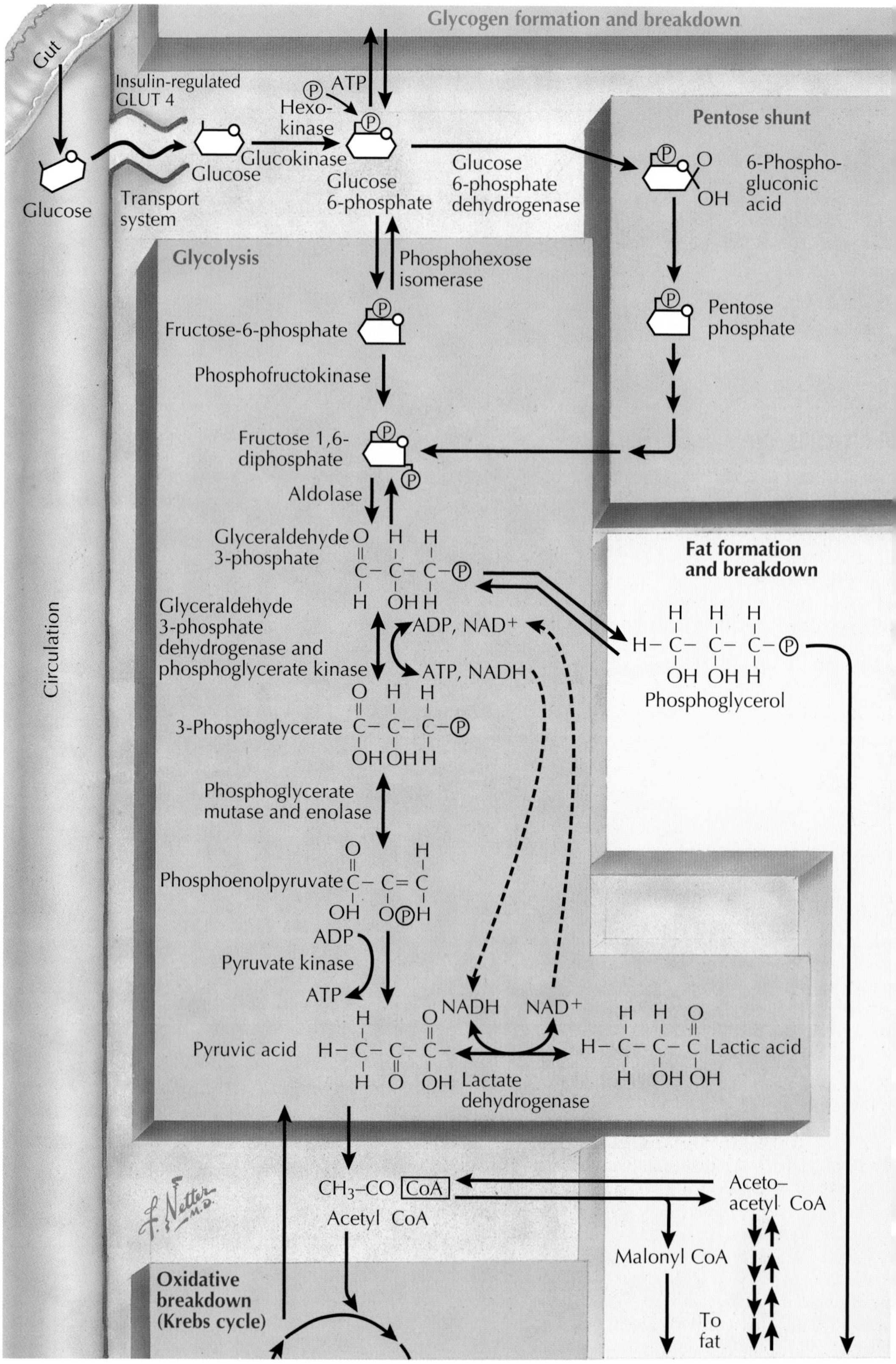

The coupling of these two reactions allows the provision of energy by carbohydrates in the absence of oxygen, albeit at the expense of considerable amounts of carbohydrate. Under aerobic conditions, approximately 30 molecules of ATP are generated per molecule of glucose that is oxidized to CO$_2$ and H$_2$O, but only two molecules of ATP when oxygen is absent. Glycolysis is regulated by the three enzymes that catalyze nonequilibrium reactions: hexokinase, phosphofructokinase, and pyruvate kinase.

Plate 5-7

Pancreas

TRICARBOXYLIC ACID CYCLE

The tricarboxylic acid (TCA) cycle, also referred to as the citric acid cycle or the Krebs cycle, is the final common pathway for oxidation of carbohydrate, lipid, and protein. Most of these nutrients are metabolized to acetyl-coenzyme A (acetyl-CoA) or one of the intermediates in the TCA cycle. For example, in protein catabolism, proteins are broken down by proteases into their constituent amino acids. The carbon backbone of these amino acids can become a source of energy by being converted to acetyl-CoA and entering into the TCA cycle. The TCA cycle also provides carbon skeletons for gluconeogenesis and fatty acid synthesis.

The TCA cycle starts with a reaction between the acetyl moiety of acetyl-CoA and the 4-carbon dicarboxylic acid, oxaloacetate, to form a 6-carbon tricarboxylic acid, citrate. In the reactions that follow, two molecules of CO_2 are released and oxaloacetate is regenerated. This process is aerobic and requires oxygen as the final oxidant of the reduced coenzymes.

From one molecule of glucose, glycolysis (see Plate 5-6) provides two molecules of pyruvate. Pyruvate is split to acetyl-CoA and CO_2 by pyruvate dehydrogenase, a step that generates one molecule of reduced nicotinamide adenine dinucleotide (NADH). Citrate synthase catalyzes the initial reaction between acetyl-CoA and oxaloacetate. Citrate is then isomerized to isocitrate by aconitase. Isocitrate is dehydrogenated by isocitrate dehydrogenase to form oxalosuccinate and then α-ketoglutarate. α-Ketoglutarate then undergoes oxidative decarboxylation to form succinyl-CoA, a step that is catalyzed by a multienzyme complex referred to as the *α-ketoglutarate dehydrogenase complex*. Succinate thiokinase converts succinyl-CoA to succinate. Succinate is then dehydrogenated to fumarate by succinate dehydrogenase. Fumarase catalyzes the addition of water across the double bond of fumarate to form malate. Malate is converted to oxaloacetate by malate dehydrogenase. Oxaloacetate can then reenter the TCA cycle.

Because of the oxidations catalyzed by the dehydrogenases in the TCA cycle, three molecules of the reduced form of NADH and one molecule of flavin adenine dinucleotide H_2 (FADH$_2$) are produced for each molecule of acetyl-CoA catabolized in one turn of the cycle.

$$\text{Acetyl-CoA} + 3\ NAD^+ + FAD + ADP + P_i + 2\ H_2O \rightarrow \text{CoA-SH} + 3\ NADH + 3\ H^+ + FADH_2 + ATP + 2\ CO_2$$

In addition, the pyruvate dehydrogenase step provides one molecule of NADH. These reducing equivalents are transferred to the respiratory chain, and reoxidation of each NADH results in approximately 2.5 adenosine triphosphate (ATP) molecules and each FADH$_2$ translates to approximately 1.5 ATP molecules. In addition, one ATP equivalent is generated from the phosphorylation step of succinyl-CoA catalyzed by succinate thiokinase. Thus, including the pyruvate dehydrogenase step, approximately 12 ATP molecules are formed per turn of the TCA cycle.

Four of the B vitamins have key roles in the TCA cycle. Riboflavin (vitamin B$_2$) in the form of FAD is a cofactor for succinate dehydrogenase. Niacin (vitamin B$_3$) in the form of NAD is the electron acceptor for

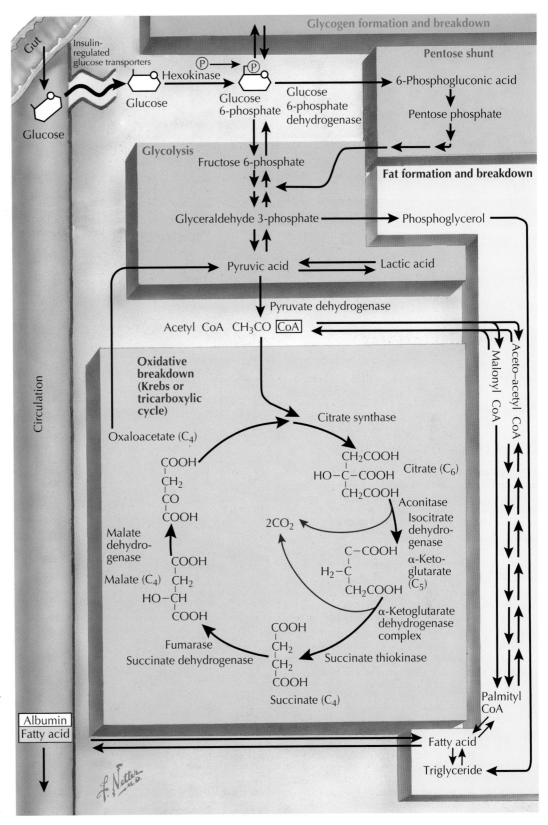

isocitrate dehydrogenase, α-ketoglutarate dehydrogenase, and malate dehydrogenase. Pantothenic acid (vitamin B$_5$) is part of CoA. Thiamine (vitamin B$_1$) serves as the coenzyme for decarboxylation of the α-ketoglutarate dehydrogenase step.

Recent studies have shown a link between intermediates of the TCA cycle and the regulation of hypoxia-inducible factors (HIFs). HIFs have a key role in the regulation of oxygen homeostasis. HIFs are transcription factors that have broad targets, which include apoptosis, angiogenesis, vascular remodeling, glucose use, and iron transport. Dysregulation of HIFs appears central to the development of paragangliomas and pheochromocytomas in individuals with von Hippel–Lindau syndrome, where the *VHL* tumor suppressor gene encodes a protein that regulates hypoxia-induced proteins (see Plate 8-4). In addition, the familial paraganglioma syndromes are associated with mutations in the genes that encode key subunits of succinate dehydrogenase (*SDHB, SDHD, SDHC, SDHA, SDHAF2*).

Plate 5-8

Endocrine System

GLYCOGEN METABOLISM

Glycogen is a branched polymer of α-D-glucose and is the major depot of carbohydrates in the body, primarily in muscle and liver. Glycogen is the analog of starch, which is a less branched glucose polymer in plants.

GLYCOGENESIS

Glycogenesis occurs mainly in the liver and muscle. Catalyzed by glucokinase in the liver and hexokinase in the muscle, glucose is phosphorylated to glucose 6-phosphate. Glucose 6-phosphate is isomerized to glucose 1-phosphate by the action of phosphogluco-mutase. Glucose 1-phosphate interacts with uridine triphosphate (UTP) to form uridine diphosphate glucose (UDPGlc) and pyrophosphate in a reaction catalyzed by UDPGlc pyrophosphorylase. Glycogen synthase catalyzes the bond between C_1 of the glucose of UDPGlc with the C_4 terminal glucose residue (1→4 linkage) of glycogen and uridine diphosphate (UDP) liberated in the process. This step keeps repeating until the glycogen chain is at least 11 glucose residues long; at that point, branching enzyme transfers six or more glucose residues to a neighboring chain to form a 1→6 linkage to establish a branch point.

GLYCOGENOLYSIS

The rate-limiting step of glycogenolysis is the cleavage of the 1→4 linkages of glycogen by glycogen phospho-rylase to produce glucose 1-phosphate. This cleaving starts at the terminal glucosyl residues until 4 glucose residues remain on either side of a 1→6 linkage, at which point glucan transferase transfers a trisaccharide unit from one branch to the other to expose the 1→6 linkage. Debranching enzyme can then hydrolyze the 1→6 linkage, and further phosphorylase actions proceed to completely convert the glycogen chain to glucose 1-phosphate. The glucose 6-phosphate molecules have three possible fates: (1) transformation to glucose 1-phosphate by phosphoglucomutase and proceeding to glycogenesis; (2) hydrolyzation by glucose 6-phosphatase in the liver and kidney to produce glucose for release into the bloodstream; or (3) proceeding on to the glycolysis or the pentose phosphate (pentose shunt) pathways.

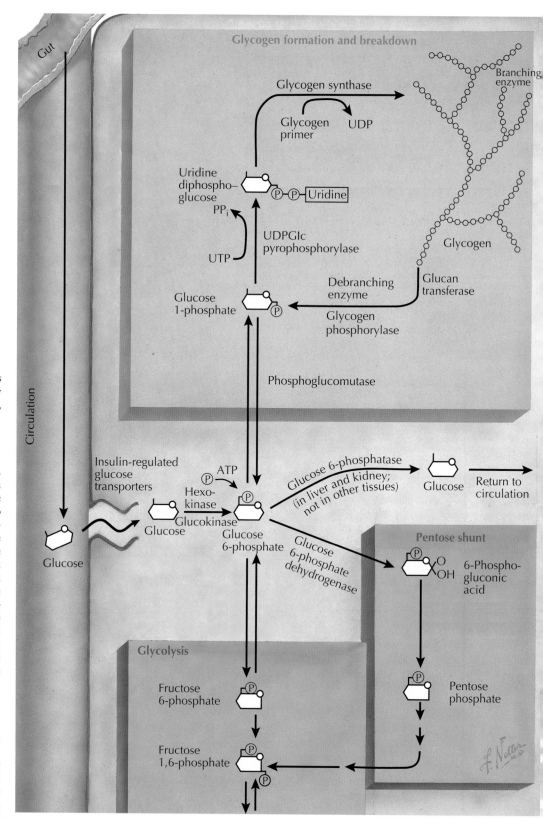

REGULATION OF GLYCOGENESIS AND GLYCOGENOLYSIS

The rate-limiting enzymes are glycogen synthase and glycogen phosphorylase. Glycogen serves as a rapid and short-term source of glucose. The liver releases glycogen-derived glucose during fasting. After ingesting a meal containing carbohydrates, blood glucose concentrations rise and stimulate the pancreas to release insulin. Insulin-regulated glucose transporters provide glucose to the hepatocyte. Insulin also stimulates glycogen synthase. Glucose continues to be added to the glycogen chains as long as glucose and insulin are supplied. After food digestion, blood glucose concentrations fall, and insulin release is decreased, leading to a cessation in glycogen synthesis. Approximately 4 hours after a meal, because of decreasing blood glucose levels, the pancreas begins to secrete glucagon. Glucagon and epinephrine are the main hormones that activate glycogenolysis.

Plate 5-9

Pancreas

CONSEQUENCES OF INSULIN DEPRIVATION

The absence of insulin is incompatible with life. Insulin deprivation can result from surgical removal (pancreatectomy) or autoimmune destruction of β-cells (type 1 diabetes mellitus); both lead to absence or severe curtailment of insulin production and release. In these settings, insulin-sensitive tissues (e.g., muscle, adipose tissue, liver) are deprived of insulin and its actions. Cell membranes are impermeable to hydrophilic molecules such as glucose and require a carrier system (e.g., GLUT 1, 2, 3, 4) to transport glucose across the lipid bilayer cell membrane. Because of decreased insulin-induced activation of the cell membrane glucose transporters, the transit of glucose from the blood into cells is diminished. At the same time, in the absence of insulin, glycogenesis is slowed. The suppressive effect of insulin on glucagon is removed, and glucagon enhances hepatic gluconeogenesis, which is fueled by the increased availability of precursors (e.g., glycerol and alanine) from accelerated fat and muscle breakdown. Thus, in the setting of insulin deprivation, there is impaired glucose utilization in peripheral tissues, increased glycogenolysis, and increased gluconeogenesis.

When the blood glucose concentration increases above 200 mg/dL, the renal tubules begin to exceed their capacity for glucose reabsorption (renal threshold). Excess glucose is lost in the urine (glucosuria) which, because of osmotic forces, takes water and sodium with it. Weight loss, thirst, polyuria, and hunger occur. Patients with indolent uncontrolled diabetes over months can present with wasting and cachexia similar to that seen in those with advanced malignancies.

In insulin-sensitive tissues, metabolic adjustments occur as a consequence of the curtailed glucose supply. Proteins are broken down faster than they can be synthesized; hence, amino acids are liberated from muscle, brought to the liver, and transformed to urea. The nonprotein nitrogen excreted in the urine rises and a negative nitrogen balance results.

Lipolysis is enhanced in the setting of insulin deprivation. There is a net liberation of stored fat as free fatty acids, which are used by many tissues for energy production. Hepatic uptake and metabolism of fatty acids lead to excess production of the ketones acetoacetate and β-hydroxybutyrate, strong organic acids that lead to ketoacidosis (see Plate 5-10). Ketones provide an alternate energy source when the utilization of glucose is impaired. The circulating β-hydroxybutyrate and acetoacetate obtain their sodium from NaHCO₃, thus leading to a metabolic acidosis. In addition, acetoacetate and β-hydroxybutyrate are excreted readily by the kidney, accompanied by base, and fixed base is lost. The severity of the metabolic acidosis depends on the rate and duration of ketoacid production.

Insulin deprivation also leads to deficits in minerals. A potassium deficit results from urinary losses with the glucose osmotic diuresis and in an effort to maintain

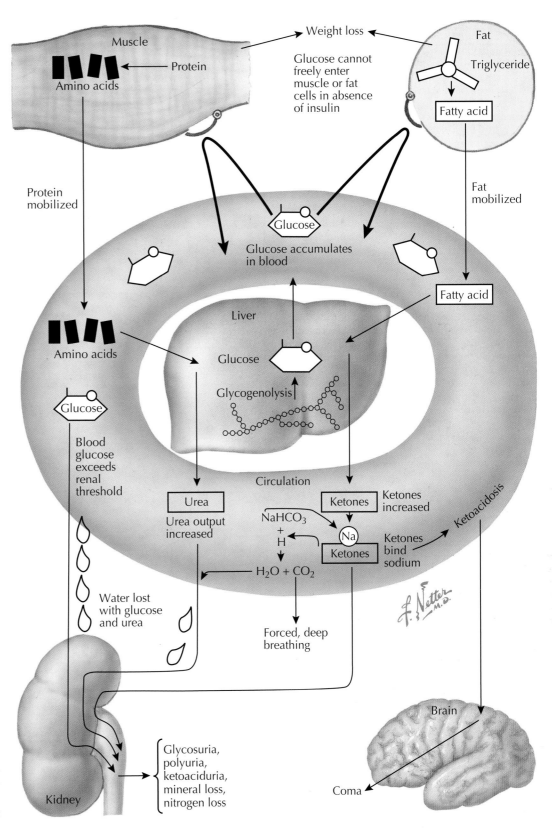

electroneutrality as ketoacid anions are excreted. A negative phosphate balance is a result of phosphaturia caused by hyperglycemic-induced osmotic diuresis.

The outcomes of severe insulin deprivation include negative nitrogen balance, weight loss, ketosis, and acidosis. These are the hallmarks of the most severe state of metabolic decompensation characteristic of insulin deprivation in individuals with no endogenous source of insulin (e.g., type 1 diabetes mellitus). Acidosis, when

not compensated for, exerts its major effect on brain function. In addition, acidosis affects the contractile responses of the small blood vessels throughout the body that, when coupled with osmotic diuresis-induced volume loss, results in hypotension and vascular collapse. Thus, diabetic coma and death—the fate of all those with type 1 diabetes mellitus before the advent of insulin replacement therapy—are the end result of uncompensated and untreated insulin deprivation.

Plate 5-10

Endocrine System

DIABETIC KETOACIDOSIS

Diabetic ketoacidosis (DKA) is serious complication of diabetes mellitus characterized by the triad of hyperglycemia, anion gap metabolic acidosis, and ketonemia. DKA results from severe insulin deficiency with resultant hyperglycemia, excessive lipolysis, increased fatty acid oxidation, and excess ketone body production. The deficiency of insulin and the excess secretion of glucagon, catecholamines, glucocorticoids, and growth hormone stimulate glycogenolysis and gluconeogenesis while simultaneously impairing glucose disposal. DKA is primarily a complication of type 1 diabetes mellitus because it is usually only seen in the setting of severe insulin deficiency. DKA may be the initial presentation of new-onset type 1 diabetes mellitus.

Most patients with DKA have preceding symptoms of polyuria, polydipsia, and weight loss that result from a partially compensated state. However, with absolute insulin deficiency, metabolic decompensation can intervene rapidly over 24 hours. Typical DKA presenting symptoms include nausea; emesis; abdominal pain; lethargy; and hyperventilation with slow, deep breaths (Kussmaul respirations). On physical examination, most patients with DKA have a low-normal blood pressure, increased heart rate, increased respiratory rate, signs of volume depletion (e.g., decreased skin turgor, low jugular venous pressure, and dry oral mucosa), and breath that smells of acetone (a fruity odor similar to nail polish remover). With profound dehydration, patients may be obtunded or comatose.

The laboratory profile in patients with DKA includes low serum bicarbonate (HCO_3) concentration (<10 mEq/L); increased serum concentrations of ketoacids (acetoacetate, β-hydroxybutyrate); increased anion gap (calculated by subtracting the sum of the serum concentrations of chloride and bicarbonate from that of sodium; reference range, <14 mEq/L; DKA usually >20 mEq/L); increased serum glucose concentration (500–900 mg/dL); and decreased arterial pH (<7.3).

The differential diagnosis of DKA includes other causes of metabolic acidosis (e.g., lactic acidosis, starvation ketosis, alcoholic ketoacidosis, uremic acidosis, and toxin ingestion [e.g., salicylate intoxication]).

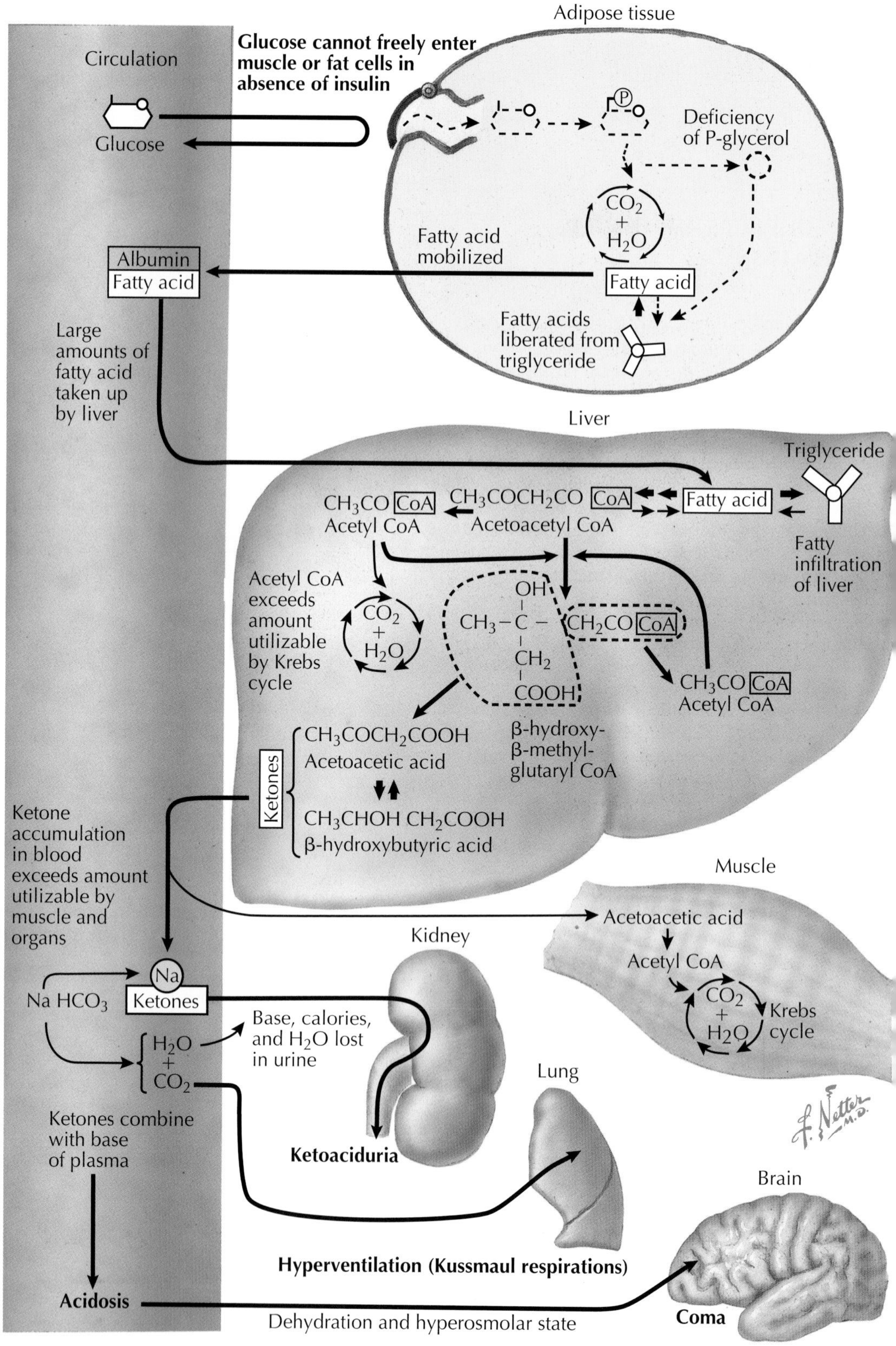

TREATMENT

Keys to successful outcomes in DKA are prompt recognition and management. The three main thrusts of treatment are fluid repletion, insulin administration, and management of electrolyte abnormalities. All patients with DKA have some degree of volume contraction, which contributes to decreased renal clearance of ketone bodies and glucose. Most patients with DKA should be treated with 1 L of normal saline over the first hour followed by 200 to 500 mL per hour until volume repletion. The rate and type of volume repletion should be guided by clinical and laboratory responses. Insulin should be administered intravenously to avoid slow absorption from hypoperfused subcutaneous tissues. Insulin is usually started with a 10-U priming dose and followed by a low-dose continuous infusion (e.g., 0.1 U/kg body weight/h). Serum glucose usually decreases by 50 to 75 mg/dL per hour. As the serum glucose concentration decreases to approximately 200 mg/dL, the insulin infusion rate should be decreased so that hypoglycemia and cerebral edema are avoided (the latter can result from too rapid a correction from the hyperosmolar state). With volume repletion, resolving acidosis, and improving blood glucose concentrations, an underlying potassium deficit usually becomes evident and should be replaced when the serum potassium concentration decreases below 5.3 mEq/L.

Most patients with DKA should be admitted to an intensive care unit setting in the hospital to facilitate close monitoring with continuous electrocardiography and hourly measurement of blood concentrations of glucose, potassium, chloride, and bicarbonate. Other blood parameters should be monitored every 2 hours (e.g., calcium, magnesium, and phosphate). DKA can be corrected in most patients over 12 to 36 hours.

It is important to address the cause of DKA. The most common cause is noncompliance with insulin therapy in a patient with known type 1 diabetes mellitus. Underlying infection (e.g., pneumonia, meningitis, or urinary tract infection) or severe illness (e.g., myocardial infarction, cerebrovascular accident, or pancreatitis) may be a trigger for DKA in a patient with type 1 diabetes.

Plate 5-15

Pancreas

DIABETIC NEPHROPATHY

Diabetic nephropathy is a major cause of morbidity and mortality in patients with type 1 or type 2 diabetes mellitus. Diabetic nephropathy is characterized as the triad of proteinuria, hypertension, and renal impairment. Approximately 40% of patients with type 1 diabetes and 20% of patients with type 2 diabetes develop some degree of diabetic nephropathy. Diabetes is the single most common cause of end-stage renal disease (ESRD).

Diabetic nephropathy can be considered in five stages or phases. The initial phase of diabetic nephropathy is hyperfiltration with increased capillary glomerular pressure and elevated glomerular filtration rate (GFR) (e.g., >150 mL/min). The glomerular hyperfiltration is associated with glomerular hypertrophy and increased renal size. The second stage is termed the *silent stage*. In this stage, although the GFR is normal and there is no proteinuria, glomerular basement membrane thickening and mesangial expansion are occurring. The third stage is termed *incipient nephropathy*, during which the urinary albumin excretion rate becomes abnormal (e.g., 30–300 mg/24 hr). Also at this stage, systemic hypertension may become evident. The fourth stage of diabetic nephropathy is the *overt nephropathy* or *macroalbuminuria* stage. In this stage, the 24-hour urinary albumin excretion is more than 300 mg, and creatinine levels in the blood rise. The majority of patients at this stage have systemic hypertension. Untreated hypertension can accelerate the decline in GFR, which in turn accelerates systemic hypertension. The fifth and final stage is *uremia*, the effective treatment of which requires renal replacement therapy.

As with diabetic retinopathy, the pathogenesis of diabetic nephropathy is complex and related to a hyperglycemia-triggered cascade of mechanisms. Chronic hyperglycemia causes impaired autoregulation of renal blood flow with intraglomerular hypertension, accumulation of advanced glycosylation end products, generation of mitochondrial reactive oxygen species, activation of protein kinase C, and accumulation of sorbitol. Improved glycemic control in patients with diabetes can slow the development of nephropathy.

Glomerular basement membrane thickening and mesangial expansion are prominent glomerular abnormalities in diabetes that progress to nodular (Kimmelstiel-Wilson lesion) or diffuse glomerulosclerosis. Nodular glomerulosclerosis is associated with hyaline deposits in the glomerular arterioles. A diabetic tubulopathy can also develop and may result in a type IV renal tubular acidosis with hyperkalemia and hyperchloremic metabolic acidosis, an outcome associated with hyporeninemic hypoaldosteronism.

The cornerstones of treatment for diabetic nephropathy are optimizing glycemic control and hypertension management. Decreases in glycosylated hemoglobin are associated with a decreased risk of development of microalbuminuria and decreased rate of progression through the stages of diabetic nephropathy. Angiotensin-converting enzyme (ACE) inhibitors and angiotensin receptor blockers (ARBs) are the antihypertensive drug classes of choice because these agents appear to have renoprotective effects that exceed their antihypertensive effects. ACE inhibitors and ARBs decrease urinary albumin excretion by more than 30% and retard the progression from microalbuminuria to overt proteinuria. In addition, exposure to agents that have adverse effects on blood pressure or renal function should be avoided. For example, nonsteroidal

GLOMERULOSCLEROSIS

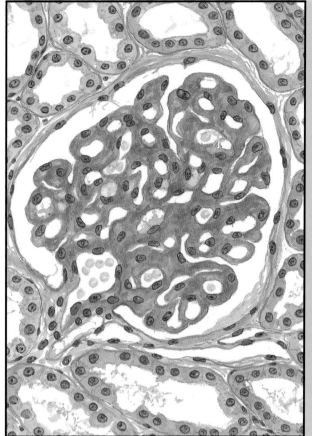

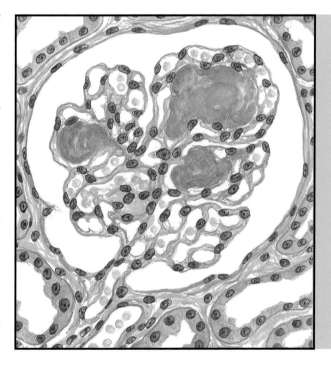

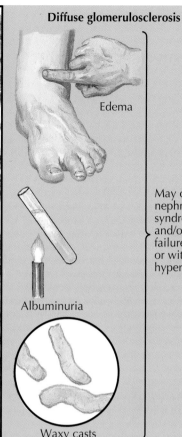

Diffuse glomerulosclerosis

Edema

Albuminuria

Waxy casts

May cause nephrotic syndrome and/or renal failure, with or without hypertension

Nodular glomerulosclerosis

This nodular component (Kimmelstiel-Wilson nodules) associated with hyaline deposits in the glomerular arterioles is pathognomonic for diabetic nephropathy

antiinflammatory drugs and cyclo-oxygenase-2 inhibitors should be avoided because of their adverse impact on hypertension. In addition, radiographic contrast dye should be avoided because of its adverse impact on renal function and risk for acute renal failure.

Progressive diabetic nephropathy may result in severe proteinuria and associated symptoms that are referred to as the *nephrotic syndrome*. Nephrotic syndrome is defined by urinary protein excretion of more than 3.5 g/1.73 m² per 24 hours, hypoalbuminemia (serum albumin concentration <3 g/dL), and peripheral edema. Microscopic examination of the urine sediment may show waxy casts (degenerated cellular casts of collecting tubules), which are found in patients with severe chronic renal disease. For patients who progress to ESRD, renal replacement options include hemodialysis, peritoneal dialysis, renal transplantation, and combined pancreas–kidney transplantation.

Plate 5-16

Endocrine System

DIABETIC NEUROPATHY

Approximately 50% of those with diabetes of more than 25 years' duration develop symptomatic diabetic neuropathy. Diabetic neuropathy is not a single disorder, but rather multiple disorders depending on the types of nerve fibers involved.

FOCAL NEUROPATHIES

In general, mononeuropathies occur in older patients with diabetes. Mononeuropathies are a result of vascular obstruction and are typically acute in onset, associated with pain and motor weakness, and self-limited (most resolve over 2 months). Nerves that are commonly involved include cranial nerves III, VI, and VII; the ulnar nerve; and the peroneal nerve. Patients may present with wrist drop or ankle drop. With third cranial nerve involvement, patients complain of diplopia, and examination shows ptosis and ophthalmoplegia. Diabetic polyradiculopathy is characterized by severe pain in the distribution of one or more nerve roots and may be accompanied by motor weakness. For example, intercostal or truncal radiculopathy presents with pain over the thorax or abdomen. Diabetic polyradiculopathy is usually self-limited and resolves over 1 year.

PROXIMAL MOTOR NEUROPATHIES

Proximal motor neuropathies (also known as diabetic amyotrophy, proximal neuropathy, femoral neuropathy, diabetic neuropathic cachexia, and Ellenberg cachexia) affect primarily older patients with type 2 diabetes. Symptoms usually start with thigh and pelvic girdle pains that progress to marked atrophy of the quadriceps muscles. Patients present with symptoms caused by lower extremity proximal muscle weakness (e.g., must use arms to assist them when rising from a chair). The signs and symptoms may start unilaterally but usually progress to bilateral involvement. Pain may be a predominant component of the clinical presentation, and profound weight loss and depression are common. Axonal loss is the primary pathophysiologic process, and electromyography shows lumbosacral plexopathy. Most of these patients prove to have chronic inflammatory demyelinating polyneuropathy, monoclonal gammopathy, ganglioside antibody syndrome, or an inflammatory vasculitis.

DISTAL SYMMETRIC POLYNEUROPATHY

Distal symmetric polyneuropathy (DSPN) is the most common form of diabetic neuropathy. The onset of DSPN is usually slow and involves small and/or large fibers of either sensory and/or motor nerves. Small fiber neuropathy usually manifests as paresthesia, hyperalgesia (increased pain response to a normally painful stimulus), allodynia (pain response from a stimulus that is not normally painful), or hypesthesia involving the feet and lower extremities. The pain is usually described as burning. The paresthesias are described as pins and needles, numbness, tingling, cold, or burning. Physical examination usually reveals reduced pinprick and light tough sensations and loss of thermal sensitivity. An acute painful small fiber neuropathy may develop with the initiation of therapy to improve glycemic control.

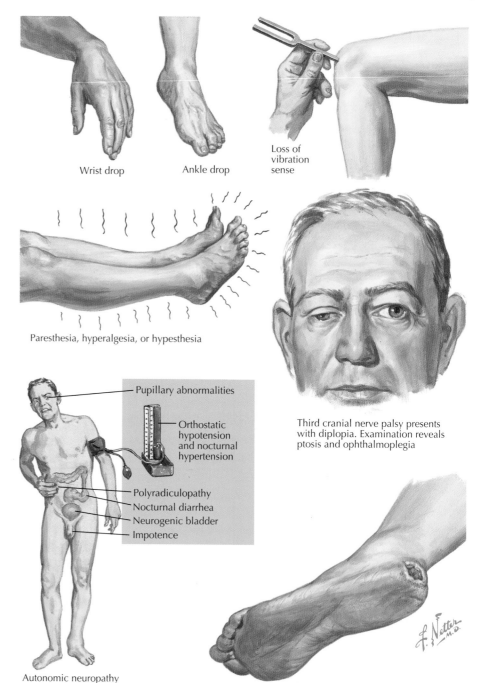

Wrist drop

Ankle drop

Loss of vibration sense

Paresthesia, hyperalgesia, or hypesthesia

Third cranial nerve palsy presents with diplopia. Examination reveals ptosis and ophthalmoplegia

Pupillary abnormalities

Orthostatic hypotension and nocturnal hypertension

Polyradiculopathy
Nocturnal diarrhea
Neurogenic bladder
Impotence

Autonomic neuropathy

Neuropathic (painless) ulcer

Large-fiber neuropathies involve the myelinated and rapidly conducting sensory or motor nerves that are normally responsible for vibration perception, cold thermal perception, position sense, and motor function. Typical initial symptoms include a sensation of walking on pebbles or cotton, inability to discriminate among coins, and trouble turning pages of a book. Large-fiber neuropathies are easily detected on physical examination (e.g., loss of vibration sense, loss of proprioception, loss of deep tendon reflexes). There may be wasting of the small muscles in the feet and hands.

Usually DSPN presents with signs and symptoms of both small- and large-fiber nerve damage. The longer nerves are especially vulnerable, and most patients have a stocking-and-glove type sensory loss that may spread proximally. Neuropathic foot ulcers and Charcot's arthropathy (neurogenic arthropathy) can result from loss of proprioception, pain, and temperature perceptions (see Plate 5-18).

AUTONOMIC NEUROPATHY

Dysfunction of the sympathetic and parasympathetic nervous systems has the potential to cause malfunction of almost all body systems. Examples of organ systems that may be affected by autonomic neuropathy include pupillary abnormalities with Argyll-Robertson-type pupil and decreased diameter of dark-adapted pupil; cardiovascular system with orthostatic hypotension, nocturnal hypertension, resting tachycardia, silent myocardial infarction, and heat and exercise intolerance; genitourinary system with erectile dysfunction, retrograde ejaculation, and neurogenic bladder with urinary retention; gastrointestinal system with gastroparesis, constipation, nocturnal diarrhea, and fecal incontinence; sweating disturbances with gustatory sweating, hyperhidrosis, and anhidrosis; and blunted adrenomedullary response to hypoglycemia, leading to hypoglycemic unawareness.

Plate 5-23

Pancreas

PRIMARY PANCREATIC β-CELL HYPERPLASIA

Primary pancreatic β-cell hyperplasia is a rare cause of hypoglycemia in children and adults. The hyperplastic process may be focal or diffuse. Nesidioblastosis, the neoformation of islets of Langerhans from pancreatic duct epithelium, is present in some patients with pancreatic β-cell hyperplasia.

CONGENITAL HYPERINSULINISM

Congenital hyperinsulinism is a rare (one in 50,000 live births) autosomal dominant or autosomal recessive disorder usually caused by mutations in the genes that encode the adenosine triphosphate–sensitive potassium channels (e.g., sulfonylurea receptor type 1 subunit [SUR1], potassium channel subunit [Kir6.2]). These loss-of-function mutations result in closure of the potassium channel and persistent β-cell membrane depolarization and insulin release despite the prevailing hypoglycemia. Diffuse β-cell hyperplasia and intractable hypoglycemia result. Congenital hyperinsulinism may also be caused by activating mutations in the genes that encode glutamate dehydrogenase or glucokinase.

Focal adenomatous islet-cell hyperplasia may result from focal loss of the normal maternally inherited allele and somatic expression of the paternally inherited abnormal genes encoding SUR1 or Kir6.2 (*ABCC8* and *KCNJ11*, respectively), which cause β-cell hyperplasia only in the involved cells. Whereas focal islet-cell hyperplasia can be cured by resection of the focally hyperplastic areas of the pancreas, diffuse hyperplasia may require more extensive pancreatic resections.

Signs of hypoglycemia in neonates include changes in level of consciousness, tremor, hypotonia, seizures, apnea, and cyanotic spells. Symptoms are usually evident in the first days after birth. Detection may be delayed until later in childhood in those with partial or mild defects in the *ABCC8* or *KCNJ11* genes. Early diagnosis can prevent neurologic damage from recurrent episodes of hypoglycemia. Macrosomia is common in newborns with congenital hyperinsulinism.

The differential diagnosis of hypoglycemia in infancy and childhood includes hyperinsulinism (congenital hyperinsulinism, nesidioblastosis, insulinoma, infant of a diabetic mother, maternal drugs [e.g., sulfonylurea]); drugs; severe illness; transient intolerance of fasting; lack of counterregulatory hormones (e.g., hypopituitarism); Beckwith-Wiedemann syndrome; or enzymatic defects in the metabolism of carbohydrate (e.g., glycogen storage diseases, glycogen synthase deficiency), protein (e.g., branched-chain α-keto acid dehydrogenase complex deficiency), or fat (e.g., defects in fatty acid oxidation). Transient intolerance of fasting is seen in premature infants and relates to incomplete development of glycogen stores and gluconeogenic mechanisms.

NONINSULINOMA PANCREATOGENOUS HYPOGLYCEMIA SYNDROME AND POST–GASTRIC BYPASS HYPOGLYCEMIA

Noninsulinoma pancreatogenous hypoglycemia syndrome (NIPHS) is a form of islet-cell hyperplasia that presents with postprandial symptoms caused by hyperinsulinemic hypoglycemia. The signs and symptoms are cured with partial pancreatectomy. Pathologic examination shows β-cell hypertrophy with or without

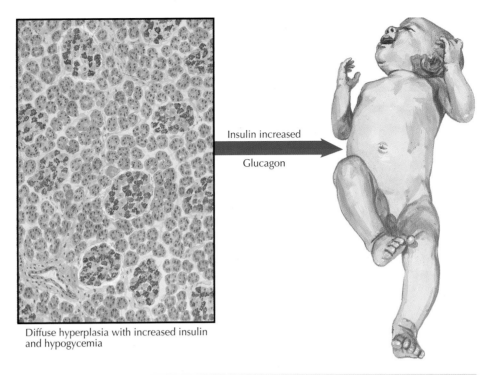

Insulin increased

Glucagon

Diffuse hyperplasia with increased insulin and hypoglycemia

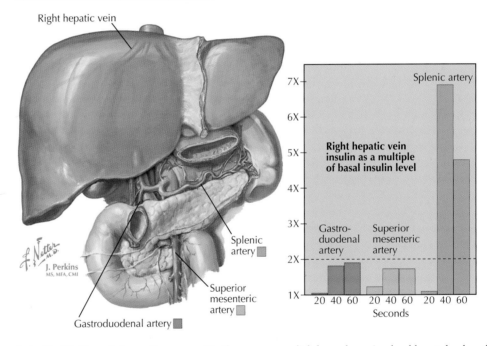

Selective arterial calcium stimulation test

Right hepatic vein

Splenic artery

Superior mesenteric artery

Gastroduodenal artery

J. Netter m.d.

J. Perkins
MS, MFA, CMI

Splenic artery

Right hepatic vein insulin as a multiple of basal insulin level

Gastro-duodenal artery

Superior mesenteric artery

Seconds

hyperplasia. Nesidioblastosis is usually present. Similar presentation and pathologic findings have been found after Roux-en-Y gastric bypass surgery for obesity, in which symptomatic postprandial hypoglycemia can develop 6 months to 8 years after surgery. The underlying pathophysiology is uncertain but may relate to decreased ghrelin, unidentified small intestine factors, or an inability to reset from the preoperative state of insulin-resistant hyperinsulinemia.

EVALUATION

Islet-cell hyperplasia may predispose to hypoglycemia, primarily in the postprandial state rather than in the fasting state as is seen with insulinoma. With the exception of the timing of hypoglycemia, the laboratory abnormalities are identical to those of patients with insulinomas (see Plate 5-22). The diagnosis of postprandial hypoglycemia should not be based on results of oral glucose tolerance testing but rather on results after a mixed meal.

β-Cell hyperplasia may be diffuse, asymmetric, or focal. Imaging studies are usually not helpful in localizing β-cell hyperplasia. Selective arterial calcium stimulation with hepatic venous sampling can regionalize the dysfunctional β-cells to arterial distributions within the pancreas. Calcium gluconate is selectively injected into the gastroduodenal, splenic, and superior mesenteric arteries, with timed hepatic venous sampling for measurement of insulin. Calcium stimulates the release of insulin from abnormal β-cells but not from normal β-cells. An abnormal result is defined as more than a two- to threefold increase from baseline in hepatic venous insulin concentrations. The selective arterial calcium stimulation test can lead to a gradient-guided partial pancreatectomy.

BONE AND CALCIUM

Plate 6-1

Endocrine System

HISTOLOGY OF THE NORMAL PARATHYROID GLANDS

The parathyroid glands are derived from branchial pouches III and IV and number between two to six glands, although four is the usual number. In adults, each of these ovoid (bean-shaped) glands measures 4 to 6 mm × by 2 to 4 mm × 0.5 to 2 mm and weighs approximately 30 mg (the lower parathyroid glands are generally larger than the upper glands). They vary in color from yellow to tan, depending on vascularity and percentage of oxyphil cells and stromal fat.

In infants and children, the glands are composed of sheets of closely packed chief cells, with little intervening stroma. Oxyphil (or oncocytic) cells first make their appearance at the time of puberty. Fat cells begin to appear in the stroma in late childhood. Both the oxyphil cells and the fat cells increase in number until they may occupy more than 50% of the volume of the glands during the fifth and sixth decades of life.

In adults, the glands are composed of cords, sheets, and acini of chief cells in a loose areolar stroma containing numerous mature fat cells. Chief cells appear in an active synthetic phase ("dark chief cell") with well-formed endoplasmic reticulum and prominent Golgi apparatus or in a resting phase ("light chief cell") with less well-developed endoplasmic reticulum. Scattered individually or in groups among these chief cells are the oxyphil cells. The chief cell measures approximately 8 μm in diameter. It has a well-defined cell membrane and a 4- to 5-μm centrally located nucleus. The chromatin is densely packed, appearing almost pyknotic, or it is finely fibrillar with peripheral margination. Nucleoli are rare. The cell cytoplasm is clear and amphophilic in hematoxylin and eosin (H&E) preparations. The periodic acid–Schiff (PAS) reaction reveals abundant glycogen in these cells. Chief cells also contain abundant intracytoplasmic neutral lipid droplets demonstrated with azure B or Erie garnet A procedures or with oil red O or Sudan IV stains. Immunohistochemical studies show stronger staining for parathyroid hormone in chief cells than in oxyphilic cells.

The oxyphilic cells are larger than chief cells (12–20 μm in diameter) and are polygonal in shape. The cell membranes are usually clear, and the nucleus is identical to that of the chief cell. The cytoplasm is composed of highly eosinophilic fine granules, which stain carmine with Bensley acid aniline fuchsin (BAAF) and dark blue with phosphotungstic acid hematoxylin. These cells contain tightly packed mitochondria filling the cytoplasm and have high levels of oxidative enzymes. Unlike chief cells, the oxyphilic cells have very little intracytoplasmic lipid or glycogen. Variants of the oxyphilic cells include transitional oxyphilic cells, which are smaller and contain less eosinophilic cytoplasm.

The ultrastructure of the active form of the chief cell and the mode of secretion are schematized in the

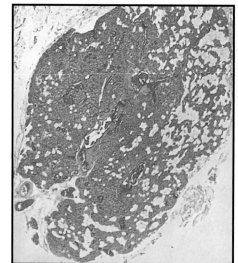

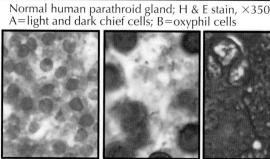

Normal human parathroid gland; H & E stain, ×350
A=light and dark chief cells; B=oxyphil cells

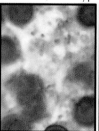

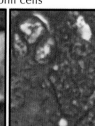

Normal human parathroid gland; H & E stain, ×17.5

PAS stain, ×675 Glycogen in chief cells

Bodian stain, ×1800 Secretory granules in chief cells

BAAF stain, ×1350 Mitochondria in oxyphil cells

Ultrastructure of parathyroid gland

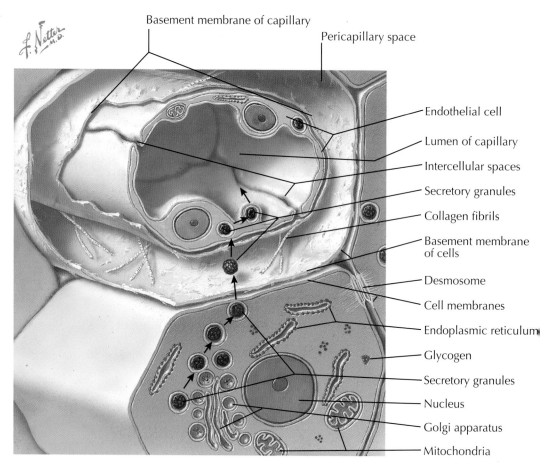

Basement membrane of capillary

Pericapillary space

Endothelial cell

Lumen of capillary

Intercellular spaces

Secretory granules

Collagen fibrils

Basement membrane of cells

Desmosome

Cell membranes

Endoplasmic reticulum

Glycogen

Secretory granules

Nucleus

Golgi apparatus

Mitochondria

illustration. The chief cells are arranged in cords and nests and separated from the interstitium by basal laminae. The chief cells have straight plasma membranes and are attached to other cells by desmosomes. During the active phase, in addition to the usual organelles, the Golgi apparatus enlarges, numerous vacuoles and vesicles appear in the Golgi apparatus, and many mature secretory granules (50–300 nm in diameter) appear in the cell. The mature secretory granule is oval to dumbbell-shaped and has a single membrane surrounding a thin clear space inside of which is a dense area composed of short rodlike profiles. The granule migrates out of the cell through the basement membrane into the wide pericapillary space. It then goes through the capillary basement membrane and into the fenestrated endothelial cells that line the capillaries, from which parathyroid hormone is liberated into the bloodstream.

Plate 6-2

Bone and Calcium

PHYSIOLOGY OF THE PARATHYROID GLANDS

Secretion of parathyroid hormone (PTH) from the four parathyroid glands is regulated by the blood level of ionized calcium (Ca2+). Serum ionized calcium concentrations below the reference range stimulate PTH secretion, and levels above the reference range inhibit PTH secretion. The principal action of PTH is the regulation and maintenance of a normal serum total calcium level between 8.9 and 10.1 mg/dL. The calcium-sensing receptors (CaSRs) in the parathyroid glands are responsible for maintaining this calcium-dependent regulation of PTH secretion. The CaSRs in the kidneys serve to adjust tubular calcium reabsorption independent of PTH.

A normal serum concentration of ionized calcium is critical for many extracellular and cellular functions, and it is normally maintained in the very narrow range through a tightly regulated calcium–PTH homeostatic system. Neuromuscular activity is just one function that is dependent on calcium homeostasis; cytosolic free calcium serves as a key second messenger. Thus, disturbances in extracellular calcium concentration result in symptoms of abnormal neuromuscular activity. For example, hypercalcemia may cause muscle weakness and areflexia, anorexia, constipation, vomiting, drowsiness, depression, confusion, or coma. Hypocalcemia may result in anxiety, muscle twitching, Chvostek and Trousseau signs, carpal or pedal spasm, seizures, stridor, bronchospasm, or intestinal cramps.

The daily dietary calcium intake ranges between 300 and 1500 mg/d; total net gastrointestinal (GI) calcium absorption averages 200 mg/d. The urinary calcium excretion averages 200 mg/d (2% of the filtered load). Although the urinary calcium excretion is rather constant, the excretion of calcium in the stool depends greatly on the body's need and the dietary intake; normally, 500 to 700 mg of calcium is excreted per 24 hours (100–200 mg/d is endogenous fecal calcium that is unaffected by dietary or serum calcium). The average dietary intake of phosphate is 800 to 900 mg/d. GI tract phosphate absorption is enhanced by 1,25-dihydroxyvitamin D (1,25[OH]2D). Phosphate absorption is impaired by increasing dietary calcium. Whereas the fecal excretion of inorganic phosphate (Pi) is roughly 30% of dietary intake, the urinary phosphate excretion varies widely with intake and serum PTH concentration.

If dietary calcium is restricted in healthy individuals, a decrease in the blood calcium concentration leads to a compensatory increase in intestinal calcium absorption. This occurs because a small decrease in serum ionized calcium triggers the CaSR, and there is a prompt increase in PTH secretion. The increased blood PTH concentration leads to increased renal 1α hydroxylation of 25-hydroxyvitamin D (25[OH]D) to the more potent 1,25(OH)2D (calcitriol). Calcitriol acts on enterocytes to increase active transport of calcium. In addition, renal tubular calcium reabsorption is increased both by PTH and by a direct effect of hypocalcemia via the CaSRs in the loop of Henle. The direct actions of PTH and calcitriol at bone increase bone resorption and calcium release. Because of these three mechanisms of action, the serum ionized calcium concentration increases, and the serum PTH concentration decreases.

With increased dietary calcium exposure, there is suppression of PTH secretion, inhibition of the 1α hydroxylation of 25(OH)D, decreased intestinal absorption of calcium, increased renal excretion of

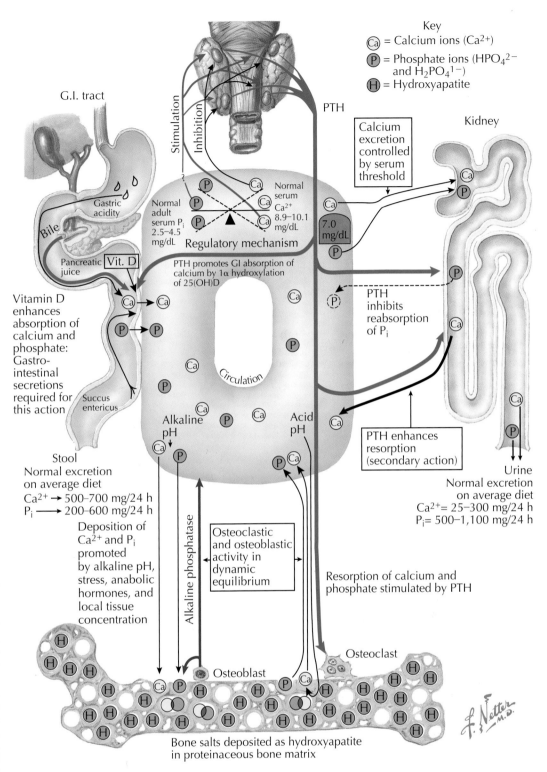

Matrix growth requires protein, vitamin C, anabolic hormones (androgens, estrogen, IGF-1) + stress of mobility. Matrix resorption favored by catabolic hormones (11-oxysteroids [cortisol], thyroid), parathyroid hormone + immobilization

calcium, decreased renal excretion of phosphate, and decreased bone resorption.

If the parathyroid glands are not functioning properly or are absent, the serum calcium level decreases, usually below the renal threshold of 7 mg/dL, and urinary calcium is absent. The presence of a large reservoir of calcium in the skeleton (~1000 g) as hydroxyapatite (Ca10[PO4]6 [OH]2), however, prevents the serum calcium from falling below 5 mg/dL even in the absence of the parathyroid glands.

In states of excessive PTH secretion, resorption of calcium and phosphate from bone matrix occurs through stimulation of the osteoclasts. The osteoclastic overresponse then evokes a tendency for the osteoblasts to become overactive and leads to bone repair, with the subsequent rise of the alkaline phosphatase level in the serum. Bone repair is promoted by enhanced absorption of calcium and phosphate from the GI tract facilitated in part by the increased serum concentration of 1,25(OH)2D.

Plate 6-3

Endocrine System

BONE REMODELING UNIT

Bone is composed of a collagen matrix, distributed in a lamellar pattern and strengthened by pyridinoline crosslinks between the triple-helical collagen molecules, on which calcium and phosphorus are deposited to form hydroxyapatite. The bone matrix also includes calcium-binding proteins such as osteocalcin. The resulting bone mineral is complex crystals of hydroxyapatite that contain fluoride and carbonate.

Bone modeling is the process of change in bone size and shape in childhood, where linear growth is the result of cartilaginous growth at the epiphyses, and bone width enlargement results from endosteal resorption and periosteal apposition. During puberty and early adulthood, endosteal apposition occurs, and peak bone mass is achieved.

Bone remodeling is the lifelong process of bone repair, which has three phases: resorption, reversal, and formation. The bone remodeling unit (osteon) involves a cycle of coupled osteoclastic and osteoblastic activities.

Osteoblasts develop from determined osteoblast progenitor cells that originate from mesenchymal stem cells. The osteoblast progenitor cells are localized to the periosteum and bone marrow. Osteoblasts have receptors for parathyroid hormone, 1, 25-dihydroxyvitamin D, testosterone, estrogen, glucocorticoids, growth hormone, thyroid hormone, and insulinlike growth factors. After osteoblasts lay down collagen and noncollagen proteins, some of the osteoblasts become osteocytes that are buried in the bone matrix. The remaining osteoblasts either become the less metabolically active, flattened lining cells or undergo apoptosis.

Osteoclasts, derived from monocytes and macrophages, are multinucleated, large cells that dissolve bone mineral and degrade matrix. Osteoclast progenitors can be found in the bone marrow and the spleen. Osteoclastic differentiation is triggered by the production of macrophage colony–stimulation factor. Excessive osteoclastic activity is associated with Paget disease, hyperparathyroidism, and a subset of osteoporosis.

RESORPTION

The bone remodeling cycle is activated by osteoblast cells that release collagenase, macrophage colony–stimulating factor, and receptor activator of NF-κ B (RANK) ligand. RANK ligand interacts with the RANK receptor and activates osteoclast formation and the initiation of bone resorption. RANK ligand also binds to osteoprotegerin, which is an osteoclastogenesis inhibitory factor. Macrophage colony–stimulating factor is also required for normal osteoclast activation. This initial osteoblast activation of osteoclasts can be affected by multiple hormones and factors. For example, parathyroid hormone induces the osteoblastic production of RANK ligand and inhibits production of osteoprotegerin. Vitamin D also increases the production of RANK ligand.

Osteoclasts enzymatically degrade bone matrix protein and remove mineral within cortical bone or on the trabecular surfaces. This process is self limited—perhaps by high local concentrations of calcium or bone matrix substances—and is completed over 2 weeks.

REVERSAL

After osteoclastic resorption, the reversal phase is initiated by mononuclear cells that lay down a

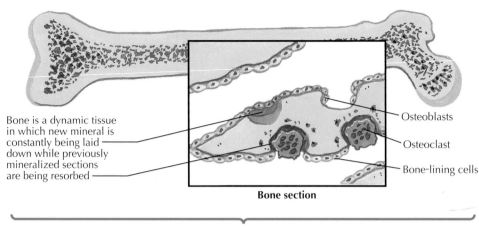

Bone is a dynamic tissue in which new mineral is constantly being laid down while previously mineralized sections are being resorbed

Osteoblasts

Osteoclast

Bone-lining cells

Bone section

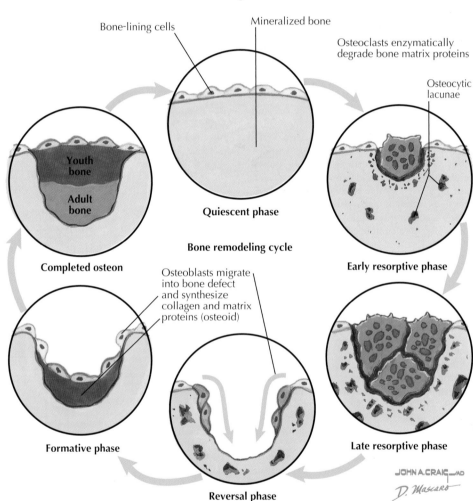

Bone-lining cells

Mineralized bone

Osteoclasts enzymatically degrade bone matrix proteins

Osteocytic lacunae

Quiescent phase

Bone remodeling cycle

Early resorptive phase

Youth bone

Adult bone

Completed osteon

Osteoblasts migrate into bone defect and synthesize collagen and matrix proteins (osteoid)

Late resorptive phase

Formative phase

Reversal phase

JOHN A. CRAIG—MD
D. Mascaro

glycoprotein-rich material (cement) on the resorbed surface and signal for osteoblast differentiation. The new osteoblasts adhere to this material. The reversal phase is approximately 4 weeks in duration.

FORMATION

During the formation phase, osteoblasts lay down osteoid (collagen and matrix proteins) until the resorbed bone is completely replaced. The formation phase takes approximately 16 weeks to complete. Normally, the new bone formed is equivalent to what was resorbed. When the formation phase is complete, the bone surface is covered with bone-lining cells, and very little cellular activity occurs until another bone remodeling cycle begins.

DEFECTIVE BONE REMODELING

In a normal bone remodeling unit, resorption and formation are tightly coupled. However, a mismatch between resorption and formation can lead to abnormally thin or dense bones. For example, if the osteoclastic resorption depth is excessive, it can perforate and weaken trabecular structure; if the osteoblasts do not completely fill the deep resorption cavity, bone density and quality decline. If the resorptive process is incomplete because the osteoclasts are not fully activated (e.g., with macrophage colony–stimulating factor deficiency) or if they are dysfunctional, excessively dense bones may result (osteopetrosis).

Plate 6-4

PATHOPHYSIOLOGY OF PRIMARY HYPERPARATHYROIDISM

The annual incidence of primary hyperparathyroidism (HPT) is approximately four in 100,000. HPT is twice as common in women, and most patients are diagnosed after age 45 years. Primary HPT is caused by a single parathyroid adenoma (89%), multiple ("double") parathyroid adenomas (4%), multigland parathyroid hyperplasia (6%), or parathyroid carcinoma (1%). The distinction between these forms of primary HPT directs the surgical approach.

Most parathyroid adenomas are encapsulated and arise from chief cells; the others are composed of oxyphilic cells. Parathyroid adenomas are usually localized to the neck, but ectopic parathyroid tumors may arise anywhere in the anterior mediastinum or even in the posterior mediastinum. The cells in the adenomas are monoclonal and are a result of somatic mutations in genes that control growth. For example, the cyclin D1 proto-oncogene (CCND1) encodes a major regulator of the cell cycle. Overexpression of cyclin D1 is found in approximately 30% of parathyroid adenomas. Multiple endocrine neoplasia (MEN) type 1 (see Plate 8-1) is caused by germline mutations in MEN1, a tumor suppressor gene, and somatic mutations are found in approximately 15% of sporadic parathyroid adenomas.

Multiple-gland hyperplasia, characterized by enlargement of all four glands, is occasionally mistaken for multiple adenomas. Chief cell hyperplasia is much more common than clear cell hyperplasia (the latter is associated with hyperplasia primarily of the superior parathyroid glands). Parathyroid hyperplasia may be sporadic or associated with a familial syndrome (e.g., MEN 1, MEN 2A, HPT–jaw tumor syndrome, or familial isolated hyperparathyroidism). Distinguishing between parathyroid gland hyperplasia and normal parathyroid tissue can be difficult for the pathologist. In general, abnormal parathyroid glands are increased in size and contain less fat. Primary HPT affects almost all patients with MEN 1, and the hypercalcemia is typically present by the third decade of life, but primary HPT affects only 10% of patients with MEN 2A and tends to occur later in life. Parathyroid adenomas and hyperplasia are multiple and cystic in patients with HPT–jaw tumor syndrome. The jaw tumor is usually fibrous in nature.

The diagnosis of parathyroid carcinoma is based on local invasion of contiguous tissues or metastases (lymph node or distant). Both sporadic and germline inactivating mutations in CDC73 (previously known as HRPT2) are responsible for HPT–jaw tumor syndrome, which is associated with an increased risk for parathyroid carcinoma.

A normal serum concentration of ionized calcium (Ca^{2+}) is critical for many extracellular and cellular functions, and it is normally maintained in the very narrow range through a tightly regulated calcium–PTH homeostatic system. In healthy individuals, a small decrease in serum ionized calcium triggers the calcium-sensing receptor, and there is a prompt increase in PTH secretion. The increased blood PTH concentration leads to an immediate increase in bone resorption and renal 1α-hydroxylation of 25-hydroxyvitamin D to the more potent 1, 25-dihydroxyvitamin D (calcitriol). Calcitriol leads to increased intestinal calcium absorption over several days. Finally, PTH leads to an immediate decrease in urinary calcium excretion by stimulating calcium reabsorption at the distal renal tubule. Because

of these three mechanisms of action, the serum ionized calcium concentration increases, and the serum PTH concentration decreases.

Patients with primary HPT have abnormal regulation of PTH secretion by calcium, a finding partly caused by an elevation in the set point. The set point for calcium-dependent feedback suppression of PTH release is 15% to 30% above normal. It is important to note that PTH secretion in primary HPT is not completely autonomous and can usually be partially inhibited by a further rise in serum calcium. The excessive production of PTH leads to hypercalcemia by increased stimulation of the osteoclastic activity of bone (with the release of calcium and phosphate), increased absorption of calcium from the gut, and increased reabsorption of calcium by the renal tubules. In addition, PTH inhibits

the tubular reabsorption of inorganic phosphate (P$_i$), causing an excessive loss of phosphate. The net effect of these chemical changes is an increase in serum calcium and a decrease in serum phosphate, with increasing amounts of both calcium and phosphate being excreted in the urine. This predisposes to the formation of calcium phosphate and calcium oxalate renal stones. At times, there may be precipitation of calcium in the soft tissues of the kidneys, producing nephrocalcinosis.

Roughly 25% of patients with primary HPT have evidence of bone disease, with marked bone resorption and a compensatory increase in osteoblastic activity. Bone mineral is formed by small hydroxyapatite crystals that contain carbonate, magnesium, sodium, and potassium.

| Adenoma (93% of cases) | Hyperplasia (6% of cases) | Carcinoma (1% of cases) |

Skin

Gut — Ca^{2+} / P$_i$ — Vit. D — Liver — 25(OH)D

Parathyroid hormone (PTH) elevated

Ca^{2+} / P$_i$

Serum and extracellular fluid

High 1,25(OH)$_2$D promotes absorption of Ca^{2+} from gut

Serum Ca^{2+} increased; fails to suppress PTH secretion

Renal tubule

↑Ca^{2+} filtered into tubule exceeds its resorptive capacity and results in hypercalciuria

Ca^{2+}

P$_i$

Serum P$_i$ low or normal

25(OH)D normal

1,25(OH)$_2$D elevated

PTH

Ca^{2+} / P$_i$

Ca^{2+} / P$_i$

High PTH promotes Ca^{2+} reabsorption, inhibits P$_i$ reabsorption. Also promotes conversion of 25(OH)D to active metabolite 1,25(OH)$_2$D

Compensatory increase in osteoblastic activity with variable rise in serum alkaline phosphatase

Ca^{2+} / P$_i$

Ca^{2+} P$_i$

High PTH stimulates osteoclastic resorption of bone (Ca^{2+}, P$_i$, and matrix)

Nephrocalcinosis

Calculi

Urine Ca^{2+} elevated

Variable reduction in bone density. In rare, severe cases, cysts and brown tumors (due to osteitis fibrosa cystica) and subperiosteal resorption

Plate 6-5

Endocrine System

PATHOLOGY AND CLINICAL MANIFESTATIONS OF PRIMARY HYPERPARATHYROIDISM

Approximately 80% of patients with primary hyperparathyroidism (HPT) are asymptomatic, and hypercalcemia is detected by routine biochemical testing. Less commonly, primary HPT is diagnosed during the evaluation of symptomatic hypercalcemia, renal lithiasis, osteoporosis, or osteitis fibrosa cystica. Although most patients with primary HPT do not have overt symptoms, it may be responsible for more subtle symptomatology (e.g., weakness, fatigue, depressed mood, or mild cognitive dysfunction).

The more overt signs and symptoms of long-standing, untreated primary HPT have been referred to as "bones, stones, abdominal moans, and groans." The "stones" refer to nephrolithiasis, which occurs in 20% of patients with primary HPT. The nephrolithiasis is caused by the hypercalciuria (a result of increased filtered calcium in the setting of hypercalcemia) that predisposes to the development of calcium oxalate stones. The most common effect on bones is osteopenia and osteoporosis. Less common bone-related sequelae of severe, long-standing primary HPT include absence of the lamina dura around the teeth; subperiosteal resorption of the bone, especially around the radial margins of the phalanges, around the sternal end of the clavicle, and along the margins of other bones; diffuse "salt-and-pepper" decalcification of the skull, resembling multiple myeloma; fractures of the terminal phalanges with telescoping, giving the appearance of pseudoclubbing (the phalangeal joints may show increased flexibility); large bone cysts (osteitis fibrosa cystica) in various locations (fractures through these cysts or fractures through rarefied bone may occur); diffuse demineralization of the skeleton, especially of the spine, with "codfishing" of the vertebral bodies; and brown tumors (also known as giant cell tumors, osteoclastoma, or epulis), which are radiolucent bone tumors that may develop in the jaw and other bones.

Hypercalcemia may also cause nausea, anorexia, constipation, nephrogenic diabetes insipidus (polyuria and polydipsia), glucose intolerance, peptic ulcer disease, pancreatitis, and hypertension. Parathyroid crisis occurs with severe hypercalcemia (calcium >15 mg/dL), and affected patients present with central nervous system dysfunction (e.g., confusion, coma). Parathyroid crisis—typically precipitated by volume depletion—is treated with volume repletion with isotonic saline and an agent to decrease bone resorption (e.g., a bisphosphonate).

Physical examination typically reveals no specific findings for primary HPT. Parathyroid adenomas are not palpable; when a parathyroid tumor is palpable, it is usually parathyroid carcinoma. With a slit-lamp examination of the eyes, calcium phosphate deposition may be seen in a semicircular form around the limbus of the cornea and is termed *band keratopathy*.

Laboratory abnormalities in patients with primary HPT include increased serum total and ionized calcium concentrations, decreased serum phosphorus concentration (parathyroid hormone [PTH] inhibits the proximal renal tubular reabsorption of phosphate), serum PTH concentration that is either above the reference range or inappropriately (in the setting of hypercalcemia) within the reference range, and increased serum

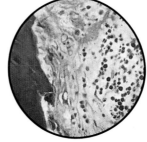

Nephrolithiasis

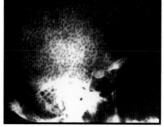

Nephrocalcinosis

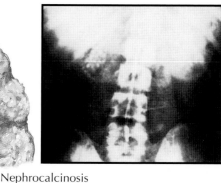

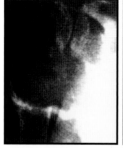

"Salt and pepper" skull

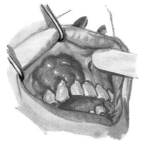

Bone biopsy (focal resorption)

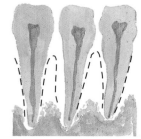

Absence of lamina dura (*broken line* indicates normal contour)

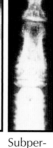

Bone rarefaction; cysts fractures

Subperiosteal resorption

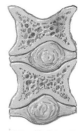

Brown tumor (giant cell tumor or osteoclastoma)

"Codfishing" of vertebrae

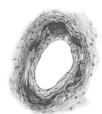

Calcium deposits in blood vessels; hypertension

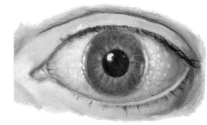

Limbus keratopathy

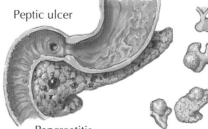

Peptic ulcer

Pancreatitis

MEN 1 with parathyroid gland hyperplasia and multiple adenomas (pituitary, thyroid, pancreas, adrenals)

calcitriol concentration (a result of PTH-stimulated renal hydroxylation of 25-hydroxyvitamin D). Serum creatinine concentrations can be increased in patients with marked and long-standing primary HPT and can be associated with nephrocalcinosis. Patients with severe primary HPT may also have a normochromic normocytic anemia.

Vitamin D deficiency is frequently present in patients with primary HPT, a state that can attenuate the degree of hypercalcemia. Treating the vitamin D deficiency in this setting can aggravate the hypercalcemia and hypercalciuria.

The treatment of primary HPT rests on the surgical removal of the parathyroid adenoma (for single-gland disease) or, rarely, of 3.5 hyperplastic parathyroid glands in the setting of diffuse parathyroid hyperplasia (e.g., with multiple endocrine neoplasia [MEN] type 1).

Plate 6-20

Bone and Calcium

HYPOPHOSPHATEMIC RICKETS

Hypophosphatemic rickets is caused by renal inorganic phosphate (P_i) wasting, either in isolation or as a component of a more generalized renal disorder (e.g., Fanconi syndrome). The usual biochemical profile includes hypophosphatemia, normal serum calcium concentration, normal serum parathyroid hormone (PTH) concentration, and increased blood concentration of fibroblast growth factor 23 (FGF23). The most common hereditary form of hypophosphatemic rickets is X-linked followed by autosomal dominant forms (associated with activating mutations in the *FGF23* gene), autosomal recessive forms (associated with inactivating mutations in the dentin matrix protein 1 gene [*DMP1*] that result in increased *FGF23* expression), and forms associated with hypercalciuria (e.g., Dent disease). If the onset of hypophosphatemia is delayed until adolescence, the differential diagnosis should include tumor-induced osteomalacia (see following text).

X-LINKED HYPOPHOSPHATEMIC RICKETS

The incidence of X-linked hypophosphatemic rickets is approximately one case per 20,000 live births. Mutations in the phosphate regulating endopeptidase homolog on the X chromosome gene (*PHEX*) are responsible for this disorder. Although penetrance is 100%, the expression is variable, even in affected individuals from the same kindred. *PHEX* regulates the degradation and production of FGF23. Excess circulating levels of FGF23 mediate renal phosphate wasting by inhibiting phosphate reabsorption by the renal sodium–phosphate cotransporter. Children with X-linked hypophosphatemic rickets usually present with typical signs and symptoms of osteomalacia (see Plate 6-21) and retarded linear growth. Additional findings unique to X-linked hypophosphatemic rickets include calcification of ligaments and tendons (enthesopathy) and abnormal dentin predisposing to early tooth decay and tooth abscesses. Typical laboratory findings include low serum concentrations of phosphorus and calcitriol (the effects of FGF23 at the renal tubule also impair calcitriol synthesis), increased serum FGF23 concentration and 24-hour urinary phosphate excretion, normal to increased blood concentrations of PTH and alkaline phosphatase, and normal blood concentrations of calcium and calcidiol. The diagnosis can be confirmed with molecular genetic testing for germline mutations in *PHEX*.

In children, treatment includes orally administered phosphate (sodium phosphate or potassium phosphate) and calcitriol. Calcitriol therapy is needed to prevent the secondary hyperparathyroidism (which can cause further renal phosphate wasting) that occurs with phosphate replacement therapy. The goals of therapy in children are resolution of bone and joint pain and normal growth. Laboratory parameters that should be followed during treatment include blood concentrations of phosphorus, calcium, alkaline phosphatase, creatinine, and PTH and urinary calcium excretion. Periodic radiographs of the hand and wrist should be obtained to document bone age and to identify any recurrence of rickets. In adults, the goals of therapy are to prevent bone pain and fractures. In patients who are not closely monitored, hypercalcemia and hypercalciuria may result in calcium–phosphate deposition in the renal tubules (nephrocalcinosis) and renal tubular acidosis.

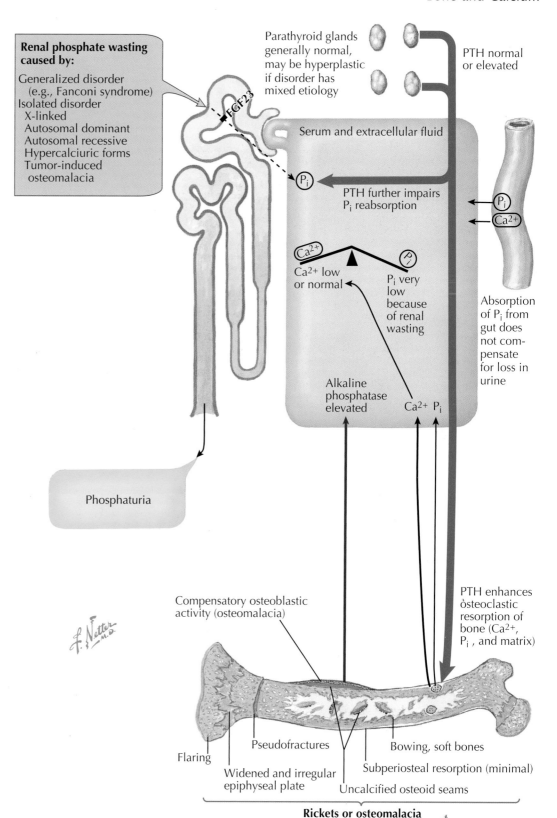

Renal phosphate wasting caused by:

Generalized disorder (e.g., Fanconi syndrome)
Isolated disorder
 X-linked
 Autosomal dominant
 Autosomal recessive
 Hypercalciuric forms
Tumor-induced osteomalacia

Parathyroid glands generally normal, may be hyperplastic if disorder has mixed etiology

PTH normal or elevated

Serum and extracellular fluid

PTH further impairs P_i reabsorption

Ca^{2+} low or normal

P_i very low because of renal wasting

Absorption of P_i from gut does not compensate for loss in urine

Alkaline phosphatase elevated

Ca^{2+} P_i

Phosphaturia

Compensatory osteoblastic activity (osteomalacia)

PTH enhances osteoclastic resorption of bone (Ca^{2+}, P_i, and matrix)

Flaring

Pseudofractures

Bowing, soft bones

Subperiosteal resorption (minimal)

Widened and irregular epiphyseal plate

Uncalcified osteoid seams

Rickets or osteomalacia

TUMOR-INDUCED OSTEOMALACIA

Tumor-induced osteomalacia is an acquired disorder caused by small, benign mesenchymal tumors (e.g., sclerosing type of hemangiopericytoma) that hypersecrete FGF23. The clinician should suspect tumor-induced osteomalacia in patients who present with signs, symptoms, and laboratory profiles identical to those observed in patients with X-linked hypophosphatemic rickets but who do not have a personal or family history of the genetic disorder. The main challenge is to localize the small tumor; it may be a small subcutaneous lesion on an extremity or more centrally located. Localization studies usually include somatostatin receptor imaging with indium In 111-diethylenetriamine pentaacetic acid-pentetreotide and total body magnetic resonance imaging. Tumor resection corrects all biochemical abnormalities.

Plate 6-21

Endocrine System

CLINICAL MANIFESTATIONS OF RICKETS IN CHILDHOOD

Rickets, a result of chronic hypocalcemia or hypophosphatemia, occurs before closure of the epiphyses and is usually most evident at sites of rapid bone growth (e.g., knees, costochondral junctions, distal forearm). Enlargement of the costochondral junctions results in visible nodules—the "rachitic rosary"—and chest wall deformities (e.g., tunnel chest). The wrist enlarges, and there is bowing of the distal ulna and radius. Impaired mineralization causes weak long bones, leading to weight-bearing–dependent skeletal deformities. For example, whereas an affected infant may have posterior bowing of the distal tibia, children who can walk may have lateral bowing of the femur and tibia (genu varum). In infants, the closure of the fontanelles may be delayed, and parietal and frontal bossing and evidence of soft skull bones (craniotabes) may be present. The "Harrison groove" refers to the indentation that results from the muscular pull of the diaphragmatic attachments to the lower ribs.

The clinical presentation of rickets is dominated by skeletal pain, skeletal deformity, fracture, slippage of epiphyses, and retarded growth. Hip pain and deformity may result in a waddling or antalgic gait. In patients with hypocalcemic rickets, extraskeletal symptoms may include decreased muscle tone, proximal myopathy, hypocalcemic seizures, hyperhidrosis, and predisposition to infections.

A uniform component of the laboratory profile in patients with rickets is a marked increase in the blood concentration of alkaline phosphatase. The serum calcium concentration is low in patients with hypocalcemic rickets and is either normal or slightly depressed in those with hypophosphatemic rickets; serum phosphorus is low in both hypocalcemic and hypophosphatemic rickets. The serum parathyroid hormone (PTH) concentration is above the reference range in patients with hypocalcemic rickets and is normal in those with hypophosphatemic rickets.

Radiographs of the distal ulna usually show findings of impaired mineralization, widening of the epiphyseal plates, irregular trabeculation, thin cortices, subperiosteal erosions (caused by the marked secondary hyperparathyroidism), and increased axial width of the epiphyseal line. Similar findings are evident in radiographs of the knees, which show flaring of the metaphyseal ends of the tibia and femur and thick and irregular growth plates. The zones of provisional calcification at the epiphyseal–metaphyseal interface are fuzzy and indistinct. With advanced rickets, the epiphyseal plates become more irregular and cupped. Osteopenia is evident in the long bones. Pelvic radiographs may disclose variegated rarefaction of the pelvic bones, coxa vara (where the angle between the ball and the shaft of the femur is reduced to <120 degrees, resulting in a shortened leg), deepened acetabula, pathologic fractures, and pseudofractures (Looser zones). Pseudofractures are narrow (2–4 mm) radiolucent lines with sclerotic borders that are perpendicular to the cortical bone margin and a few millimeters to several centimeters in length. Pseudofractures are frequently bilateral and symmetric and can be seen in the pubic rami, ischial rami, medial part of the femoral shaft, femoral neck, outer edge of the scapula, clavicle, ulna, and ribs. Pseudofractures appear at sites where major arteries cross the bone and may be caused by the mechanical forces of normal arterial pulsation on poorly mineralized bone (see Plate 6-22).

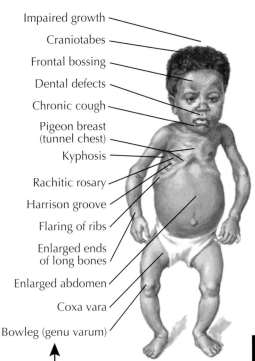

Impaired growth
Craniotabes
Frontal bossing
Dental defects
Chronic cough
Pigeon breast (tunnel chest)
Kyphosis
Rachitic rosary
Harrison groove
Flaring of ribs
Enlarged ends of long bones
Enlarged abdomen
Coxa vara
Bowleg (genu varum)

Clinical findings (all or some present in variable degree)

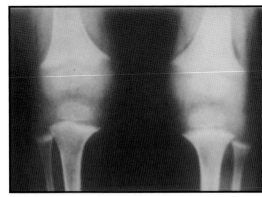

Flaring of metaphyseal ends of tibia and femur. Growth plates thickened, irregular, cupped, and axially widened. Zones of provisional calcification fuzzy and indistinct. Bone cortices thinned and medullae rarefied

Radiographic findings

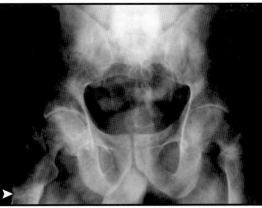

Radiograph shows variegated rarefaction of pelvic bones, coxa vara, deepened acetabula, and subtrochanteric pseudofracture of right femur

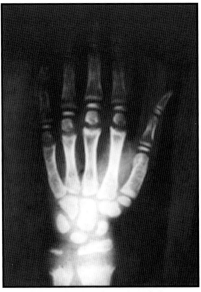

Radiograph of rachitic hand shows decreased bone density, irregular trabeculation, and thin cortices of metacarpal and proximal phalanges. Note increased axial width of epiphyseal line, especially in radius and ulna

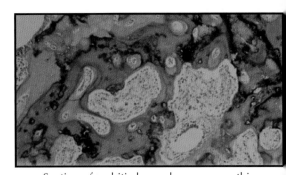

Section of rachitic bone shows sparse, thin trabeculae surrounded by much uncalcified osteoid (osteoid seams) and cavities caused by increased resorption

In children with suspected rickets, obtaining thorough dietary (e.g., calcium and vitamin D) and medication histories is key. Initial laboratory studies should exclude renal failure and hepatic disease. Laboratory testing should include measurement of blood concentrations of calcium, phosphorus, PTH, and 25-hydroxyvitamin D. For a description of the typical laboratory findings in patients with nutritional-deficiency rickets, pseudovitamin D–deficient rickets, and hypophosphatemic rickets, see Plates 6-18, 6-19,

and 6-20. Although bone biopsies are usually not needed to confirm rickets, they show sparse, thin trabeculae; thick layers of uncalcified osteoid (osteoid seams); and large bone resorption cavities.

Effective treatment of patients with rickets is determined by the underlying cause. Deformities that occur before age 4 years usually slowly correct themselves with effective therapy. When deformities occur after age 4 years (e.g., bowleg, knock-knee), they may be permanent.

Plate 6-22

Bone and Calcium

CLINICAL MANIFESTATIONS OF OSTEOMALACIA IN ADULTS

Osteomalacia is a disorder of impaired mineralization of newly formed osteoid in adults. Bone is composed of a collagen matrix (osteoid) distributed in a lamellar pattern and strengthened by pyridinoline crosslinks between the triple-helical collagen molecules, on which alkaline phosphate facilitates the deposition of calcium and phosphorus to form hydroxyapatite (see Plate 6-3). Bone remodeling is a continuous process, and new bone formation requires osteoid production from osteoblasts followed by mineralization of the osteoid. The mineralization step requires an adequate supply of calcium and phosphorus in extracellular fluid and normal bioactivity of alkaline phosphatase. Hypophosphatemia is the most common cause of osteomalacia (see Plate 6-20). Hypophosphatasia, a rare inherited disorder, is associated with low concentrations of alkaline phosphatase in serum and bone that cause defective bone and tooth mineralization, resulting in osteomalacia and severe periodontal disease (see Plate 6-27).

The clinical presentation of osteomalacia ranges from incidental detection of osteopenia on radiographs to markedly symptomatic patients with diffuse bone pain (most prominent in the pelvis, lower extremities, and lower spine), proximal muscle weakness, muscle wasting, hypotonia, and waddling gait. Low-impact fractures of the ribs and vertebral bodies may also be the initial presentation.

Radiographs typically show osteopenia with thinning of the cortex and loss of vertebral body trabeculae. With advanced vertebral body softening, end-plate concavities develop ("codfish" deformities) (see Plate 6-17). Looser zones (pseudofractures) are narrow (2-4 mm) radiolucent lines with sclerotic borders that are perpendicular to the cortical bone margin and a few millimeters to several centimeters in length. Pseudofractures are frequently bilateral and symmetric and can be seen in the pubic rami, ischial rami, medial part of the femoral shaft, femoral neck, outer edge of the scapula, clavicle, ulna, and ribs. Pseudofractures appear at sites where major arteries cross the bone and may be caused by the mechanical forces of normal arterial pulsation on poorly mineralized bone. Pseudofractures appear as hot spots on bone scintigraphy. Because Milkman initially recognized pseudofractures in 1930, the term *Milkman syndrome* has been used when a patient with osteomalacia has multiple, bilateral, symmetric pseudofractures. If secondary hyperparathyroidism is present, additional radiographic findings may be evident (e.g., subperiosteal resorption, bone cysts). With severe and long-standing osteomalacia, bowing of the tibia, radius, and ulna, as well as coxa profunda hip deformities, may occur.

The findings on laboratory testing in adults with osteomalacia depend on the underlying pathophysiology. For example, the typical laboratory profile in patients with osteomalacia caused by nutritional vitamin D deficiency includes hypocalcemia, hypophosphatemia, low blood concentration of 25-hydroxyvitamin D, and increased blood concentration of parathyroid hormone (see Plate 6-18).

If there is doubt about the diagnosis of osteomalacia, a bone biopsy using double labeling with tetracycline

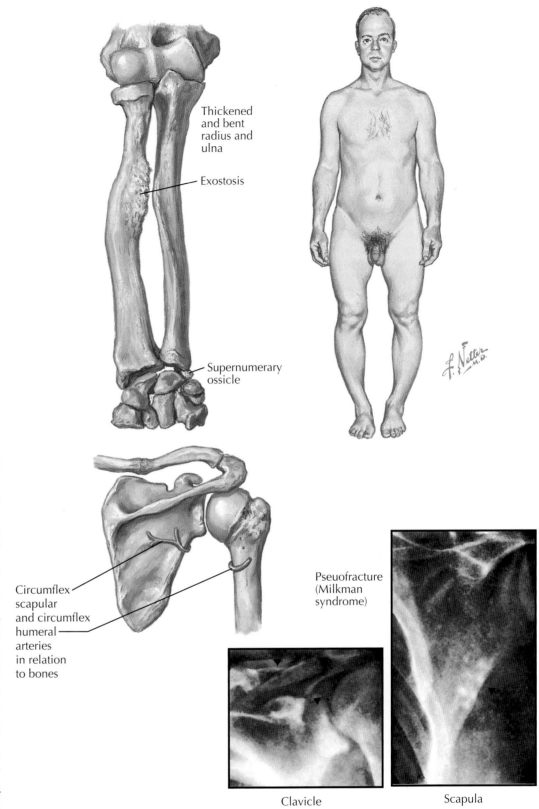

Thickened and bent radius and ulna

Exostosis

Supernumerary ossicle

Circumflex scapular and circumflex humeral arteries in relation to bones

Pseuofracture (Milkman syndrome)

Clavicle

Scapula

can be performed. Tetracyclines are fluorescent; they are deposited in a band at the mineralization front and are easily seen with a fluorescence microscope. A tetracycline is administered for 3 days, and the dosing is repeated 11 to 14 days later. An iliac crest bone biopsy is performed 3 to 5 days after the second tetracycline course is completed. The bone growth rate can be estimated on the basis of the distance between the two bands of deposited tetracycline. Normal bone growth rate is 1 µm per day. In patients with osteomalacia, the bone growth rate is slow, and there are large amounts of unmineralized osteoid.

The treatment of osteomalacia is guided by the underlying cause. For example, patients with vitamin D deficiency should be treated with vitamin D and calcium supplementation.

Plate 6-23

Endocrine System

PAGET DISEASE OF THE BONE

Paget disease of the bone (osteitis deformans) is a localized skeletal disorder of uncontrolled, highly active, large osteoclasts that results in increased bone resorption, which triggers intense and chaotic osteoblastic bone formation. Increased local bone blood flow is observed, and fibrous tissue develops in the adjacent bone marrow. The new bone lacks the usual lamellar structure and is disorganized. This disorder affects approximately 3% of adults older than 40 years; it is usually asymptomatic and evolves slowly.

Although the prevalence of Paget disease is the same in men and women, it is more commonly symptomatic in men. The typical age at the time of detection is in the sixth decade of life. The method of detection is frequently incidental (e.g., increased serum alkaline phosphatase observed on routine blood testing or evidence seen on a radiograph done for other reasons). When symptomatic, the primary symptom is pain caused by periosteal stretching or microfractures. The bone pain is aggravated by weight bearing. The skin may be warm over pagetic bone because of the increased blood flow. Paget disease can affect one bone (monostotic) or multiple bones (polyostotic). The most common bones to be involved are the pelvis, spine, femur, skull, and tibia. With femur or tibia involvement, bowing of the legs is common. The bowing deformities in the bones of the lower extremities lead to gait changes. Transverse traumatic and pathologic bone fractures are common complications.

Spine involvement can lead to kyphosis and symptoms related to spinal cord compression. Hearing loss (caused by compression of the eighth cranial nerve or pagetic involvement of the middle ear ossicles) and skull deformities (frontal and occipital areas) are common when the skull is involved. Compression of the second, fifth, and seventh cranial nerves in the skull may result in visual symptoms and facial palsy. Skull base involvement predisposes to platybasia (invagination of the skull by cervical vertebral bodies) and hydrocephalus by compression of the cerebral aqueduct.

Other complications of Paget disease may develop over time. Bony neoplasia (giant cell tumors [osteoclastomas], fibrosarcomas, chondrosarcomas, and osteosarcoma) occurs more frequently in patients with Paget disease. Primary hyperparathyroidism is also more common. The increased blood flow to bone (when more than 20% of the skeleton is involved) can lead to high-output heart failure.

EVALUATION

A thorough history and physical examination are important. A radionuclide bone scan can be helpful in identifying the sites of involved bone; areas of pagetic bone appear as focal areas of increased uptake. Plain radiographs should be obtained of all the sites identified on the bone scan to confirm Paget disease and its extent. For patients with skull involvement, baseline and annual audiograms should be performed. Because

Manifestations of advanced, diffuse Paget disease of bone (may occur singly or in combination)

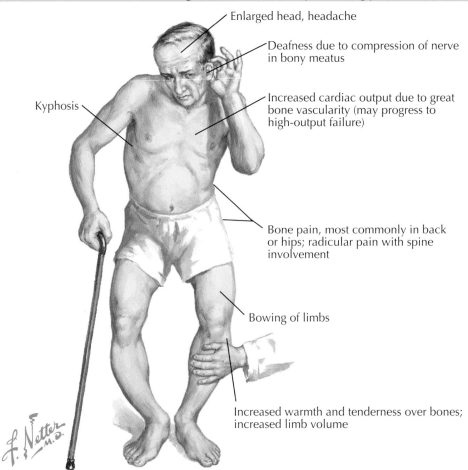

Enlarged head, headache

Deafness due to compression of nerve in bony meatus

Increased cardiac output due to great bone vascularity (may progress to high-output failure)

Kyphosis

Bone pain, most commonly in back or hips; radicular pain with spine involvement

Bowing of limbs

Increased warmth and tenderness over bones; increased limb volume

Mild cases often asymptomatic (may be discovered incidentally on radiographs taken for other reasons)

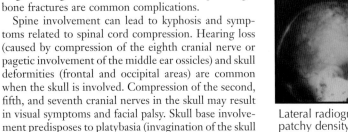

Lateral radiograph shows patchy density of skull, with areas of osteopenia (osteoporosis circumscripta cranii)

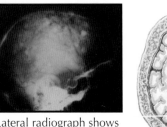

Extremely thickened skull bones, which may encroach on nerve foramina or brainstem and cause hydrocephalus (shown) by compressing cerebral aqueduct

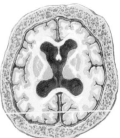

Characteristic radiographic findings in tibia include thickening, bowing, and coarse trabeculation, with advancing radiolucent wedge

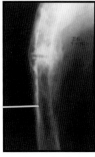

Healing chalk-stick fracture

of the increased risk of primary hyperparathyroidism, serum calcium should be measured. If the imaging studies cannot distinguish between Paget disease and metastatic neoplasm, a bone biopsy may be needed. On bone biopsy, an irregular marble bone–type pattern and giant osteoclasts are seen. Measurement of bone markers at baseline and with treatment is useful. Markers of bone formation include blood concentrations of bone-specific alkaline phosphatase (reflecting cellular activity of osteoblasts), osteocalcin (an estimate of the rate of synthesis of osteocalcin by osteoblasts), and C-terminal and N-terminal propeptides of type I collagen (reflecting changes in synthesis of new collagen). Bone resorption can be followed by measuring urinary excretion of hydroxyproline (reflecting breakdown of collagen in bone) and the collagen N-telopeptide and C-telopeptide crosslinks. Both the resorption and synthetic markers are increased in patients with untreated Paget disease and normalize with effective treatment.

LIPIDS AND NUTRITION

Plate 7-1

CHOLESTEROL SYNTHESIS AND METABOLISM

Cholesterol is a 4-ring hydrocarbon structure with an 8-carbon side chain. Cholesterol serves as a key component of cell membranes, and it is the substrate for synthesis of steroid hormones and bile acids. Cholesterol is either synthesized endogenously or obtained exogenously by ingestion of animal fats (e.g., meat, eggs, and dairy products). The biosynthesis of cholesterol starts with three molecules of acetate that are condensed to form 3-hydroxy-3-methylglutaryl coenzyme A (HMG-CoA). HMG-CoA is then converted to mevalonic acid by HMG-CoA reductase—the rate-limiting step in cholesterol biosynthesis—and mevalonic acid is converted to cholesterol. Competitive inhibitors of HMG-CoA reductase (statins) are used clinically to decrease cholesterol biosynthesis and to lower serum cholesterol concentrations.

Cholesterol is metabolized by the biliary excretion of free cholesterol or by conversion to bile acids that are secreted into the intestine. Approximately 50% of biliary cholesterol and 97% of bile acids are reabsorbed in the small intestine and recirculate to the liver (enterohepatic circulation); the remaining biliary cholesterol and bile acids are excreted in the feces.

Lipoproteins, which are composed of protein, triglycerides, cholesterol esters, and free cholesterol, are macromolecules that transport cholesterol and triglycerides in the blood to target tissues (for bile acid formation, adrenal and gonadal steroidogenesis, energy production). The 12 proteins in the lipoproteins are termed *apolipoproteins* (apo) and are given letter designations. The apolipoproteins act as ligands for receptors and as cofactors for enzymes. The lipoproteins have a nonpolar lipid core surrounded by a polar monolayer of phospholipids and the polar portions of cholesterol and apolipoproteins. Specific lipoproteins differ in the lipid core content, the proportion of lipids in the core, and the protein on the surface. Lipoproteins are classified on the basis of density as chylomicrons, very low-density lipoprotein (VLDL), low-density lipoprotein (LDL), and high-density lipoprotein (HDL).

- Chylomicrons are large, low-density particles that transport dietary lipid (see Plate 7-2). The associated apolipoproteins include apo A (I, II, IV); apo B_{48}; apo C (I, II, III), and apo E.
- VLDL transports primarily triglycerides. The associated apolipoproteins include apo B_{100}, apo C (I, II, III), and apo E.
- LDL transports primarily cholesterol esters and is associated with apo B_{100}.
- HDL also transports cholesterol esters. HDL is associated with apo A (I, II), apo C (I, II, III), and apo E.

How lipids are transported and metabolized is determined in large part by the apolipoproteins. For example, apo AI is not only a structural protein in HDL, but it also activates lecithin–cholesterol acyltransferase (LCAT). Apo AII is a structural protein of HDL and activates hepatic lipase. Apo AIV is an activator for

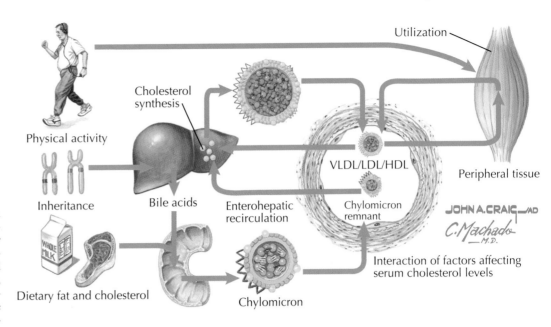

Interaction of factors affecting serum cholesterol levels

JOHN A. CRAIG—AD
C. Machado
—M.D.

Lipoprotein structure

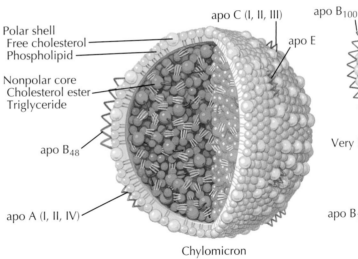

Chylomicron

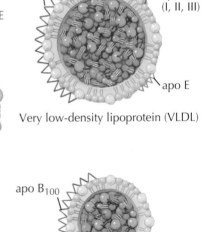

Very low-density lipoprotein (VLDL)

Low-density lipoprotein (LDL)

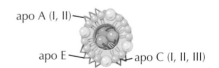

High-density lipoprotein (HDL)

Cholesterol is transported in blood as macromolecules of lipoproteins, with the nonpolar lipid core surrounded by a polar monolayer of phospholipids and the polar portion of cholesterol and apolipoproteins. Specific lipoproteins differ in lipid core content, proportion of lipids in the core, and proteins on the surface. Lipoproteins are classified by density as chylomicrons, very low-density lipoproteins (VLDLs), low-density lipoproteins (LDLs), and high-density lipoproteins (HDLs).

lipoprotein lipase (LPL) and LCAT. Apo B_{100} is a structural protein for VLDL and LDL and serves as a ligand for the LDL receptor. Apo B_{48} is critical for the formation and secretion of chylomicrons. Apo CI serves to activate LCAT. Apo CII is a key cofactor for LPL. Apo CIII inhibits the hydrolysis of triglycerides by LPL. The three genetically determined isoforms of apo E clear lipoproteins (VLDL and chylomicrons) from the circulation by serving as ligands for the VLDL remnant receptor. The presence of two copies of the apo E2

isoform (homozygous) results in less efficient clearance of chylomicrons and VLDL and is clinically referred to as *familial dysbetalipoproteinemia* (see Plate 7-9).

The cholesterol concentration in the blood is controlled by the LDL receptor. The LDL receptor mediates the endocytosis of apo B– and apo E–containing lipoproteins (LDL, chylomicron remnants, VLDL, and VLDL remnants) into cells. The number of LDL receptors on the cell surface is regulated to maintain normal intracellular cholesterol content.

Plate 7-2   Endocrine System

GASTROINTESTINAL ABSORPTION OF CHOLESTEROL AND TRIGLYCERIDES

Dietary fat digestion starts in the stomach and is completed in the small intestine. Most dietary lipid is in the form of long-chain triglycerides (three fatty acids [with at least 12 carbon atoms each] that are esterified to glycerol). Other dietary lipids include phospholipids, plant sterols, cholesterol, and fat-soluble vitamins (vitamins A, D, E, and K). Gastric peristalsis and mixing serve to disperse dietary triglycerides and phospholipids into an emulsion. Intestinal (gastric) lipase acts on the oil droplets in the emulsion to generate free fatty acids and diglycerides. The presence of fatty acids in the small intestine leads to the secretion of cholecystokinin. Cholecystokinin promotes the secretion and release of pancreatic enzymes into the intestinal lumen (see Plate 5-2); it also promotes contraction of the gallbladder, leading to release of concentrated bile. The pancreatic lipase metabolizes triglycerides to fatty acids and monoglycerides. Another pancreatic enzyme is phospholipase A$_2$, which breaks down dietary phospholipids.

By partially solubilizing water-insoluble lipids, bile salt micelles facilitate intestinal transport of lipids to the intestinal epithelial cells (enterocytes) for absorption. Specific carrier proteins facilitate diffusion of lipids across the brush border membrane. In addition, enterocytes in the duodenum and proximal jejunum directly take up long-chain fatty acids by passive transfer. Medium-chain fatty acids (six to 12 carbon atoms) are not esterified, and the enterocytes release these directly into the portal venous system along with other absorbed nutrients. Long-chain fatty acids and monoglycerides are re-esterified into triglyceride in the smooth endoplasmic reticulum of the enterocyte. In addition, cholesterol is esterified by cholesterol acyltransferase. The reassembled lipids are coated with apolipoproteins (apo) (see Plate 7-1) to produce chylomicrons in the Golgi apparatus. The primary intestinal apolipoproteins are apo B$_{48}$, apo AI, and apo AIV. Chylomicrons acquire apo C and apo E during transit in the lymph and blood. Approximately 85% of the chylomicron is composed of triglyceride. The chylomicrons are too large to cross intercellular junctions linking to capillary epithelial cells. Thus, chylomicrons are transported across the basolateral membrane by exocytosis into the

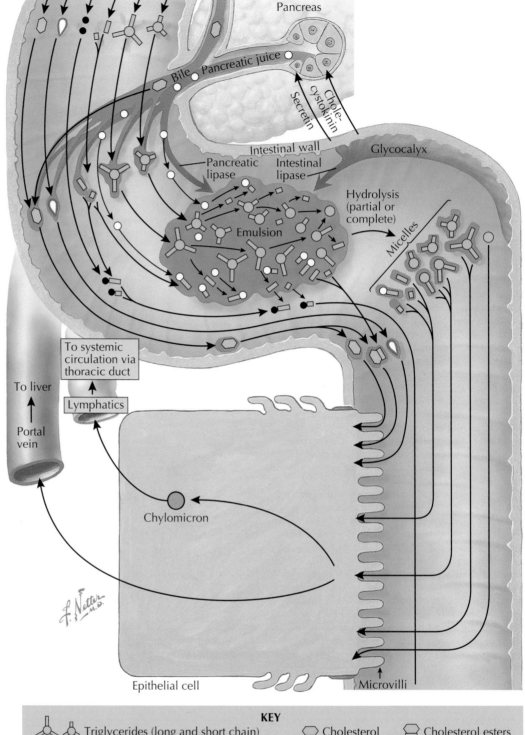

mesenteric lymphatic system that flows to the thoracic duct, where they enter the systemic circulation. Chylomicrons are therefore present in postprandial plasma but are absent with fasting. Apo CII is a cofactor for lipoprotein lipase, the enzyme that hydrolyzes the core triglycerides of the chylomicron and releases free fatty acids. Lipoprotein lipase is bound to the capillary endothelial cells in muscle, adipose, and breast tissues. The activity of lipoprotein lipase is regulated based on energy needs. For example, in the fasting state,

lipoprotein lipase activity increases in heart muscle and decreases in adipose tissue. In addition, in the postpartum state, breast lipoprotein lipase activity increases 10-fold to promote milk production. Because of the action of lipoprotein lipase, the circulating chylomicrons become progressively smaller, and triglyceride-poor chylomicron remnants are removed from the circulation in the liver, where apo E is the ligand for the hepatic low-density lipoprotein receptor–related protein.

KEY

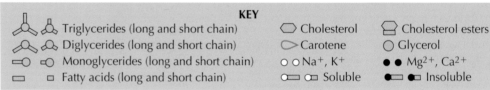

Triglycerides (long and short chain)	Cholesterol	Cholesterol esters	
Diglycerides (long and short chain)	Carotene	Glycerol	
Monoglycerides (long and short chain)	Na$^+$, K$^+$	Mg^{2+}, Ca^{2+}	
Fatty acids (long and short chain)	Soluble	Insoluble	

Plate 7-3

Lipids and Nutrition

REGULATION OF LOW-DENSITY LIPOPROTEIN RECEPTOR AND CHOLESTEROL CONTENT

The cholesterol concentration in the blood is controlled primarily by the low-density lipoprotein (LDL) pathway. Approximately 70% of total plasma cholesterol is LDL. The LDL receptor—located on the surface of all cells—facilitates the internalization of lipoproteins. Approximately 75% of LDL is taken up by hepatocytes. The number of LDL receptors on each cell is in flux and is tightly regulated to keep the intracellular cholesterol concentration constant. Sterol regulatory element–binding protein (SREBP) mediates LDL receptor synthesis. Thus, when a cell's cholesterol content is in positive balance, LDL receptor expression is downregulated by decreased expression of SREBP. In addition, with increased cellular cholesterol, the cholesterol synthetic enzyme 3-hydroxy-3-methylglutaryl coenzyme A (HMG-CoA) reductase is also downregulated. When a cell's cholesterol content is in negative balance, increased expression of SREBP leads to increased numbers of LDL receptors and enhanced cholesterol uptake from the circulation.

The LDL receptor binds lipoproteins that contain the apolipoproteins (apo) apo B_{100} and apo E (e.g., LDL, chylomicron remnants, very low-density lipoprotein [VLDL], and VLDL remnants). The lipoprotein–LDL receptor complex localizes to an area of the cell membrane referred to as the "coated pit." The coated pit contains clathrin that facilitates the clustering of LDL receptors to an area of the cell membrane that can invaginate to form an intracellular vesicle (endosome). As the endosome becomes more acidic, the LDL receptor and lipoprotein dissociate and the lipoproteins are degraded in lysosomes. The free LDL receptor returns to the cell surface in a recycling vesicle. The intracellular pool of cholesterol and cholesterol esters in the hepatocyte is dynamic. Increased intracellular cholesterol enhances acyl-CoA:cholesterol acyltransferase (ACAT) activity, increasing the esterification and storage of cholesterol. In turn, cholesterol ester hydrolase can generate free cholesterol.

The guidelines from the 2002 National Cholesterol Education Program suggest the following cutoffs for plasma total cholesterol concentrations: less than 200 mg/dL, desirable; between 200 and 240 mg/dL, borderline high; and greater than 240 mg/dL, high. Increased blood concentrations of cholesterol are related to increased production or secretion into the circulation or to decreased clearance or removal from the circulation (or both).

Familial hypercholesterolemia (FH) is an autosomal dominant disorder that increases susceptibility to coronary heart disease (CHD). FH is caused by mutations in the gene encoding the LDL receptor, leading to two- to threefold increased plasma cholesterol concentrations in heterozygous individuals (prevalence of one in 500) and a three- to sixfold increase above the upper limit of the reference range in homozygous individuals. These patients may have characteristic physical findings (see Plates 7-6 and 7-7). Familial defective apo B_{100} is a disorder caused by mutations in the gene encoding apo B_{100}. Defective apo B_{100} apolipoprotein binding to the LDL receptor results in a high plasma LDL concentration and an increased CHD risk.

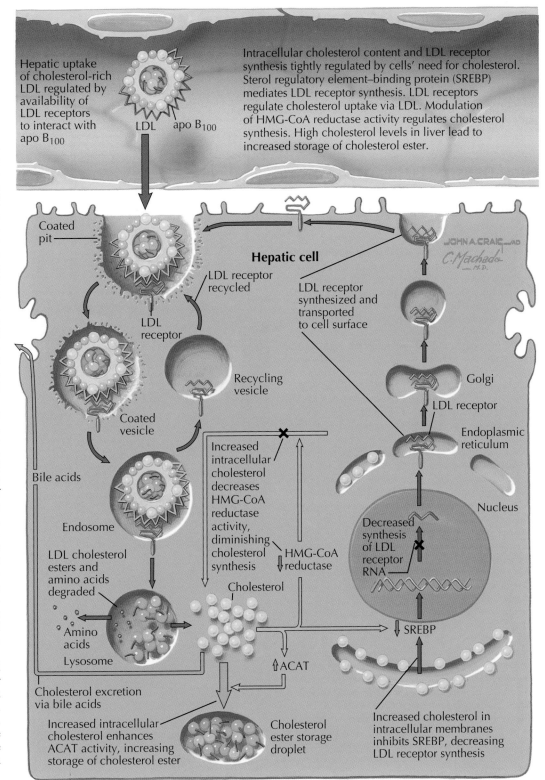

Hepatic uptake of cholesterol-rich LDL regulated by availability of LDL receptors to interact with apo B_{100}

LDL   apo B_{100}

Intracellular cholesterol content and LDL receptor synthesis tightly regulated by cells' need for cholesterol. Sterol regulatory element–binding protein (SREBP) mediates LDL receptor synthesis. LDL receptors regulate cholesterol uptake via LDL. Modulation of HMG-CoA reductase activity regulates cholesterol synthesis. High cholesterol levels in liver lead to increased storage of cholesterol ester.

Coated pit

Hepatic cell

LDL receptor recycled

LDL receptor

LDL receptor synthesized and transported to cell surface

Coated vesicle

Recycling vesicle

Golgi

LDL receptor

Bile acids

Endosome

Increased intracellular cholesterol decreases HMG-CoA reductase activity, diminishing cholesterol synthesis

HMG-CoA reductase

Endoplasmic reticulum

Nucleus

Decreased synthesis of LDL receptor RNA

LDL cholesterol esters and amino acids degraded

Cholesterol

Amino acids

Lysosome

↑ACAT

↓ SREBP

Cholesterol excretion via bile acids

Increased intracellular cholesterol enhances ACAT activity, increasing storage of cholesterol ester

Cholesterol ester storage droplet

Increased cholesterol in intracellular membranes inhibits SREBP, decreasing LDL receptor synthesis

Type III hyperlipoproteinemia (familial dysbetalipoproteinemia) is an autosomal recessive disorder characterized by moderate to severe hypercholesterolemia and hypertriglyceridemia and is the result of mutations in the gene encoding apo E, with resultant defective lipoprotein binding to the LDL receptor (see Plate 7-9).

Elevated plasma lipoprotein(a) (Lp[a]) is a disorder characterized by increased concentrations of modified LDL particles in the plasma, in which the apo B_{100} protein of LDL is covalently bonded to Lp(a). Lp(a) has structural similarity to plasminogen and can interfere with fibrinolysis. Increased plasma Lp(a) is associated with increased CHD risk.

Polygenic hypercholesterolemia refers to combinations of multiple genetic and environmental factors that contribute to hypercholesterolemia. Polygenic hypercholesterolemia is diagnosed by exclusion of other primary genetic causes, absence of tendon xanthomas, and documentation that hypercholesterolemia is present in fewer than 10% of first-degree relatives.

Plate 7-4

Endocrine System

Reverse cholesterol transport
Cholesterol from peripheral
tissues returned to liver

Direct mechanism.
Because of its apo E,
HDL$_1$ is taken up by
LDL receptors in the
liver

Indirect mechanism.
Cholesterol-rich
form of apo B$_{100}$
lipoproteins (LDL,
VLDL remnants)
taken up by liver

Nascent HDL synthesized
and secreted into circulation
by liver and gut

JOHN A. CRAIG—AD
C. Machado
—M.D.

LPL
apo C
apo E
apo A
TGRLP
(apo B$_{100}$ lipoproteins)
apo B$_{100}$

apo A, C, E
Phospholipids
Cholesterol

Acquisition and
esterification of
free cholesterol
by nascent HDL
mediated by
LCAT. HDL$_3$
formed

apo A, E
apo C II, III
CETP
Cholesterol esters
apo E
apo C II, III
Triglyc-
erides

Exchange of
cholesterol esters
in HDL$_{2a}$ for
triglycerides in
TGRLP mediated by
CETP. HDL$_{2b}$ formed,
and cholesterol-rich
form of apo B$_{100}$
lipoprotein provided
for uptake by liver

LCAT
HDL$_{2a}$
CETP

HDL cycle

apo A
LCAT
apo E
apo C
Hepatic lipase

Nascent HDL
HDL cholesterol
mobilized from
peripheral tissues

Free
cholesterol
HDL$_3$

HDL$_{2b}$ hydrolyzed by
hepatic lipase to yield
HDL$_3$ and fatty acids

HDL$_{2b}$

Free
fatty acids

Free
cholesterol

Peripheral (extrahepatic) tissues

Free
fatty acids

Adipose
tissue

Energy utilization

Trigly-
cerides

Fatty acids

Muscle

HIGH-DENSITY LIPOPROTEIN METABOLISM AND REVERSE CHOLESTEROL TRANSPORT

High-density lipoproteins (HDLs) are small particles that contain 50% lipid (phospholipid, cholesteryl esters, free cholesterol, triglyceride) and 50% protein. The main apolipoproteins (apo) are apo AI (65%), apo AII (25%), and smaller amounts of apo C and apo E. The two major subclasses of HDL are HDL$_2$ and HDL$_3$. HDL$_1$ is a minor subclass and is associated with apo E. HDLs function to redistribute lipids among cells and lipoproteins by a process referred to as *reverse cholesterol transport*, in which HDL acquires cholesterol from cells and transports it either to other cells or to the liver.

The steps in the formation and metabolism of HDL include the following: small nascent or precursor HDL disks composed of apo AI and phospholipid are synthesized in the liver and small intestine; precursor HDL disks accept free cholesterol from cells or from other lipoproteins (triglyceride-rich lipoproteins [TGRL] and chylomicron and very low-density lipoprotein [VLDL] remnants); and HDL free cholesterol is esterified by the apo AI–activated enzyme, lecithin–cholesterol acyltransferase (LCAT). The esterified cholesterol increases its hydrophobicity, and it moves away from the surface of the disk to form a cholesteryl ester–rich core and changes the HDL shape from a disk to a sphere. The spherical, mature HDL$_2$ particles function to remove excess cholesterol, and as they enlarge, the particle is termed *HDL$_3$*. HDL acquires cholesterol by aqueous transfer from cells (passive desorption) or by transport that is facilitated by cell surface–binding proteins. Several cell surface proteins facilitate the efflux of free cholesterol. For example, ABCA1 binds apo AI and facilitates the transfer of free cholesterol and phospholipids onto HDL. Mutations in the gene that encodes ABCA1 can prevent this transfer process, resulting in a lipid disorder called Tangier disease (see Plate 7-8).

Because of its apo E, HDL$_1$ is taken up by LDL receptors in the liver. In addition, cholesteryl ester transfer protein (CETP) transfers cholesteryl esters (in exchange for triglycerides) from HDL$_2$ to TGRL (e.g., VLDL, LDL, and remnants), which are then delivered to the liver. An additional pathway of cholesterol redistribution from HDL is via scavenger receptor B1 (SR-B1) facilitation of selective uptake of cholesteryl esters by the adrenal glands, gonads, and liver. The HDL$_2$ particles that have been partially depleted of cholesteryl esters and enriched with triglycerides by CETP can be converted back to HDL$_3$ by the action of hepatic lipase that hydrolyzes the triglycerides.

Reverse cholesterol transport—with a redistribution of cholesterol from cells with excess (e.g., arterial walls) to cells requiring cholesterol or to the liver for excretion—is antiatherogenic. There is an inverse relationship between plasma HDL concentration and cardiovascular risk. In addition to reverse cholesterol transport, HDL has other antiatherogenic properties. For example, the HDL-associated enzyme paraoxonase serves to inhibit oxidation of LDL. In addition, HDL and apo AI stabilize the erythrocyte cell membrane and prevent transbilayer diffusion of anionic lipids, a step that is required for prothrombin activation and thrombus formation.

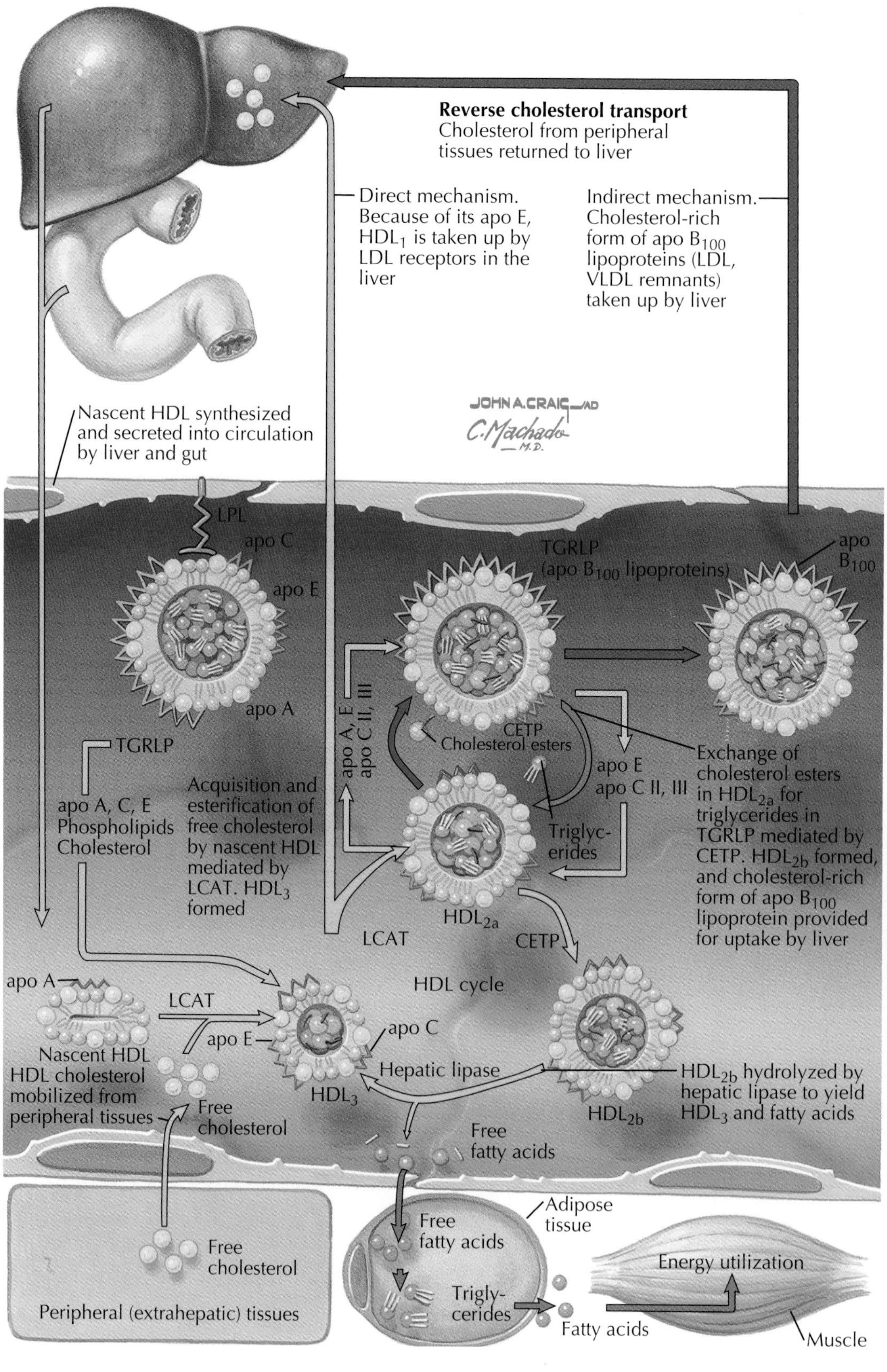

Several alterations in the HDL pathway can result in low or high plasma HDL concentrations. For example, mutations in the gene encoding apo AI can decrease HDL formation because of lack of LCAT activation; resultant plasma concentrations are less than 10 mg/dL (reference ranges: low, less than 40 mg/dL; normal, 40 to 60 mg/dL; desirable, greater than 60 mg/dL). Increased plasma HDL concentrations are found in individuals with CETP deficiency because of the decreased transfer of cholesteryl esters from HDL to apo B-containing lipoproteins. CETP deficiency homozygotes have HDL concentrations greater than 100 mg/dL.

Plate 7-5

Lipids and Nutrition

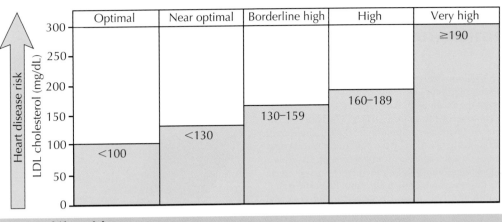

Optimal	Near optimal	Borderline high	High	Very high
<100	<130	130–159	160–189	≥190

Heart disease risk — LDL cholesterol (mg/dL)

Multifactorial causes

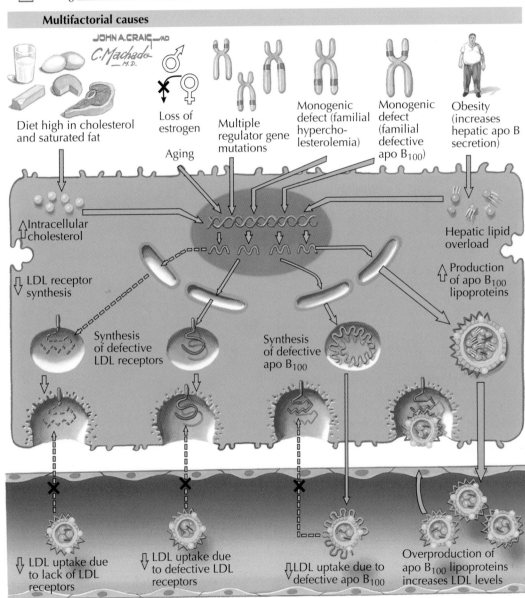

JOHN A. CRAIG—MD
C. Machado—M.D.

Diet high in cholesterol and saturated fat

Loss of estrogen

Aging

Multiple regulator gene mutations

Monogenic defect (familial hypercholesterolemia)

Monogenic defect (familial defective apo B_{100})

Obesity (increases hepatic apo B secretion)

↑Intracellular cholesterol

Hepatic lipid overload

⇓ LDL receptor synthesis

↑ Production of apo B_{100} lipoproteins

Synthesis of defective LDL receptors

Synthesis of defective apo B_{100}

⇓ LDL uptake due to lack of LDL receptors

⇓ LDL uptake due to defective LDL receptors

⇓LDL uptake due to defective apo B_{100}

Overproduction of apo B_{100} lipoproteins increases LDL levels

HYPERCHOLESTEROLEMIA

Cholesterol has a chief role in the function of cell membranes and serves as a precursor of steroid hormones. However, when blood concentrations of low-density lipoprotein (LDL) cholesterol exceed certain levels, it is termed *hypercholesterolemia*. Hypercholesterolemia can predispose to atherosclerosis and increase the risk for vascular disease (e.g., coronary heart disease [CHD], cerebrovascular disease, and peripheral vascular disease).

The National Heart Lung and Blood Institute of the National Institutes of Health has published a series of three guidelines (1988, 1993, 2002), each updating the existing recommendations for clinical management of high blood cholesterol. The Third Report of the Expert Panel on Detection, Evaluation, and Treatment of High Blood Cholesterol in Adults is termed the Adult Treatment Panel III (ATP III) and is the most recent version from the National Cholesterol Education Program (NCEP). ATP III set cutoffs for blood LDL cholesterol concentrations on the basis of cardiovascular risk. For example, a plasma LDL concentration less than 100 mg/dL is considered optimal. As plasma LDL levels increase, cardiovascular risk increases. The presence of risk factors (e.g., cigarette smoking, hypertension, low plasma concentration of high-density lipoprotein [HDL] cholesterol, family history of premature CHD, age [men, ≥45 years; women, ≥55 years]) should modify the target for LDL cholesterol. For example, the presence of CHD or CHD risk equivalents (e.g., diabetes mellitus) decreases the LDL cholesterol goal to less than 100 mg/dL; if there are two or more risk factors, the LDL cholesterol goal should be less than 130 mg/dL; if there is zero to one risk factor, the LDL cholesterol goal should be less than 160 mg/dL. These targets may be modified when NCEP ATP IV guidelines are published in the fall of 2011.

Many factors contribute to high plasma LDL concentrations. For example, diets high in saturated fats and cholesterol lead to increased blood cholesterol concentrations. Although the level of cholesterol in the blood is controlled at multiple sites, the primary regulator is the LDL receptor pathway. LDL receptors are present on the cell surface of most cells and mediate the uptake of lipoproteins that contain the apolipoproteins (apo) apo B_{100} and apo E (e.g., LDL, chylomicron remnants, very low-density lipoproteins [VLDL], VLDL remnants, and HDL_1).

Familial hypercholesterolemia is a relatively common disorder caused by mutations in the gene that encodes the LDL receptor. Decreased synthesis or synthesis of defective LDL receptors leads to increased plasma concentrations of LDL cholesterol (three- and sixfold increased above the reference range in heterozygotes and homozygotes, respectively) (see Plates 7-6 and 7-7).

Mutations in the gene that encodes apo B_{100} are relatively common and lead to defective binding of LDL cholesterol to the LDL receptor. The clinical findings

and the blood lipid profile are similar to those of familial hypercholesterolemia (see Plates 7-6 and 7-7).

Familial hyperapobetalipoproteinemia (with overproduction of apo B_{100}) and familial combined hyperlipidemia are both inherited in an autosomal dominant fashion. Although the genetic defects underlying these conditions have yet to be identified (probably multiple genetic defects), they are relatively common disorders and are associated with elevations of plasma LDL cholesterol and triglyceride concentrations and increased

susceptibility to CHD. Other associations include moderate decrease in plasma HDL cholesterol concentrations, fasting hyperglycemia, obesity, and hyperuricemia. Familial combined hyperlipidemia should be suspected in individuals with moderate hypercholesterolemia in combination with moderate hypertriglyceridemia in the setting of a family history of premature CHD. Xanthomas are not seen in individuals with familial hyperapobetalipoproteinemia or with familial combined hyperlipidemia.

Plate 7-6

Endocrine System

HYPERCHOLESTEROLEMIC XANTHOMATOSIS

Severe hypercholesterolemia can lead to cutaneous and tendinous xanthomas. These cutaneous protuberances represent the accumulation of large (10–20 μm in diameter), cholesterol-filled macrophages. The high concentrations of low-density lipoprotein (LDL) cholesterol in the blood are taken up by the nonsaturable scavenger receptors on macrophages. Xanthelasma of the eyelids is frequently accompanied by premature arcus corneae (i.e., in persons younger than 40 years). Plain and tuberous xanthomas are most frequently found over the elbows, knees, and buttocks, possibly related to continuous irritation by garments. Tuberous xanthomas are seen most frequently in individuals with homozygous mutations in the gene that encodes the LDL receptor (see the following text).

The characteristic lesions of tendinous xanthoma are actually part of the tendon, from which they cannot be mechanically separated. The nodules are found in the extensor tendons of the hands, Achilles tendons, and patellar tendons. This type of nodular lesion may be easily confused with the nodules of rheumatoid arthritis, but it can readily be distinguished because a xanthoma is not painful, and patients with rheumatoid arthritis lack the marked increased in blood LDL cholesterol concentrations that are seen in patients with xanthomas.

In the first phase, atherosclerotic lesions consist of cushionlike elevations of lipid-filled macrophages (foam cells) beneath the intima. Later, they become sclerotic (see Plates 7-12 and 7-13). The atheroma of the arterial intima is the most dangerous feature of familial hypercholesterolemic xanthomatosis because of its frequent occurrence in the coronary vessels, which may cause angina and myocardial infarction at an early age.

Hypercholesterolemic xanthomatosis is a manifestation of either familial hypercholesterolemia (FH) (an autosomal dominant disorder caused by mutations in the gene that encodes the LDL receptor) or familial defective apolipoprotein apo B_{100} (caused by mutations in the gene that encodes apo B_{100}).

FAMILIAL HYPERCHOLESTEROLEMIA— LOW-DENSITY LIPOPROTEIN RECEPTOR MUTATIONS

FH is a monogenic disorder caused by mutations in the gene that encodes the LDL receptor. Thus, LDL cholesterol is not effectively cleared from the circulation, and plasma concentrations of LDL cholesterol are increased. There is increased uptake of LDL cholesterol by the macrophage scavenger receptors, with marked lipid accumulation in the macrophages (foam cells). More than 900 different mutations in the LDL receptor have been identified to cause FH. The types of mutations in the gene that encodes the LDL receptor include mutations that cause the following: decreased LDL receptor synthesis, decreased intracellular transport of the LDL receptor from the endoplasmic reticulum to the Golgi apparatus, defective binding of LDL cholesterol to the LDL receptor, and a defect in the internalization of the LDL receptor after binding LDL cholesterol. Thus, the impact of the LDL receptor mutation on plasma LDL cholesterol concentrations and coronary heart disease (CHD) risk is very dependent on the specific mutation. In addition, individuals with homozygous LDL receptor mutations are much more severely affected than heterozygous individuals.

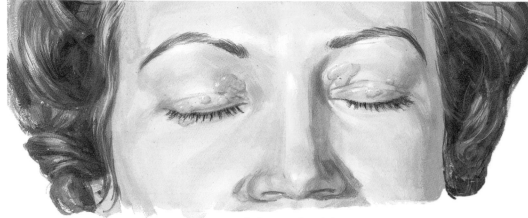

Xanthelasma of eyelids

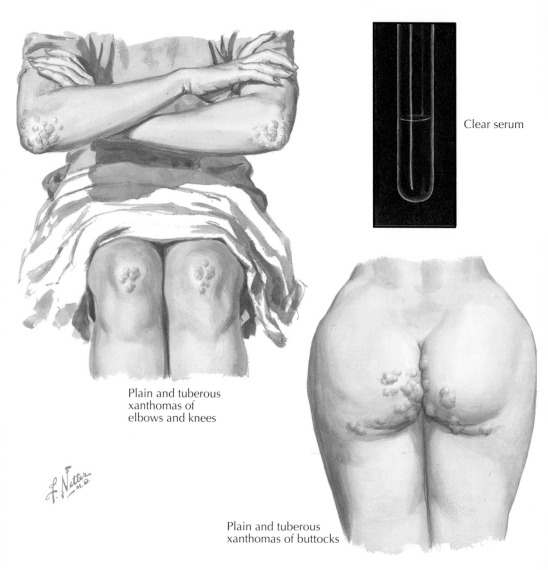

Clear serum

Plain and tuberous xanthomas of elbows and knees

Plain and tuberous xanthomas of buttocks

Heterozygous FH is a relatively common disorder, affecting one in 500 persons, and its manifestations are present from birth. In individuals with heterozygous FH, the plasma total cholesterol concentrations are typically more than 300 mg/dL, and the LDL cholesterol concentrations are more than 250 mg/dL. Plasma triglycerides are not elevated in this condition. Approximately 75% of patients with heterozygous FH have xanthelasma and tendon xanthomas. Also, premature CHD and heart valvular disease occurring before age 45 years are common. Heterozygous FH should be suspected in individuals with high plasma concentrations of LDL cholesterol, normal plasma triglyceride concentrations, tendon xanthomas, and a family history of premature CHD. The diagnosis of heterozygous FH is made on clinical grounds. Because of the large number of potential mutations, germline mutation testing for abnormalities in the gene that encodes the LDL receptor is not routinely done.

Plate 7-7

Lipids and Nutrition

HYPERCHOLESTEROLEMIC XANTHOMATOSIS *(Continued)*

Fortunately, homozygous FH is rare. These individuals come to clinical attention either because of a family history of premature CHD or the appearance of xanthomas at a young age (i.e., younger than 10 years). Typical plasma total cholesterol concentrations range from 600 to 1000 mg/dL; plasma LDL cholesterol concentrations range from 550 to 950 mg/dL. Tuberous xanthomas usually develop before age 6 years and are unique to homozygous FH; these individuals also develop the xanthelasma and tendon xanthomas that are common in individuals who are heterozygous for mutations in the LDL receptor gene. Symptomatic CHD can occur before age 10 years, and fatal myocardial infarction usually occurs before age 20 years if the hypercholesterolemia is not treated. Aortic valvular disease (e.g., aortic stenosis) is more common (occurring in ~50% of affected individuals) and is more severe in homozygous FH than in heterozygous FH. The diagnosis of homozygous FH should be suspected when the plasma LDL cholesterol concentration is more than 500 mg/dL.

Treatment of individuals with heterozygous FH includes a low-cholesterol diet and pharmacologic therapy with a 3-hydroxy-3-methylglutaryl coenzyme A (HMG-CoA) reductase inhibitor. Some patients may require the addition of a bile acid sequestrant or an intestinal cholesterol absorption inhibitor.

Treatment of individuals with homozygous FH is problematic. Because of very little residual LDL cholesterol binding, pharmacologic therapy with HMG-CoA reductase inhibitors, bile acid sequestrants, and intestinal cholesterol absorption inhibitors is suboptimally effective. The most effective therapy involves the periodic (i.e., every 1–3 weeks) selective removal of LDL cholesterol by extracorporeal apheresis.

FAMILIAL DEFECTIVE APOLIPOPROTEIN B$_{100}$

Familial defective apo B$_{100}$ is relatively common disorder affecting in one in 500 persons that is caused by a mutation in the gene encoding apo B$_{100}$. To date, most affected patients have the same single point mutation at nucleotide number 3500. Apo B$_{100}$ is the ligand that binds LDL cholesterol to the LDL receptor; thus, biochemical and clinical phenotypes are very similar to those in individuals with LDL receptor mutations. These individuals have isolated elevations in plasma LDL cholesterol concentrations, xanthelasma, tendon xanthomas, and premature CHD. In general, the clinical presentations of heterozygous and homozygous familial defective apo B$_{100}$ are less severe than those of the heterozygous and homozygous forms of FH, respectively. Clinically, familial defective apo B$_{100}$ cannot be distinguished from FH; germline mutation testing is the only method currently available to make this distinction.

Treatment of familial defective apo B$_{100}$ is similar to that of heterozygous FH, with emphasis on a low-cholesterol diet and pharmacologic therapy with HMG-CoA reductase inhibitors, bile acid sequestrants, and intestinal cholesterol absorption inhibitors.

SITOSTEROLEMIA AND CEREBROTENDINOUS XANTHOMATOSIS

Tendon xanthomas and premature CHD can also occur independently of an abnormality in LDL cholesterol

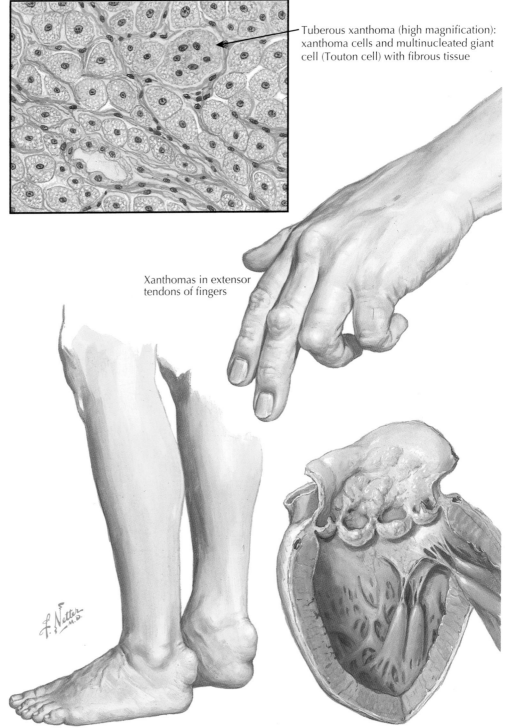

Tuberous xanthoma (high magnification): xanthoma cells and multinucleated giant cell (Touton cell) with fibrous tissue

Xanthomas in extensor tendons of fingers

Large xanthomas of both Achilles tendons

Xanthomatous infiltration of aortic valve and aortic intima around coronary orifice

metabolism. Sitosterolemia is an autosomal recessive disorder resulting from mutations in the genes encoding the adenosine triphosphate–binding cassettes G5 and G8 that normally limit plant sterol absorption. There is a resultant increase in gastrointestinal absorption of cholesterol and plant sterols. The plant sterols and LDL cholesterol accumulate in the plasma and peripheral tissues, leading to premature CHD and tendon xanthomas. Plasma levels of LDL cholesterol are high. Gas-liquid chromatography shows high levels of plant sterols.

Cerebrotendinous xanthomatosis (CTX) is an autosomal recessive lipid storage disease and a form of leukodystrophy. CTX is caused by a block in bile acid synthesis because of absent 27-hydroxylase (caused by mutations in *CYP27A1*), resulting in an accumulation of cholesterol and cholestanol in all tissues. The plasma lipid levels in individuals with CTX are normal. Xanthomas develop in the central nervous system, tendons, skin, bones, and lungs. Because of the associated defects in synthesis and maintenance of the myelin sheath of nerves, CTX has dominant effects on the central nervous system with resultant cerebellar ataxia and pyramidal tract signs.

Plate 7-8

Endocrine System

ABETALIPOPROTEINEMIA AND TANGIER DISEASE

Two familial syndromes are characterized by severe deficiency or absence of specific lipoproteins: abetalipoproteinemia and Tangier disease.

ABETALIPOPROTEINEMIA

Abetalipoproteinemia (OMIM 200100) is a rare autosomal recessive disorder that usually presents in infancy with fat malabsorption, hypocholesterolemia, and acanthocytosis. Later in life, deficiencies in fat-soluble vitamins result in atypical retinitis pigmentosa, posterior column neuropathy, and myopathy. Abetalipoproteinemia is caused by mutations in the gene encoding the large subunit of microsomal triglyceride transfer protein, resulting in abnormal production and secretion of apolipoprotein B (apo B) and apo B–containing lipoproteins. Microsomal triglyceride transfer protein is key in the transfer of triglycerides and phospholipids into the lumen of the endoplasmic reticulum of the enterocyte for the assembly of very low-density lipoprotein (VLDL), a step required for normal hepatic secretion of apo B$_{100}$. Insufficient lipidation of these nascent particles prevents synthesis and secretion of chylomicrons and VLDL by the intestine and liver. This defect results in gastrointestinal fat malabsorption and extremely low plasma concentrations of cholesterol and VLDL triglycerides and absent betalipoprotein.

The absence of apo B results in steatorrhea, symptoms associated with deficiency of fat-soluble vitamins (vitamins A, D, E, and K), neurologic manifestations (e.g., retinitis pigmentosa, peripheral neuropathy, ataxia, lordosis caused by muscular weakness, sensory motor neuropathy, mental retardation), and acanthocytosis (crenated appearance of erythrocytes). In individuals who are homozygous for mutations in the disease-causing gene, there may be deficient adrenocortical glucocorticoid production. The neurologic manifestations may dominate the clinical presentation with early onset (e.g., age 1–2 years) of generalized weakness, distal muscular atrophy, loss of proprioception, posterior column degeneration with sensory neuropathy, and cerebellar atrophy with ataxia and nystagmus. Children with abetalipoproteinemia appear malnourished and have growth retardation. Some patients may have hepatic steatosis and cirrhosis, which can result from treatment with medium-chain triglycerides. In one patient who underwent liver transplantation for hepatic cirrhosis, the serum lipoprotein profile normalized but gastrointestinal fat malabsorption persisted.

Laboratory studies show the absence of plasma apo B–containing proteins and extremely low levels of total cholesterol (<50 mg/dL). Early diagnosis and treatment are key to avoid growth retardation and neuroretinal complications. Treatment includes a lipid-poor diet (e.g., 5 g/d in children) to treat digestive intolerance and allow normal absorption of carbohydrates and proteins, provision of dietary essential fatty acids in the form of vegetable oils, and high doses of fat-soluble vitamins (vitamins A, D, E, and K).

TANGIER DISEASE

Tangier disease (OMIM 205400) is an autosomal dominant disorder that results in low serum concentrations of high-density lipoprotein (HDL) cholesterol. Tangier disease was originally described and named on the basis

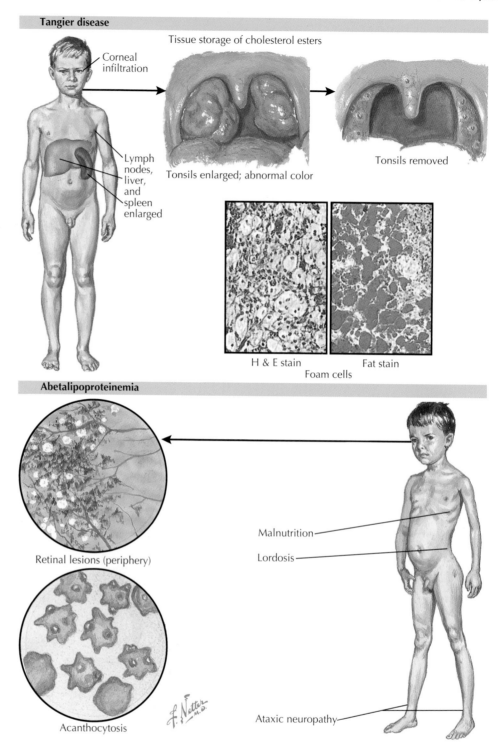

Tangier disease

Corneal infiltration

Tissue storage of cholesterol esters

Lymph nodes, liver, and spleen enlarged

Tonsils enlarged; abnormal color

Tonsils removed

H & E stain

Fat stain

Foam cells

Abetalipoproteinemia

Retinal lesions (periphery)

Acanthocytosis

Malnutrition

Lordosis

Ataxic neuropathy

of a kindred living on Tangier Island in Chesapeake Bay. Tangier disease is caused by mutations in the adenosine triphosphate–binding cassette transporter-1 gene (*ABCA1*), which encodes the cholesterol efflux regulatory protein. *ABCA1* is critical for intracellular cholesterol transport, the impairment of which results in decreased cholesterol efflux onto nascent HDL particles, leading to lipid-depleted particles that are then rapidly catabolized. Thus, the inability of newly synthesized apolipoproteins to acquire cellular lipids by the *ABCA1* pathway leads to their rapid degradation and an overaccumulation of cholesterol in macrophages. *ABCA1* has a critical role in modulating flux of tissue cholesterol and phospholipids into the reverse cholesterol transport pathway. The impaired HDL-mediated

cholesterol efflux from macrophages leads to massive accumulation of cholesteryl esters (foam cells) throughout the body and resultant hepatosplenomegaly. These individuals frequently develop premature coronary disease. Individuals with homozygous mutations in *ABCA1* have absent plasma HDL, and heterozygotes have HDL concentrations about 50% of those in individuals with two normal alleles.

Findings on physical examination include orange tonsils (caused by cholesterol deposits), corneal opacities, hepatosplenomegaly, and peripheral neuropathy. Findings from laboratory studies show absent HDL cholesterol and low total cholesterol concentrations. Currently, there is no disease-specific treatment for Tangier disease.

Plate 7-9

Lipids and Nutrition

HYPERTRIGLYCERIDEMIA

Based on coronary risk, serum triglyceride concentrations can be stratified as follows: normal, less than 150 mg/dL; borderline high, 150 to 199 mg/dL; high, 200 to 499 mg/dL; and very high, 500 mg/dL or greater. Serum triglyceride concentrations greater than 199 mg/dL are termed hypertriglyceridemia and are associated with an increased risk of cardiovascular disease. Hypertriglyceridemia can be caused by or exacerbated by obesity, poorly controlled diabetes mellitus, nephrotic syndrome, hypothyroidism, and orally administered estrogen therapy.

Hypertriglyceridemia results from the accumulation of triglyceride-rich lipoproteins (e.g., very low-density lipoproteins [VLDL], VLDL remnants, and chylomicrons) in blood. Hypertriglyceridemia is associated with variable degrees of hypercholesterolemia because the triglyceride-rich lipoproteins also transport cholesterol. Triglycerides in chylomicrons and VLDL are hydrolyzed by lipoprotein lipase (LPL), and the free fatty acid molecules are used as an energy source. LPL also facilitates the transfer of cholesterol to high-density lipoprotein (HDL) cholesterol. Thus, when LPL activity is deficient, hypertriglyceridemia and low blood HDL cholesterol concentrations occur.

Disorders in lipid metabolism can be categorized by the Fredrickson hyperlipoproteinemia phenotype classification, which is based on the pattern of lipoproteins on electrophoresis or ultracentrifugation:

- Phenotype I (LPL deficiency): increased serum chylomicron concentration and markedly increased serum triglyceride concentration. The serum has a creamy top layer.
- Phenotype IIa (familial hypercholesterolemia): increased serum LDL cholesterol and total cholesterol concentrations. The serum is clear.
- Phenotype IIb: increased serum concentrations of LDL and VLDL cholesterol. The serum is clear.
- Phenotype III (familial dysbetalipoproteinemia): increased serum concentrations of VLDL remnants and chylomicrons. The serum is turbid.
- Phenotype IV (familial hypertriglyceridemia): increased serum concentrations of VLDL. The serum is turbid.
- Phenotype V (mixed hypertriglyceridemia): increased serum concentrations of chylomicrons and VLDL. The serum has a creamy top layer and a turbid bottom layer.

The type I hyperlipoproteinemia phenotype is caused by rare recessive disorders and is associated with complete absence of either LPL activity or apolipoprotein (apo) CII (the ligand for LPL on chylomicrons and VLDL). Severe hypertriglyceridemia results because the clearance of triglyceride-rich lipoproteins from plasma is blocked. Chylomicronemia syndrome is a frequent finding in patients with type I hyperlipoproteinemia (see Plates 7-10 and 7-11).

Type IIa hyperlipoproteinemia is familial hypercholesterolemia and is associated with LDL receptor deficiency, resulting in markedly increased serum concentrations of LDL (see Plates 7-6 and 7-7). Type IIb hyperlipoproteinemia is combined hyperlipidemia caused by decreased LDL receptor availability or function and increased apo B, resulting in increased blood levels of LDL cholesterol and VLDL (see Plate 7-5).

Familial dysbetalipoproteinemia, also termed type III hyperlipoproteinemia, is associated with specific isoforms of the *APOE* gene; however, other genetic and

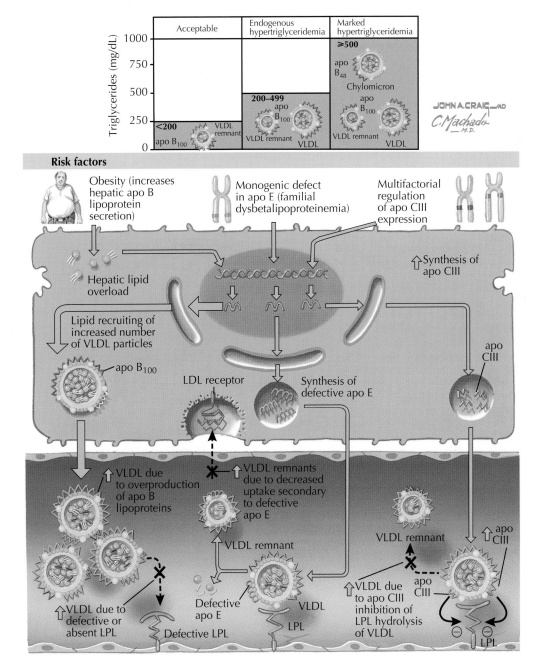

environmental factors probably contribute to disease development and severity. Apo E is required for receptor-mediated clearance of chylomicron and VLDL remnants. The most common *APOE* genotype is *APOE*E3/APOE*E3*. The E2 isoform has lower affinity for the LDL receptor than the E3 isoform, which leads to poor clearance of VLDL and chylomicron remnants that contain the E2 isoform. Familial dysbetalipoproteinemia occurs when individuals are homozygous for the E2 allele. This defect leads to premature coronary heart disease and peripheral vascular disease. Tuberoeruptive xanthomas may be evident on physical examination (see Plates 7-6 and 7-7).

Familial hypertriglyceridemia (type IV hyperlipoproteinemia phenotype) is an autosomal dominant disorder caused by inactivating mutations in the gene encoding LPL and is associated with moderately increased serum triglyceride concentrations (200–500 mg/dL), normal serum LDL cholesterol concentrations, and low serum HDL cholesterol concentrations. The degree of hypertriglyceridemia can be aggravated by exogenous

agents (e.g., orally administered estrogen replacement therapy). Familial hypertriglyceridemia is usually associated with obesity, insulin resistance, hyperglycemia, and hypertension.

Mixed hypertriglyceridemia (type V hyperlipoproteinemia phenotype) is characterized by triglyceride levels above the 99th percentile of normal. The plasma supernatant is creamy, and there are increased concentrations of chylomicrons and VLDL. The clinical manifestations include hepatosplenomegaly and eruptive xanthomas.

Familial combined hyperlipidemia is a genetically heterogenous disorder caused by overproduction of hepatically derived apolipoprotein B_{100} associated with VLDL. Affected patients typically present with hypercholesterolemia and hypertriglyceridemia.

The C apolipoproteins also regulate triglyceride metabolism. Apo CI and apo CIII modulate the uptake of triglyceride-rich lipoproteins (chylomicron remnants, VLDL) by interfering with the ability of apo E to mediate binding to lipoprotein receptor pathways.

Plate 7-10

Endocrine System

CLINICAL MANIFESTATIONS OF HYPERTRIGLYCERIDEMIA

Hypertriglyceridemia is usually asymptomatic. However, serum triglyceride concentrations higher than 1000 mg/dL may result in chylomicronemia syndrome. Signs and symptoms associated with chylomicronemia syndrome include abdominal pain, pancreatitis, eruptive xanthoma, flushing with alcohol intake, memory loss, and lipemia retinalis. The acute pancreatitis can be life threatening, and the patients most commonly affected are those with poorly controlled diabetes mellitus or alcoholism. Serum triglyceride values higher than 1000 mg/dL result in opalescent serum caused by an increase in very low-density lipoprotein (VLDL). At markedly increased levels, the serum may be milky because of hyperchylomicronemia.

Triglycerides in chylomicrons and VLDL are hydrolyzed by lipoprotein lipase (LPL), and the free fatty acid molecules are used as an energy source in muscle for triglyceride synthesis or for storage in adipocytes or formation of hepatic VLDL. LPL is synthesized by adipocytes, myocytes, and macrophages. LPL attaches to heparan sulfate proteoglycans on the surface of capillary endothelial cells, where it interacts with circulating chylomicrons and VLDL. Apolipoprotein (apo) CII is a cofactor for LPL. Mutations that inactivate LPL or apo CII result in severe hypertriglyceridemia (see following text).

Hepatic lipase is synthesized by hepatocytes and is found in capillary endothelial cells of the liver, adrenals, and gonads. Hepatic lipase—activated by androgens and suppressed by estrogens—functions to release lipids from lipoproteins by hydrolyzing triglycerides in the processing of chylomicron remnants and also to convert high-density lipoprotein (HDL) cholesterol from HDL_2 to HDL_3 by removing phospholipid and triglyceride from HDL_2. Thus, when the hepatic lipase activity is high, serum concentrations of total HDL cholesterol levels are low. Unlike LPL, apo CII is not a cofactor for hepatic lipase. Defects or deficiencies in hepatic lipase result in an accumulation of remnant lipoproteins and HDL_2.

LIPOPROTEIN LIPASE DEFICIENCY

Mutations in the gene encoding LPL can result in deficient LPL activity, a rare autosomal recessive disorder that manifests with severe hypertriglyceridemia because the clearance of triglyceride-rich lipoproteins from the plasma is blocked. Individuals heterozygous for a mutation in the *LPL* gene (approximate frequency of one in 500) may have LPL activity that is 50% of normal, leading to mild hypertriglyceridemia.

Normally, chylomicrons are cleared from plasma within 8 hours of eating. In persons with complete LPL deficiency, the chylomicrons can take days to be cleared after a single meal. Chylomicronemia syndrome results when there are massive accumulations of these lipoproteins in the blood. LPL deficiency is usually diagnosed in infancy or childhood when individuals present with chylomicronemia syndrome. Manifestations of chylomicronemia syndrome include recurrent abdominal pain, pancreatitis, hepatosplenomegaly caused by the accumulation of triglycerides in reticuloendothelial cells, eruptive xanthomas, lipemia retinalis, lipemic plasma, neurologic manifestations, dyspnea, and severe hypertriglyceridemia (>2000 mg/dL). The pancreatitis resulting from chemical irritation by fatty acids and

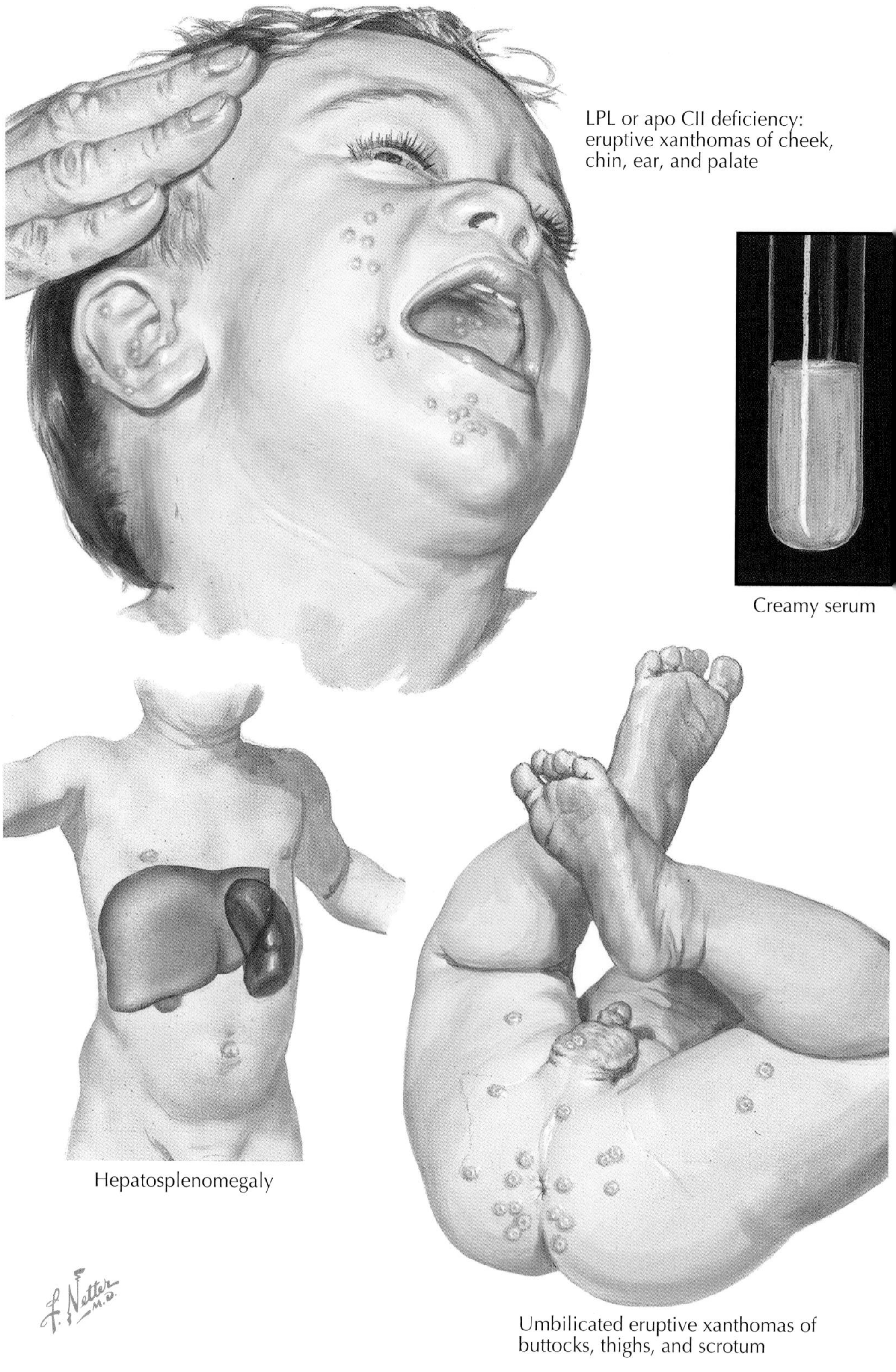

LPL or apo CII deficiency: eruptive xanthomas of cheek, chin, ear, and palate

Creamy serum

Hepatosplenomegaly

Umbilicated eruptive xanthomas of buttocks, thighs, and scrotum

lysolecithin can be life threatening. Chylomicrons are usually present whenever the triglyceride concentration is higher than 1000 mg/dL in a fasting blood sample. The serum appears creamy. Because of the effect on blood volume, severe hypertriglyceridemia can lead to measurement errors in serum electrolytes. For example, if serum is not cleared of triglyceride-rich lipoproteins by centrifugation, serum sodium may appear low (pseudohyponatremia).

LPL deficiency should be suspected in infants and children with recurrent abdominal pain and pancreatitis. Eruptive xanthomas are usually present in this setting, especially when serum triglyceride concentrations are higher than 2000 mg/dL. LPL deficiency can be confirmed with the heparin infusion test. Heparin displaces LPL from heparan sulfate proteoglycans on the surface of capillary endothelial cells, and LPL activity can be assayed in plasma.

Plate 7-11

Lipids and Nutrition

CLINICAL MANIFESTATIONS OF HYPERTRIGLYCERIDEMIA
(Continued)

When patients with LPL deficiency present with pancreatitis, the initial treatment should include a fat-free diet. Long term, patients with LPL deficiency should be treated with a fat-restricted diet, with fat accounting for less than 10% of total calories. The therapeutic goal is to maintain serum triglyceride concentrations at less than 1000 mg/dL. Pharmacologic options are limited for patients with LPL deficiency (see following text).

APOLIPOPROTEIN CII DEFICIENCY

Apo CII deficiency is another rare autosomal recessive disorder that can cause the chylomicronemia syndrome. The clinical presentation is identical to that of LPL deficiency. The lack of apo CII, an activating cofactor for LPL, results in a functional LDL deficiency. Apo CII deficiency can be confirmed by the absence of apo CII on electrophoresis of plasma apolipoproteins. The treatment of apo CII deficiency is identical to that of LPL deficiency.

FAMILIAL HYPERTRIGLYCERIDEMIA

Individuals with familial hypertriglyceridemia overproduce VLDL triglycerides, resulting in serum triglyceride concentrations in the range of 200 to 500 mg/dL and normal LDL cholesterol concentrations. The hypertriglyceridemia typically occurs in concert with low serum HDL cholesterol levels and obesity. Because of the relative mild degree of hypertriglyceridemia and the lack of associated symptomatology, most affected patients are not diagnosed until adulthood. The degree of hypertriglyceridemia is usually less than 1000 mg/dL unless aggravated by alcohol use, orally administered estrogen, or hypothyroidism. Treatment of individuals with familial hypertriglyceridemia includes avoidance of alcohol and orally administered estrogens, as well as implementation of some of the nonpharmacologic and pharmacologic approaches outlined in the following text.

TREATMENT

Hypertriglyceridemia promotes atherosclerosis, and treatment should be considered when serum triglyceride concentrations are higher than 200 mg/dL. Nonpharmacologic treatment options include weight loss in obese patients, a regular isotonic exercise program, improved glycemic control in patients with diabetes mellitus, limitation of alcohol intake, and avoidance of free carbohydrates in the diet. Pharmacologic therapy is indicated when hypertriglyceridemia persists despite nonpharmacologic interventions.

When serum LDL cholesterol concentrations are elevated in concert with serum triglycerides, a 3-hydroxy-3-methylglutaryl coenzyme A (HMG-CoA) reductase inhibitor may lower the blood triglyceride concentration, as well as the LDL cholesterol concentration. When the main lipid profile anomaly is hypertriglyceridemia, it can be treated with a fibric acid

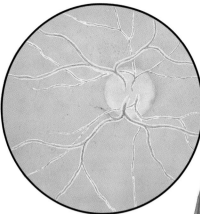

Hyperlipemia retinalis

Chylomicronemia syndrome:
▶ Recurrent abdominal pain
▶ Pancreatitis
▶ Hepatosplenomegaly
▶ Eruptive xanthomas
▶ Lipemia retinalis
▶ Lipemic plasma
▶ Severe hypertriglyceridemia
  (e.g., >2000 mg/dL)

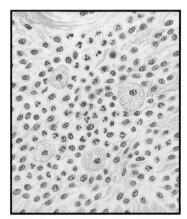

Hyperlipemic xanthomatous nodule (high magnification): few foam cells amid inflammatory exudate

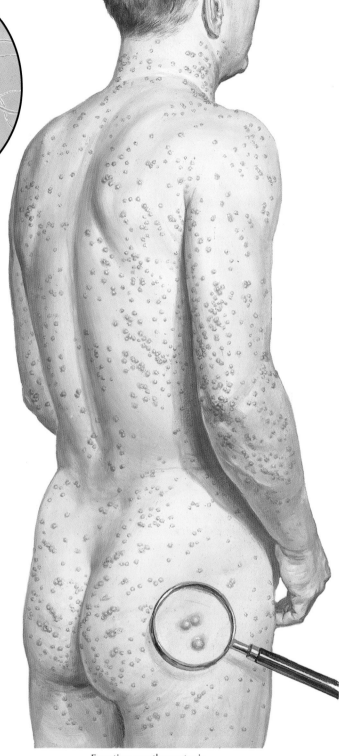

Eruptive xanthomatosis

derivative (i.e., fenofibrate or gemfibrozil), nicotinic acid, or omega-3 fatty acids (e.g., fish oil at doses >3 g/d). Fish oil decreases VLDL production and can lower serum triglyceride concentrations by as much as 50%. Nicotinic acid may cause hyperglycemia and should be avoided in patients with hyperglycemia or impaired glucose tolerance. Gemfibrozil may increase the risk for HMG-CoA reductase inhibitor–related myositis and should be avoided in these patients. Orlistat may be helpful in patients with type V

hyperlipoproteinemia and very high serum triglyceride levels that are refractory to the aforementioned therapies because it inhibits gastrointestinal fat absorption and decreases intestinal chylomicron synthesis.

When the serum triglyceride concentration is very high (≥500 mg/dL), the first goal is to avoid pancreatitis. Prompt institution of pharmacologic therapy with nicotinic acid or a fibrate is indicated. For example, gemfibrozil can lower serum triglyceride concentrations in this setting by as much as 70%.

Plate 7-12

Endocrine System

ATHEROGENESIS: FATTY STREAK FORMATION

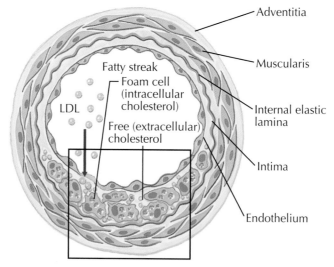

Adventitia

Muscularis

Fatty streak
Foam cell
(intracellular
cholesterol)

LDL

Internal elastic
lamina

Free (extracellular)
cholesterol

Intima

Endothelium

Extracellular cholesterol and cholesterol-filled macrophages (foam cells) accumulate in subendothelial space. Subsequent structural modifications of LDL particles render them more atherogenic. Oxidation of subendothelial LDL attracts monocytes, which enter subendothelium and change into macrophages. Macrophages may take up oxidized LDL to form foam cells.

JOHN A. CRAIG—AD
C. Machado
—M.D.

Circulating monocyte

Circulating LDL

Monocyte adheres to endothelium

Monocyte migrates into subendothelium

LDL migrates into subendothelium

Insoluble LDL aggregates form

Monocyte transforms into macrophage

Cytotoxicity

Monocyte chemo-attraction

Macrophage differentiation

Oxidation

Uptake of oxidized LDL by macrophage

Oxidized LDL

Dena-turation

Free radicals

H_2O_2

Intimal LDL

O_2

Foam cell forms

Glycation

Cholesterol released

Free cholesterol

Interaction with proteo-glycans

Macrophage

Extracellular cholesterol

Cholesterol ester

ATHEROSCLEROSIS

Atherogenesis starts in the arterial wall and eventually may lead to vascular disease (coronary heart disease [CHD], peripheral vascular disease, or cerebrovascular disease). Occlusive arterial disease resulting from atherosclerosis is a leading cause of disability and death. Atherosclerosis, a result of a chronic inflammatory response to vascular injury, is the buildup of plaque in the walls of arteries that is composed of lipoproteins, inflammatory cells, extracellular matrix, vascular smooth muscle cells, and calcium. The sites of atherosclerosis are typically those parts of the arterial vascular tree associated with increased turbulent blood flow (bifurcations and curvatures). Typical locations for symptomatic atherosclerotic lesions are the proximal left anterior descending coronary artery, proximal renal arteries, and carotid bifurcations. These sites have an upregulation of proinflammatory adhesion molecules for inflammatory cells (e.g., monocytes and T cells). Risk factors for endothelial dysfunction and injury include increased serum concentrations of low-density lipoprotein (LDL) cholesterol, decreased serum concentrations of high-density lipoprotein (HDL) cholesterol, increased oxidant stress (e.g., cigarette smoking, hypertension, diabetes mellitus), and aging. The serum concentration of LDL cholesterol is a strong predictor of CHD and atherosclerosis; more than 70% of individuals with premature CHD have hyperlipidemia. Total serum cholesterol concentrations less than 160 mg/dL markedly decrease CHD risk.

Atherogenesis is a slow process that occurs over years. The clinical manifestations of atherosclerosis may be chronic (e.g., stable angina pectoris or intermittent claudication) or acute (e.g., myocardial infarction, stroke). However, most atheromata produce no symptoms. The normal arterial wall is composed of the endothelial cell layer, intima and subendothelial space, internal elastic lamina, media (muscularis layer formed by smooth muscle cells), and adventitia (loose connective tissue). The initial events in atherosclerosis involve movement of electronegative LDL cholesterol and other apolipoprotein (apo) B_{100}–containing lipoproteins (e.g., very low-density lipoprotein, lipoprotein[a]) from the blood into the subendothelial space where they are retained because of a charge-mediated interaction with the positively charged proteoglycans. Small LDL particles penetrate the endothelial barrier more effectively than large LDL particles. LDL cholesterol in the subendothelial space becomes oxidized. The presence of oxidized LDL promotes synthesis of monocyte

chemoattractant protein 1 and other chemoattractants by endothelial and smooth muscle cells. Circulating monocytes then attach to the surface of endothelial cells and subsequently migrate between these cells to enter the subendothelial space, where they differentiate into macrophages. The activated macrophage releases mitogens and chemoattractants, which recruit more macrophages and smooth muscle cells. The macrophages take up the oxidized LDL cholesterol in an unregulated fashion by scavenger receptors. The

internalization of oxidized LDL cholesterol leads to formation of lipid peroxides and facilitates the accumulation of cholesterol esters, resulting in foam cell formation. As foam cells accumulate, they form a visible atherosclerotic lesion—the fatty streak. Fatty streaks, the initial lesion of atherosclerosis, can be seen in infants and young children. The fatty streak may resolve (based on HDL cholesterol reverse cholesterol transport) or may mature into a fibrous plaque that extends into the vessel lumen.

Plate 7-13

Lipids and Nutrition

ATHEROGENESIS: FIBROUS PLAQUE FORMATION

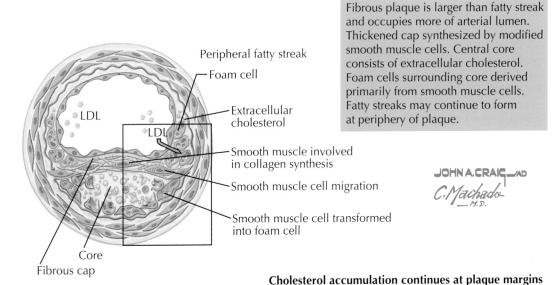

Fibrous plaque is larger than fatty streak and occupies more of arterial lumen. Thickened cap synthesized by modified smooth muscle cells. Central core consists of extracellular cholesterol. Foam cells surrounding core derived primarily from smooth muscle cells. Fatty streaks may continue to form at periphery of plaque.

Peripheral fatty streak
Foam cell
LDL
LDL
Extracellular cholesterol
Smooth muscle involved in collagen synthesis
Smooth muscle cell migration
Smooth muscle cell transformed into foam cell
Core
Fibrous cap

JOHN A. CRAIG ━AD
C. Machado ━M.D.

Cholesterol accumulation continues at plaque margins

Fibrous cap forms over core

Monocyte
apo B₁₀₀
LDL
Oxidized LDL
Macrophage
Foam cell
Fibrous cap
Collagen synthesis and secretion form fibrous cap
Central core of free (extra-cellular) cholesterol
Foam cell death releases cholesterol into intima
Smooth muscle transformed into foam cell
Smooth muscle migrates into intima

ATHEROSCLEROSIS (Continued)

As fibrous plaques enlarge and age, foam cells necrose and release oxidized LDL, intracellular enzymes, and oxygen free radicals that can damage the vessel wall. Oxidized LDL induces apoptosis of endothelial cells and vascular smooth muscle cells. The extracellular cholesterol deposition and continued inflammatory response promote smooth muscle cell proliferation and migration and collagen synthesis. Smooth muscle cells become the main cell type, lying in parallel layers with proteoglycan and basement membrane in between. Continued inflammation results in the recruitment of increased numbers of macrophages and lymphocytes that release proteolytic enzymes, cytokines, chemokines, and growth factors. Focal necrosis develops, and free cholesterol forms the central lipid core of the fibrous plaque. Some smooth muscle cells accumulate lipid to become foam cells. Cycles of accumulation of mononuclear cells, migration and proliferation of smooth muscle cells, and formation of fibrous tissue lead to a continuous restructuring of the atherosclerotic lesion. A fibrous cap develops that overlies the core of lipid and necrotic tissue.

With progression of an atherosclerotic lesion, new microvessels arise from the arterial vasa vasorum. The microvessels provide a portal of entry for monocytes and lymphocytes into the developing plaque. The microvessels are fragile and are prone to rupture, resulting in small focal hemorrhages within the plaque. Calcification may occur as a late event in fibrous plaques, and the elasticity of the arterial wall becomes limited. Bone-related proteins (e.g., osteopontin and osteocalcin) can be found in atherosclerotic plaques. Coronary calcification is a marker of atherosclerosis that can be quantified with the use of cardiac computed tomography (CT), and it is proportional to the extent and severity of atherosclerotic disease. Cardiac CT is a noninvasive tool to assess the presence of coronary artery disease. Increased cardiac CT calcium scores indicate higher risk for CHD in both asymptomatic and symptomatic individuals and can be used to guide

management decisions. For example, aggressive preventive medical therapy (see Plate 7-17) and risk factor modification (see Plate 7-14) should be considered for asymptomatic individuals with high cardiac CT calcium scores.

The plaque can progress to a complicated lesion, where the surface endothelial cells may be lost, and the fibrous cap ruptures to expose the subendothelial space. Platelets adhere to the exposed surface, and thrombus formation is initiated. Platelets release their granules,

which contain cytokines, growth factors, and thrombin, resulting in further proliferation and migration of smooth muscle cells and monocytes. A large thrombus may form in unstable ruptured plaques where blood dissects into the artery wall. The plaque rupture and thrombosis can lead to acute ischemic syndromes and sudden cardiac death. Plaque rupture is responsible for approximately 75% of fatal coronary thrombi; these plaques tend to have thin fibrous caps, increased macrophage content, and large lipid cores.

Plate 7-14

Endocrine System

ATHEROSCLEROSIS RISK FACTORS

The main modifiable cardiovascular risk factors are hypercholesterolemia with increased low-density lipoprotein (LDL) cholesterol, hypertension, cigarette smoking, and diabetes mellitus.

HYPERLIPIDEMIA

The Third Report of the Expert Panel on Detection, Evaluation, and Treatment of High Blood Cholesterol in Adults is termed the Adult Treatment Panel III (ATP III) and is the most recent version from the National Cholesterol Education Program (NCEP). ATP III guidelines recommend lipid screening (total cholesterol, triglycerides, LDL cholesterol, and high-density lipoprotein [HDL] cholesterol) every 5 years in all adults older than 20 years. The 10-year risk for developing coronary heart disease (CHD) can be determined based on data from the Framingham database. The risk factors included in the Framingham calculation are age, total cholesterol, HDL cholesterol, systolic blood pressure, treatment of hypertension, and cigarette smoking. An online risk calculator is found at http://hp2010. nhlbihin.net/atpiii/calculator.asp. The intensity of treatment of hypercholesterolemia should be personalized on the basis of CHD risk. ATP III set cutoffs for blood LDL cholesterol concentrations on the basis of cardiovascular risk. For example, a plasma LDL cholesterol concentration less than 100 mg/dL is considered optimal. As plasma LDL cholesterol levels increase, cardiovascular risk increases. The presence of risk factors (cigarette smoking, hypertension, low plasma concentration of HDL cholesterol, family history of premature CHD, older age [men, ≥45 years; women, ≥55 years]) should modify the target LDL cholesterol concentration. For example, the presence of CHD or CHD risk equivalents (e.g., diabetes mellitus) decreases the LDL cholesterol goal to less than 100 mg/dL; if there are two or more risk factors, the LDL cholesterol goal should be less than 130 mg/dL; if there is zero to 1 risk factor, the LDL cholesterol goal should be less than 160 mg/dL. These targets may be modified when NCEP ATP IV guidelines are published in the fall of 2011.

Although LDL-lowering treatments do not markedly regress known obstructing coronary artery lesions, they do markedly decrease coronary events. Thus, the benefit of lipid lowering in patients with known CHD may not be plaque regression but rather plaque stabilization. In addition, the consistent benefit of LDL lowering by 3-hydroxy-3-methylglutaryl coenzyme A (HMG-CoA) reductase inhibitors (statins) may depend not only on their effects on LDL cholesterol but also on their direct influence on plaque biology.

HYPERTENSION

The cause-and-effect relationship between hypertension and CHD risk is well established. Normalization of blood pressure by nonpharmacologic measures (e.g., weight reduction, sodium-restricted diet, regular isotonic exercise) and pharmacologic measures reduces the risk of stroke, heart failure, and CHD events. The Seventh Report of the Joint National Committee on Prevention, Detection, Evaluation, and Treatment of High Blood Pressure (JNC7) determined that starting at a blood pressure of 115/75 mm Hg, cardiovascular risk doubles for each incremental increase of 20/10 mm

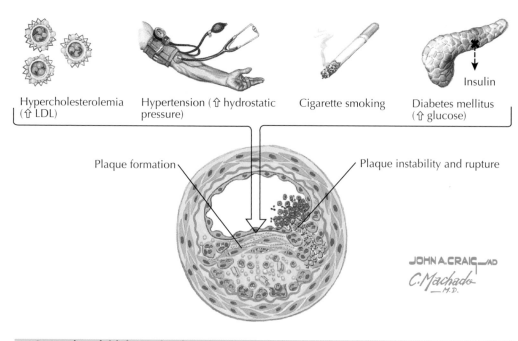

RISK FACTORS IN CORONARY HEART DISEASE

Hypercholesterolemia (⇧ LDL) Hypertension (⇧ hydrostatic pressure) Cigarette smoking Diabetes mellitus (⇧ glucose) Insulin

Plaque formation Plaque instability and rupture

JOHN A. CRAIG—AD
C. Machado—M.D.

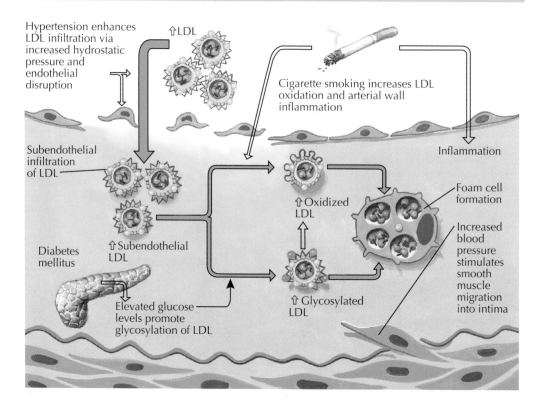

Interaction of risk factors in atherogenesis

Hypertension enhances LDL infiltration via increased hydrostatic pressure and endothelial disruption

⇧LDL

Cigarette smoking increases LDL oxidation and arterial wall inflammation

Subendothelial infiltration of LDL

Inflammation

Diabetes mellitus

⇧Subendothelial LDL

⇧Oxidized LDL

Foam cell formation

Elevated glucose levels promote glycosylation of LDL

⇧Glycosylated LDL

Increased blood pressure stimulates smooth muscle migration into intima

Hg. JNC7 recommends that prehypertensive individuals (systolic blood pressure, 120–139 mm Hg or diastolic blood pressure, 80–89 mm Hg) engage in health-promoting lifestyle modifications to prevent the progressive increase in blood pressure and the development of cardiovascular disease.

DIABETES MELLITUS

Most individuals with diabetes mellitus die of atherosclerosis complications. The increased prevalence of atherosclerosis in individuals with diabetes is partly caused by the presence of small and dense LDL

cholesterol, low serum HDL cholesterol concentrations, and increased serum triglyceride concentrations. Increased blood glucose levels also promote glycosylation of LDL cholesterol.

CIGARETTE SMOKING

The understanding of the mechanisms involved in cigarette smoking–related atherosclerosis is not complete. However, cigarette smoking clearly increases inflammation, thrombosis, and oxidation of LDL cholesterol, leading to increased oxidative stress and arterial wall inflammation.

Plate 7-15

Lipids and Nutrition

METABOLIC SYNDROME

The metabolic syndrome is characterized by insulin resistance, hyperinsulinemia, predisposition to diabetes mellitus, dyslipidemia, atherosclerotic vascular disease, and hypertension. Most individuals with the components of the metabolic syndrome are overweight (body mass index [BMI], 25–29 kg/m²) or obese (BMI ≥30 kg/m²). Excess abdominal visceral fat is very characteristic. Based on the Third Report of the Expert Panel on Detection, Evaluation, and Treatment of High Blood Cholesterol in Adults (Adult Treatment Panel III [ATP III]) guidelines, approximately 50 million people in the United States have the metabolic syndrome. Individuals with this diagnosis have a two- to fourfold increase in subsequent cardiovascular events. It is debated whether the metabolic syndrome is truly a unique entity and whether it confers risk beyond its individual components. However, identifying and treating components of the metabolic syndrome are important to decrease morbidity and mortality related to cardiovascular disease and diabetes.

Insulin resistance occurs when more than normal amounts of insulin are required to elicit a normal biologic response, a situation inferred by high fasting levels of blood insulin. Insulin resistance affects muscle, liver, and adipose tissues and results in decreased peripheral glucose and fatty acid use. Biomarkers consistent with the concept that the metabolic syndrome is a prothrombotic and proinflammatory state include increased serum levels of C-reactive protein, plasminogen activator inhibitor 1, interleukin 6, and adipocyte cytokines (e.g., adiponectin).

No single test is available to diagnose the metabolic syndrome. The ATP III diagnostic criteria include the presence of any three of the following five traits: (1) abdominal obesity defined as a waist circumference larger than 102 cm in men or larger than 88 cm in women; (2) serum triglyceride concentration above 150 mg/dL or medication therapy for hypertriglyceridemia; (3) serum high-density lipoprotein (HDL) cholesterol concentration below 40 mg/dL in men or below 50 mg/dL in women or medication therapy for low HDL cholesterol; (4) blood pressure above 130/80 mm Hg or medication therapy for hypertension; and (5) fasting plasma glucose concentration 100 mg/dL or above or medication therapy for hyperglycemia. The diagnostic criteria from the World Health Organization include insulin resistance (identified by type 2 diabetes mellitus, impaired fasting glucose, or impaired glucose tolerance) plus any two of the following five traits: (1) antihypertensive medication use or high blood pressure (i.e., ≥140/90 mm Hg); (2) serum triglyceride concentration 150 mg/dL or above; (3) serum HDL cholesterol concentration below 35 mg/dL in men or below 39 mg/dL in women; (4) BMI above 30 kg/m² or a waist-to-hip ratio above 0.9 in men or above 0.85 in women; and (5) urinary albumin excretion rate 20 µg/min or above or albumin-to-creatinine ratio 30 mg/g or above.

Clinical assessment of patients with one or more risk factors for the metabolic syndrome should include a history, physical examination (including blood pressure measurement, determination of BMI, and waist circumference measurement), fasting lipid profile, and fasting plasma glucose.

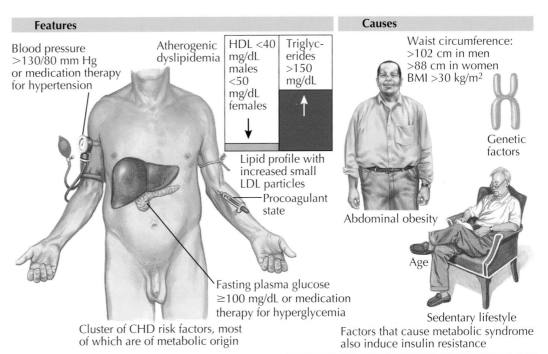

Features

Blood pressure >130/80 mm Hg or medication therapy for hypertension

Atherogenic dyslipidemia

HDL <40 mg/dL males <50 mg/dL females	Triglyc- erides >150 mg/dL

Lipid profile with increased small LDL particles

Procoagulant state

Fasting plasma glucose ≥100 mg/dL or medication therapy for hyperglycemia

Cluster of CHD risk factors, most of which are of metabolic origin

Causes

Waist circumference: >102 cm in men >88 cm in women BMI >30 kg/m²

Genetic factors

Abdominal obesity

Age

Sedentary lifestyle

Factors that cause metabolic syndrome also induce insulin resistance

Insulin resistance (biochemical basis of metabolic syndrome)

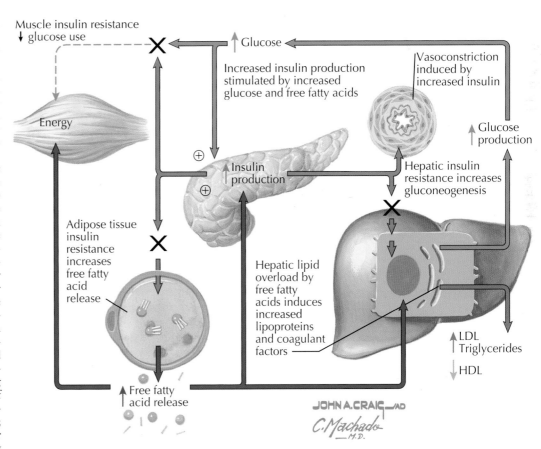

Muscle insulin resistance ↓ glucose use

↑ Glucose

Energy

Increased insulin production stimulated by increased glucose and free fatty acids

Vasoconstriction induced by increased insulin

↑ Glucose production

Insulin production

Hepatic insulin resistance increases gluconeogenesis

Adipose tissue insulin resistance increases free fatty acid release

Hepatic lipid overload by free fatty acids induces increased lipoproteins and coagulant factors

↑ LDL ↑ Triglycerides

↓ HDL

↑ Free fatty acid release

JOHN A. CRAIG—AD
C. Machado—M.D.

The cornerstone of treatment of the metabolic syndrome is lifestyle modification with weight loss and increased physical activity. Diet and exercise can delay the onset of diabetes in patients with impaired glucose tolerance. Exercise (e.g., ≥30 minutes of moderate-intensity physical activity daily) has the potential to decrease abdominal fat. Cigarette smoking should be discouraged. In patients with impaired fasting glucose or type 2 diabetes, the addition of metformin can very effectively improve glycemic control because it enhances insulin action. The overall management of diabetes in patients with the metabolic syndrome should follow clinical guidelines for diabetes (see Plate 5-20). The metabolic syndrome is a coronary risk equivalent, and serum cholesterol targets should follow clinical guidelines (see Plates 7-5 and 7-17). If the Framingham coronary artery risk score (see Plate 7-14) is more than 10%, the addition of low-dose aspirin (e.g., 81 mg/d) should also be considered.

Plate 7-16

MECHANISMS OF ACTION OF LIPID-LOWERING AGENTS

Lipid-lowering agents include cholesterol absorption inhibitors, 3-hydroxy-3-methylglutaryl coenzyme A (HMG-CoA) reductase inhibitors (statins), bile acid sequestrants, nicotinic acid, fibric acid derivatives, and fish oil. Each drug class differs with regard to mechanism of action and type of and degree of lipid lowering. The benefits seen with lipid lowering are multifaceted and extend beyond regression of atherosclerosis to include decreased thrombogenesis, reversal of endothelial dysfunction, and atherosclerotic plaque stabilization.

CHOLESTEROL ABSORPTION INHIBITORS

Ezetimibe is the first drug in a class of cholesterol absorption inhibitors that impair cholesterol absorption at the brush border of the intestine. Ezetimibe does not affect the absorption of triglycerides or fat-soluble vitamins. Its mechanism of action involves Niemann-Pick C1–like 1 proteins that have a role in intestinal cholesterol transport. Thus, there is decreased intestinal delivery of cholesterol to the liver. At a dose of 10 mg/d, ezetimibe lowers the serum low-density lipoprotein (LDL) cholesterol concentration by an average of 17%. The effect of ezetimibe is additive to that of statins.

STATINS

Statins are competitive inhibitors of HMG-CoA reductase—the rate-limiting step in cholesterol biosynthesis. The statin-induced decrease in hepatocyte cholesterol content results in increased LDL-receptor turnover and LDL-receptor cycling. Statins lower serum LDL cholesterol concentrations by 30% to 60%. In addition, statins modify the atherogenic lipoprotein phenotype by decreasing the serum concentration of small dense LDL cholesterol. Most statins lower triglyceride concentrations by 20% to 40% and increase high-density lipoprotein (HDL) cholesterol by 5% to 10%. Currently available statins include lovastatin, simvastatin, pravastatin, fluvastatin, atorvastatin, pitavastatin, and rosuvastatin.

BILE ACID SEQUESTRANTS

Bile acid sequestrants bind bile acids in the intestine and thus interrupt the usually efficient (90%) reabsorption of bile acids. The resultant reduction in intrahepatic cholesterol promotes the synthesis of LDL receptors. The increased numbers of hepatocyte LDL receptors bind LDL cholesterol from the plasma and thus reduce the serum LDL cholesterol concentration by 10% to 24%. The cholesterol-lowering effect of bile acid sequestrants is additive to that of statins. Currently available bile acid sequestrants include cholestyramine, colestipol, and colesevelam.

NICOTINIC ACID

Nicotinic acid inhibits the hepatic production of very low-density lipoproteins (VLDL), which results in reduced lipolysis to LDL cholesterol. Nicotinic acid also increases serum HDL cholesterol concentrations by up to 35% by decreasing lipid transfer of cholesterol from HDL to VLDL and by inhibiting HDL clearance. Nicotinic acid is available in immediate-release (crystalline) and sustained-release formulations.

Ezetimibe. Localizes at intestinal brush border of small intestine Blocks absorption of intestinal cholesterol

Statins (HMG-CoA reductase inhibitors). Reduce cholesterol synthesis, lowering intracellular cholesterol, which stimulates LDL receptor synthesis

Bile acid sequestrants. Bind bile acids in gut, decreasing intracellular cholesterol content, which stimulates LDL receptor synthesis

Nicotinic acid. Decreases hepatic production of VLDL

Fibric acids. Stimulate PPAR-α nuclear receptor, increasing LPL synthesis and decreasing apo CIII synthesis

JOHN A.CRAIG—AD
C.Machado—M.D.

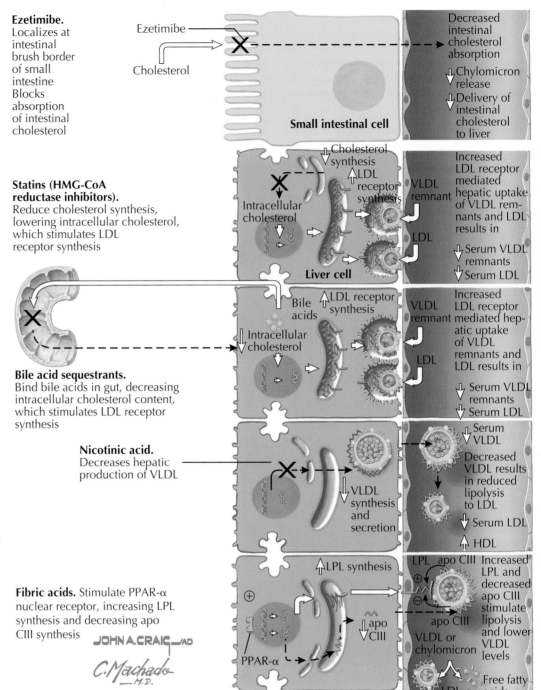

FIBRIC ACIDS

Fibric acids lower serum triglyceride concentrations and increase serum HDL cholesterol concentrations by activation of peroxisome proliferator–activated receptor-α (PPAR-α). Fibric acids reduce serum triglyceride concentrations by reducing hepatic secretion of VLDL and by stimulating lipoprotein lipase (LPL) activity that increases the clearance of triglyceride-enriched lipoproteins. These effects are also mediated by downregulation of apolipoprotein (apo) CIII gene expression. Fibric acids increase serum HDL cholesterol concentrations by stimulating synthesis of apo AI and apo AII. Fibric acid administration lowers serum triglyceride concentrations by 35% to 50%, increases serum HDL cholesterol concentrations by 15% to 25%, and lowers serum lipoprotein(a) concentrations to a variable degree. Currently available fibric acids are gemfibrozil and fenofibrate.

FISH OIL

The active components in fish oil are the long-chain omega-3 fatty acids, eicosapentaenoic acid (EPA, 20:5n-3) and docosahexaenoic acid (DHA, 22:6n-3). Ingested EPA and DHA are absorbed in the small intestine and transported to the liver as triglycerides in chylomicron particles. The liver releases EPA and DHA into the circulation as triglycerides in lipoprotein particles (e.g., LDL cholesterol and HDL cholesterol). EPA and DHA decrease the hepatic secretion of triglyceride-rich lipoproteins; the exact mechanism of this effect is not yet known. Daily intake of 3 to 4 g of EPA and DHA lowers serum triglyceride concentrations by 20% to 50%. Fish oil supplementation also increases serum HDL cholesterol concentrations by 3% and lowers the proportion of small, dense LDL cholesterol.

Plate 7-21

Lipids and Nutrition

VITAMIN C DEFICIENCY: SCURVY

Scurvy is a nutritional deficiency disorder resulting from a lack of vitamin C (ascorbic acid). Known since antiquity, during the fifteenth and sixteenth centuries scurvy became well recognized as an important disorder of seafaring men and was related to lack of fresh foods on prolonged journeys. In 1754, a British naval surgeon Dr. James Lind noted that consumption of oranges or lemons could prevent scurvy. Humans cannot synthesize ascorbic acid, and it is an essential dietary nutrient. Food sources high in ascorbic acid content include citrus fruits, tomatoes, potatoes, cabbage, spinach, Brussels sprouts, cauliflower, broccoli, and strawberries. Scurvy can occur as early as 3 months of being on an ascorbic acid–free diet.

Ascorbic acid is the enolic form of α-ketolactone and functions as a cofactor and cosubstrate in providing reducing equivalents for a number of biochemical reactions involving iron and copper. Ascorbic acid provides electrons needed to reduce molecular oxygen. For example, ascorbic acid serves as an enzymatic cofactor for carnitine synthesis. Ascorbic acid is necessary for normal collagen synthesis, where it is a cofactor for the enzymatic hydroxylation of proline and lysine. Deficiency in this hydroxylation step results in impaired wound healing, defective tooth formation, and impaired osteoblast function. Ascorbic acid is also a cofactor for dopamine β-hydroxylase that converts dopamine to norepinephrine (see Plate 3-26). Absorbed in the jejunum and ileum (see Plate 7-18), blood levels of ascorbic acid are regulated by renal excretion.

Scurvy usually develops with an insidious onset of weakness, malaise, shortness of breath, bone pain, myalgias, arthralgias, edema, neuropathy, and vasomotor instability. Impaired collagen and connective tissue functions result in dry, rough skin with impaired wound healing, hyperkeratotic papules, perifollicular hemorrhages, and follicular hyperkeratosis (hair follicles may be coiled and fragmented). Petechial hemorrhages occur in the lower extremities initially and then may involve the skin around the joints or along other irritated areas. Affected patients have positive test results for the Rumpel-Leede test for abnormal capillary fragility; after inflating the blood pressure cuff between the systolic and diastolic blood pressure for 1 minute, numerous petechial hemorrhages occur. Massive hemorrhages with ecchymoses and proptosis caused by retrobulbar hemorrhage may occur. Hemorrhages into joints result in marked pain, swelling, and immobility. Subungual "splinter" hemorrhages may be seen. Gingival tissues may become swollen, reddish-blue in color, spongy, and friable, and teeth may loosen and fall out.

Subperiosteal hemorrhages in infants with scurvy prompt a less painful "frog leg" position, and infants may have "pseudoparalysis" caused by pain. Radiographs show large periosteal calcium deposits and central epiphyseal lucency. Also in infants, the costochondral junctions may be prominent, which is termed the *scorbutic rosary*. Affected children have impaired growth because of osteoblast dysfunction.

Death may occur in individuals with scurvy because of widespread cerebral petechial hemorrhages with associated hyperpyrexia, tachycardia, cyanosis, hypotension, and Cheyne-Stokes respirations.

DIAGNOSIS

In the United States, scurvy may be seen in severely malnourished individuals. If vitamin C

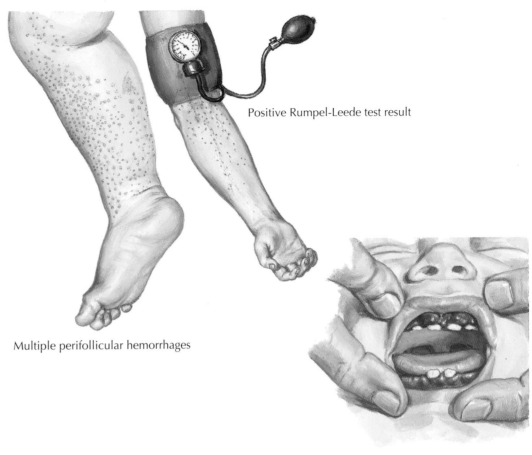

Positive Rumpel-Leede test result

Multiple perifollicular hemorrhages

Swollen, congested, bleeding gums

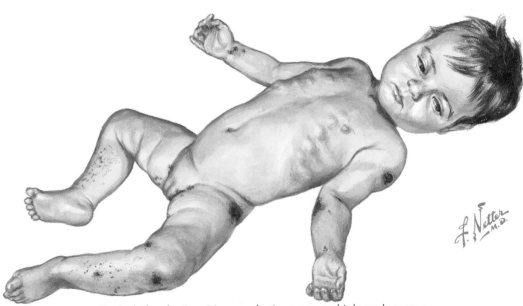

Typical "frog leg" position, scorbutic rosary, multiple ecchymoses

deficiency is suspected, a blood test for ascorbic acid may be performed (reference range, 0.6–2.0 mg/dL; values <0.3 mg/dL indicate significant deficiency).

TREATMENT

Scurvy is treated by the administration of 500 mg daily of ascorbic acid until all signs and symptoms resolve. Also, the factors that predisposed to the dietary deficiency must be addressed.

PREVENTION

The recommended daily dietary allowance of ascorbic acid is 90 mg daily for men and 75 mg daily for women (120 mg daily for pregnant or lactating women). These amounts of ascorbic acid are easily achieved with a balanced diet that includes citrus fruits and vegetables.

Plate 7-22

Endocrine System

Principal food sources of vitamin A

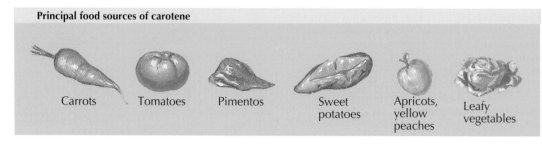

Milk Butter Egg yolk Cod liver oil Certain fish oils Liver Kidneys

VITAMIN A DEFICIENCY

Vitamin A is part of a family of lipid-soluble compounds (retinols, β-carotenes [provitamin A], and carotenoids) referred to as *retinoic acids*. Vitamin A has a major role in phototransduction and cellular differentiation of the eyes, which was recognized by the ancient Egyptians who used liver ingestion to treat poor vision in dim light (referred to as night blindness [nyctalopia]). The best food sources of vitamin A are liver, egg yolk, kidneys, fish oils, and butter. β-Carotene is found in green leafy vegetables, carrots, sweet potatoes, apricots, tomatoes, and pimentos.

β-Carotene is hydrolyzed in the gastrointestinal tract to two molecules of vitamin A. Vitamin A is absorbed in the jejunum and ileum (see Plate 7-18). The enterocytes form retinyl-esters that are incorporated into chylomicrons and released into lymph and plasma. The chylomicrons are then broken down into multiple remnants, including apolipoproteins (apo) B and apo E, which contain retinol esters. Apo B and apo E are then taken up by the liver; the retinol esters are freed and combine with retinol-binding proteins (RBPs) and are stored in vitamin A–containing lipid globules within the hepatic stellate cells. The liver stores 50% to 85% of the total body vitamin A. When released from the liver, vitamin A circulates bound to RBPs.

Vitamin A plays a key role in the function of the retina, growth and differentiation of epithelial tissue, bone growth, and immune function. The two types of retinal photoreceptor cells are cone and rod cells. The rod cells are responsible for night vision and motion detection. The cone cells are responsible for color vision in bright light. Deficiency in vitamin A leads to a deficiency in retinal 11-cis-retinol and rhodopsin, which affects rod vision more than cone vision. Xerophthalmia (keratinization of ocular tissue) is a progressive vitamin A deficiency disorder of night blindness, xerosis (dryness), and keratomalacia (corneal thinning). The xerosis is caused by both poor lacrimal gland function and the conversion of secretory epithelium (goblet mucous cells) to keratinized epithelium (basal cells). Bitot spots are distinctive triangular white patches on the sclera that represent areas of abnormal conjunctival squamous cell proliferation and keratinization. The corneal thinning can lead to perforation of the cornea and permanent blindness. Vitamin A deficiency is also associated with poor bone growth and follicular hyperkeratosis.

DIAGNOSIS

Vitamin A deficiency can occur from inadequate vitamin A ingestion or from malabsorption. When vitamin A deficiency is suspected, it can be confirmed by measuring a serum vitamin A (retinol) level (adult reference range, 325–780 μg/L; severe deficiency <100 μg/L).

Vitamin A

Principal food sources of carotene

Carrots Tomatoes Pimentos Sweet potatoes Apricots, yellow peaches Leafy vegetables

β-carotene

Principal deficiency manifestations

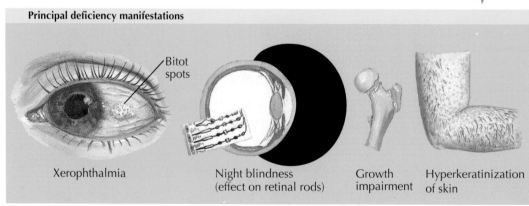

Xerophthalmia — Bitot spots

Night blindness (effect on retinal rods)

Growth impairment

Hyperkeratinization of skin

TREATMENT

Patients with xerophthalmia should be treated with 60 mg of vitamin A and repeated 1 and 14 days later. If the deficiency is not as severe and the presentation is limited (e.g., night blindness and Bitot spots), it may be treated with lower doses of vitamin A (e.g., 3 mg daily for 3 months). In both settings, the cause of the deficiency must be addressed.

PREVENTION

The recommended daily allowance for retinol in the United States is 900 μg/d for men and 700 μg/d women (1.4 mg/d during pregnancy and lactation). One μg of retinol is equivalent to 12 μg of β-carotene. The recommended daily amounts of retinol and β-carotene equivalents are easily obtained with a nutritious diet that is rich in milk, eggs, fish, butter, and yellow and dark green vegetables.

GENETICS AND ENDOCRINE NEOPLASIA

Plate 8-1

Genetics and Endocrine Neoplasia

MULTIPLE ENDOCRINE NEOPLASIA TYPE 1

Multiple endocrine neoplasia type 1 (MEN 1) is a rare (prevalence ~two per 100,000) autosomal dominant endocrine disorder that is characterized by neoplasms of the pituitary, parathyroid, and pancreas. In addition, neoplasms may arise in the adrenal glands, duodenum (gastrinoma), lung (carcinoid tumor), thymus gland (carcinoid tumor), and esophagus (leiomyoma). An MEN1 mutation is highly probable in a patient with two of the three main MEN 1 tumor types (pituitary, parathyroid, or gastroenteropancreatic [GEP] endocrine neoplasms).

Primary hyperparathyroidism is the most common manifestation of MEN 1; the penetrance is 100% by age 50 years. The diagnosis is biochemical with documentation of hypercalcemia and a nonsuppressed serum parathyroid hormone (PTH) concentration. All four (or occasionally five) of the parathyroid glands are involved, and removing 3.5 of the parathyroid glands is the treatment of choice. Recurrent hypercalcemia may require reoperation or percutaneous ethanol injection.

Pituitary adenomas are found in 20% of patients with MEN 1. Prolactinomas are the most common pituitary tumor. However, all pituitary tumor cell types have been identified in MEN 1 kindreds, including growth hormone (GH), corticotropin (adrenocorticotropic hormone [ACTH]), gonadotropin, and null cell. The management of pituitary tumors in patients with MEN 1 is the same as that for patients with sporadic pituitary neoplasms (see Plates 1-19 to 1-24).

The GEP neoplasms are the major life-threatening manifestation of MEN 1. Pancreatic islet cell (often nonfunctioning) and duodenal carcinoid tumors are frequently malignant and may metastasize. Peptic ulcer disease is the most common symptomatic presentation related to GEP tumors and is caused by gastrin-secreting neoplasms (Zollinger-Ellison syndrome). Zollinger-Ellison syndrome is the initial manifestation of MEN 1 in 40% of patients. The gastrinomas are frequently small, multifocal, and localized to the duodenum. The hypercalcemia from primary hyperparathyroidism may aggravate gastrin hypersecretion in Zollinger-Ellison syndrome. Thus, normalization of the serum calcium concentration is important in the management of patients with this syndrome. Proton pump inhibitors very effectively control the signs and symptoms related to hypergastrinemia. Removal of the gastrin-secreting duodenal carcinoids may be considered at the time of a pancreatic operation.

The pancreatic islet tumors may hypersecrete insulin, glucagon, human pancreatic polypeptide, chromogranin A, and vasoactive intestinal polypeptide. Insulinomas in MEN 1 may be small and numerous (see Plate 5-22). Cushing syndrome (see Plate 3-9) in individuals with MEN 1 may be caused by an ACTH-secreting pituitary tumor, a cortisol-secreting adrenal adenoma, or ectopic ACTH secretion from an islet cell tumor. Symptomatic islet cell tumors (e.g., insulinomas) should be resected. Pancreatic surgery should also be considered in patients with MEN 1 when a nonfunctioning pancreatic islet cell tumor is approaching 2 cm in diameter; larger islet cell tumors are more likely to be malignant and are prone to metastasize. The hormonal status of the GEP tumors can be monitored by annual measurement of gastrin, glucagon, human pancreatic polypeptide, and chromogranin A.

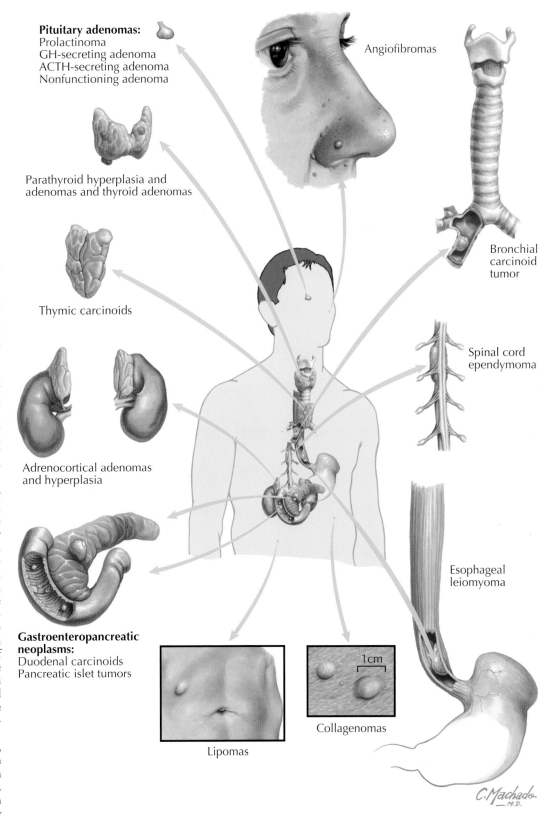

Pituitary adenomas:
Prolactinoma
GH-secreting adenoma
ACTH-secreting adenoma
Nonfunctioning adenoma

Angiofibromas

Parathyroid hyperplasia and adenomas and thyroid adenomas

Thymic carcinoids

Bronchial carcinoid tumor

Spinal cord ependymoma

Adrenocortical adenomas and hyperplasia

Esophageal leiomyoma

Gastroenteropancreatic neoplasms:
Duodenal carcinoids
Pancreatic islet tumors

Lipomas

Collagenomas

1cm

C. Machado _M.D._

Patients with MEN 1 may have several skin manifestations. Angiofibromas, collagenomas, and subcutaneous lipomas occur in about 75% of patients with MEN 1. The dermal and subcutaneous lesions are benign and should be removed only if symptomatic. Patients with MEN 1 are also at risk of developing spinal cord ependymomas.

The MEN1 protein product is menin, and most MEN1 mutations inactivate or disrupt menin function.

This tumor suppressor gene has no strong genotype–phenotype correlations. Most individuals with MEN 1 inherit 1 inactivated copy of MEN1 from an affected parent; tumorigenesis requires the subsequent somatic inactivation (e.g., gene deletion) of the remaining normal copy in a cell from a susceptible gland (e.g., parathyroid, pituitary, and pancreas). When an endocrine cell lacks menin tumor suppressor function, it begins the process of proliferation and neoplasia.

Plate 8-2

Endocrine System

MULTIPLE ENDOCRINE NEOPLASIA TYPE 2

Multiple endocrine neoplasia type 2 (MEN 2) is an autosomal dominant disorder with an estimated prevalence of 2.5 per 100,000 in the general population, and it is classified into three distinct syndromes—MEN 2A, MEN 2B, and familial medullary thyroid cancer (FMTC). MEN 2A is characterized by medullary thyroid cancer (MTC) in all patients, pheochromocytoma in 50%, primary hyperparathyroidism in 20%, and cutaneous lichen amyloidosis in 5%. MEN 2B is characterized by MTC in all patients, pheochromocytoma in 50%, mucocutaneous neuromas (typically involving the tongue, lips, and eyelids) in most patients, skeletal deformities (kyphoscoliosis or lordosis), joint laxity, myelinated corneal nerves, and intestinal ganglioneuromas (Hirschsprung disease). FMTC is a variant of MEN 2A, and the clinical presentation is limited to MTC.

MEDULLARY THYROID CARCINOMA

MTC is a neuroendocrine tumor of the parafollicular C cells of the thyroid gland and accounts for approximately 3% to 5% of all primary thyroid cancers. C cells—representing 0.1% of thyroid mass and concentrated in the upper third of the thyroid gland—are neuroendocrine cells derived from the ultimobranchial bodies. Multicentric C-cell hyperplasia is found in all patients with MEN 2, and nearly all eventually develop MTC. The C cells produce calcitonin, a 32–amino acid peptide that regulates blood calcium levels in fish. However, a physiologic role for this hormone in humans is unknown. MTC in MEN 2 is multicentric and is concentrated in the upper third of the thyroid gland, reflecting the normal distribution of C cells. Approximately 25% of all patients with MTC have a family history of this disease. whereas in MEN 2A and FMTC, the peak incidence of clinical detection of index cases is in the third decade of life, the typical age of presentation of sporadic MTC is in the fifth to sixth decades of life. When diagnosed as an index case, the clinical presentation (e.g., thyroid nodule) and manifestations (e.g., cervical adenopathy) of MEN 2–associated MTC are similar to those of sporadic MTC. Serum calcitonin concentrations have a positive correlation with tumor mass. MTC in patients with MEN 2B is earlier in onset and more aggressive (e.g., metastatic disease at a young age).

PHEOCHROMOCYTOMA

Pheochromocytomas—affecting approximately 50% of patients with MEN 2A and 2B—frequently involve both adrenal glands and are multicentric. MTC is usually detected before pheochromocytoma in patients with MEN 2. In this patient population, pheochromocytomas are typically diagnosed when asymptomatic because of routine annual case-detection testing. However, patients with MEN 2 who are not followed up regularly or who are new index cases may present with symptoms of pheochromocytoma such as paroxysms of hypertension, forceful heart beat, hyperhidrosis, headache, and pallor.

PRIMARY HYPERPARATHYROIDISM

Approximately 20% of patients with MEN 2A have primary hyperparathyroidism, and when it occurs, two or more parathyroid glands are involved.

MEN 2A

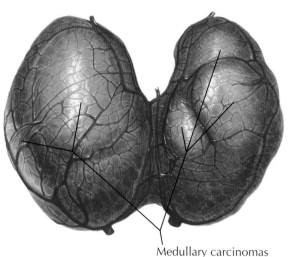

Medullary carcinomas

Multicentric C-cell hyperplasia, which eventually evolves into multicentric medullary thyroid carcinoma.

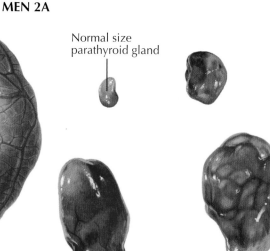

Normal size parathyroid gland

Approximately 20% of patients with MEN 2A have primary hyperparathyroidism, and when it occurs, 2 or more parathyroid glands are involved.

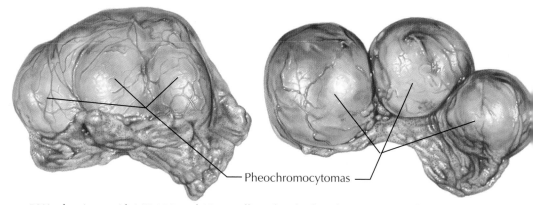

Pheochromocytomas

50% of patients with MEN 2A and 2B are affected with pheochromocytomas that are usually multicentric involve both adrenal glands

Cutaneous lichen amyloidosis is a rare, pruritic, papular, scaly, and pigmented skin lesion that is typically located in the interscapular region or on the extensor surfaces of the extremities that occurs in 5% of patients with MEN 2A.

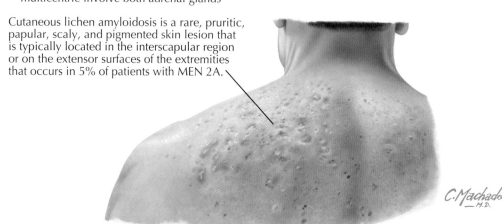

CUTANEOUS LICHEN AMYLOIDOSIS

Cutaneous lichen amyloidosis is a rare skin disorder that may occur in patients with MEN 2A. It is a pruritic, papular, scaly, and pigmented skin lesion that is typically located in the interscapular region or on the extensor surfaces of the extremities.

HIRSCHSPRUNG DISEASE

Hirschsprung disease may occur in individuals with MEN 2B and is characterized by the absence of autonomic ganglion cells within the distal colon parasympathetic plexus, resulting in chronic obstruction and megacolon.

Plate 8-3

Genetics and Endocrine Neoplasia

MULTIPLE ENDOCRINE NEOPLASIA TYPE 2 (Continued)

GENETICS

MEN 2A, MEN 2B, and FMTC are inherited in an autosomal dominant pattern with a high degree of penetrance. The mutations causing these disorders occur in the *RET* proto-oncogene on chromosome 10. The RET protein is a receptor tyrosine kinase that controls growth and differentiation signals in several tissues, including those derived from the neural crest. Interestingly, there is overlap in the specific *RET* mutations causing MEN 2A and FMTC; however, MEN 2B is caused by different *RET* mutations. Most mutations in MEN 2A kindreds (93%–98%) and in FMTC kindreds (80%–96%) involve one of six cysteine residues in the cysteine-rich region of the RET protein's extracellular domain encoded in *RET* exons 10 (codons 609, 611, 618, and 620) or 11 (codons 630 or 634).

Eighty-five percent of individuals with MEN 2A have a mutation in codon 634, particularly p.Cys634Arg. These extracellular MEN 2A/FMTC cysteine mutations lead to constitutive activation of intracellular signaling pathways. Less common mutations in MEN 2A and FMTC occur in exon 13 (codons 790 and 791). MEN 2B–associated tumors are caused by mutations in the RET protein's intracellular domain. A single methionine to threonine missense mutation in exon 16 (p.Met918Thr) is responsible for more than 95% of MEN 2B cases. Another mutation—alanine to phenylalanine at codon 883 in exon 15—has been found in 4% of MEN 2B kindreds. Other infrequent missense mutations in exons 14, 15, and 16 (codons 804, 806, 904, and 922) have been found in individuals with MEN 2B. Germline mutations in codons 768 (exon 13), 804 (exon 14), and 891 (exon 15) are found only in FMTC but account for a minority of FMTC cases.

The germline *RET* mutations causing MEN 2 and FMTC result in a gain-of-function defect; this is different from almost all other inherited neoplasia syndromes, which are caused by heritable "loss of function" mutations that inactivate tumor suppressor proteins. Other mutations in *RET* can produce disorders seemingly unrelated to MEN 2. For example, tissue-specific inactivating mutations of *RET* have been associated with Hirschsprung disease (congenital megacolon). Thus, in some families with a *RET* mutation, both Hirschsprung disease and MEN 2B are present.

There are genotype–phenotype correlations in MEN 2 that help direct clinical management. For example, the risk of MTC has been stratified into three categories according to *RET* mutations:

- Children with MEN 2B or *RET* mutations in codons 883, 918, or 922 have the highest risk of aggressive MTC and should undergo total thyroidectomy with central node dissection within the first 6 months of life.
- Children with *RET* mutations in codons 611, 618, 620, or 634 have a high risk of MTC. Total thyroidectomy should be performed before age 5 years, with or without central node dissection.
- Children with *RET* mutations in codons 609, 768, 790, 791, 804, or 891 have a less aggressive and slowly growing MTC and may be operated at a later stage. Some clinicians recommend a prophylactic thyroidectomy by age 5 years, but others suggest thyroidectomy by age 10 years.
- For individuals with other known *RET* mutations, no specific recommendations can be made at

present because there is not sufficient experience with these kindreds.

Genetic information can also be useful to assess the risk of developing pheochromocytoma. Individuals with *RET* mutations in codons 609, 611, 618, 620, 630, 634, 790, 883, 918, or 922 (or the specific mutation p.Val804Leu) should have annual biochemical screening. In contrast, it is unlikely that pheochromocytoma will develop in patients with mutations in codon 768 or in those with the mutation p.Val804Met.

Genetic testing for mutations in the *RET* protooncogene is commercially available and should be considered for patients with bilateral pheochromocytoma, family history of pheochromocytoma, or cophenotype

disorders. More than 95% of patients with MEN 2A and more than 98% of those with MEN 2B have an identifiable mutation in the *RET* protooncogene. In a family with MEN 2, a family member with a clinical diagnosis of MEN 2 should be tested first. When a *RET* mutation is found, all family members of unknown status should be offered genotyping. Genetic counseling consultation should be considered before genetic testing is performed. In families with known MEN 2, genetic testing shortly after birth facilitates prompt surgical management of the thyroid gland—an element of care especially important in MEN 2B families in which the thyroid gland should be removed in the first 6 months of life.

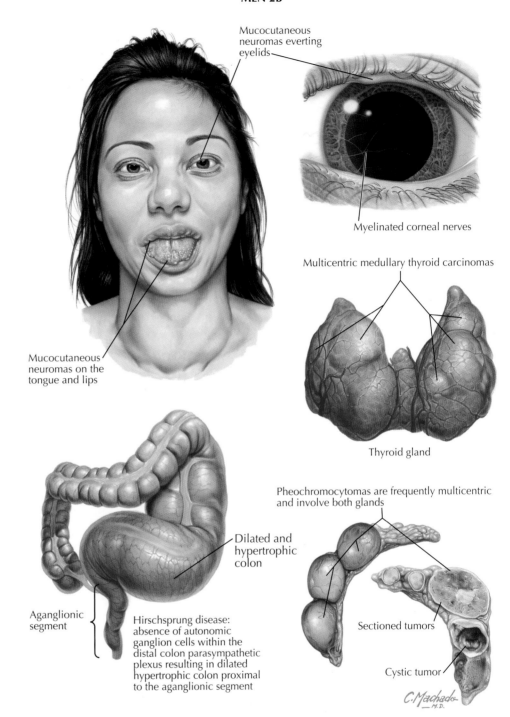

MEN 2B

Mucocutaneous neuromas everting eyelids

Myelinated corneal nerves

Multicentric medullary thyroid carcinomas

Thyroid gland

Mucocutaneous neuromas on the tongue and lips

Pheochromocytomas are frequently multicentric and involve both glands

Dilated and hypertrophic colon

Aganglionic segment

Hirschsprung disease: absence of autonomic ganglion cells within the distal colon parasympathetic plexus resulting in dilated hypertrophic colon proximal to the aganglionic segment

Sectioned tumors

Cystic tumor

Plate 8-4

Endocrine System

VON HIPPEL–LINDAU SYNDROME

von Hippel–Lindau (VHL) syndrome is an autosomal dominant disorder that may present with a variety of benign and malignant neoplasms, including pheochromocytoma (frequently bilateral), paraganglioma (mediastinal, abdominal, pelvic), hemangioblastoma (involving the cerebellum, spinal cord, or brain stem), retinal angioma, clear cell renal cell carcinoma (RCC), pancreatic neuroendocrine tumors, endolymphatic sac tumors of the middle ear, serous cystadenomas of the pancreas, and papillary cystadenomas of the epididymis and broad ligament. The average age of symptomatic presentation is 26 years. Retinal angiomas and cerebellar hemangioblastomas are usually detected in the third decade of life; RCC is typically detected in the fifth decade. Penetrance is very high; the probability of developing RCC, retinal angiomas, and cerebellar hemangioblastomas is approximately 75%. Pheochromocytoma occurs in 20% of patients with VHL syndrome, and the occurrence depends on the subtype of VHL (see following text). The most common cause of death in patients with VHL syndrome is RCC.

Patients with VHL syndrome may be divided into two groups: type I and type II. Patients from kindreds with type I syndrome do not develop pheochromocytoma, but patients from kindreds with type II syndrome are at high risk for developing pheochromocytoma. In addition, kindreds with type II VHL syndrome are subdivided into type IIA (low risk for RCC), type IIB (high risk for RCC), and type IIC (pheochromocytomas only).

The prevalence of VHL is approximately one in 35,000 persons. The *VHL* tumor suppressor gene, chromosomal location 3p25-26, encodes a protein that regulates hypoxia-induced proteins. More than 300 germline *VHL* mutations have been identified that lead to loss of function of the VHL protein. Nearly 100% of patients with VHL have an identifiable gene mutation. Genotype–phenotype correlations have been documented for this disorder, and specific mutations are associated with particular patterns of tumor formation. In up to 98% of cases, pheochromocytoma is associated with missense mutations, rather than truncating or null mutations, in the *VHL* gene. Certain missense mutations appear to be associated with the type IIC presentation of VHL (pheochromocytomas only). Genetic testing for VHL is commercially available and should be considered for patients with bilateral pheochromocytoma, family history of pheochromocytoma, diagnosis of pheochromocytoma at a young age (i.e., 30 years or younger), or cophenotype disorders.

Pheochromocytomas and paragangliomas occurring in patients with VHL produce predominately norepinephrine and normetanephrine. Patients with VHL should have annual biochemical testing for catecholamine-secreting neoplasms.

Hemangioblastomas are vascular neoplasms that are benign and usually do not invade locally or metastasize. They may be asymptomatic or cause mass-effect symptoms because of pressure on adjacent structures or hemorrhage. Annual or every 2-year imaging surveillance (e.g., magnetic resonance imaging [MRI] of brain and spine) is indicated. However, surgery or stereotactic radiotherapy (or both) is typically reserved for rapidly growing or symptomatic lesions.

RCC is typically multicentric and bilateral and may arise in conjunction with cysts or from noncystic renal parenchyma. Early tumor detection and selective resec-

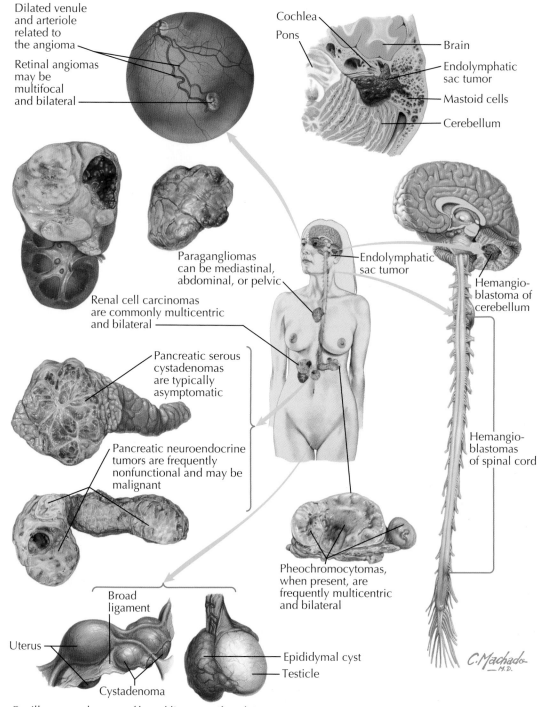

Dilated venule and arteriole related to the angioma

Retinal angiomas may be multifocal and bilateral

Cochlea
Pons
Brain
Endolymphatic sac tumor
Mastoid cells
Cerebellum

Paragangliomas can be mediastinal, abdominal, or pelvic

Renal cell carcinomas are commonly multicentric and bilateral

Endolymphatic sac tumor

Hemangioblastoma of cerebellum

Pancreatic serous cystadenomas are typically asymptomatic

Pancreatic neuroendocrine tumors are frequently nonfunctional and may be malignant

Hemangioblastomas of spinal cord

Pheochromocytomas, when present, are frequently multicentric and bilateral

Broad ligament

Uterus

Epididymal cyst
Testicle

Cystadenoma

Papillary cystadenoma of broad ligament (female) and epididymal cysts (male) are benign and frequently bilateral

tion with renal-sparing surgery or ablative therapies is the optimal management strategy. Annual imaging (e.g., computed tomography, MRI, or ultrasonography) of the kidneys is indicated.

Retinal angiomas develop in the retina and within the optic nerve and may be multifocal and bilateral. Annual ophthalmologic examinations are indicated. When left untreated, these lesions can hemorrhage and lead to vision loss. Laser photocoagulation and cryotherapy are very effective treatments for angiomas that do not involve the optic nerve.

Pancreatic abnormalities in VHL syndrome are common and include simple cysts (70%), serous cystadenomas (10%), and neuroendocrine tumors (20%). The cysts and serous cystadenomas are typically asymp-

tomatic. The neuroendocrine tumors of the pancreas are similar to those found in multiple endocrine neoplasia type 1, and they are frequently nonfunctional; however, they may cause symptoms related to hormone hypersecretion (e.g., glucagon, insulin, vasoactive intestinal polypeptide), and they can metastasize. The pancreas should be visualized at the time of annual renal imaging.

The epididymal cysts (frequently bilateral) in men and the papillary cystadenomas in the broad ligament in women are benign and usually asymptomatic. Papillary cystadenomas of the endolymphatic sac are vascular lesions arising within the posterior temporal bone, and affected patients may present with tinnitus, hearing loss, and vertigo.

GLOSSARY OF ABBREVIATIONS

$1,25[OH]_2D$ 1,25-dihydroxyvitamin D (calcitriol)
3β-HSD1 3β-hydroxysteroid dehydrogenase type I isozyme
3β-HSD2 3β-hydroxysteroid dehydrogenase type II isozyme
5-HIAA 5-hydroxyindoleacetic acid
11β-HSD1 11β-hydroxysteroid dehydrogenase type 1
11β-HSD2 11β-hydroxysteroid dehydrogenase type 2
17β-HSD1 17β-ketosteroid reductase
17β-HSD2 17β-hydroxysteroid dehydrogenase
17β-HSD3 17β-ketosteroid reductase
17-OHP 17-hydroxyprogesterone
25[OH]D 25-hydroxyvitamin D (calcidiol)
AADC aromatic L-amino acid decarboxylase
ACAT acyl-CoA: cholesterol acyltransferase
ACE angiotensin-converting enzyme
ACTH adrenocorticotropic hormone (corticotropin)
ADH antidiuretic hormone
ADP adenosine diphosphate
AGI α-glucosidase inhibitor
AIH androgen insensitivity syndrome
AIMAH adrenocorticotropic hormone–independent macronodular adrenal hyperplasia
AMH antimüllerian hormone
APA aldosterone-producing adenoma
APECED autoimmune polyendocrinopathy–candidiasis–ectodermal dystrophy
apo apolipoprotein
APS1 autoimmune polyglandular syndrome type I
APS2 autoimmune polyglandular syndrome type II
ARB angiotensin receptor blocker
ATC anaplastic thyroid carcinoma
ATP adenosine triphosphate
ATP III Adult Treatment Panel III
AVS adrenal venous sampling

BAAF Bensley acid aniline fuchsin
BMD bone mineral density
BMI body mass index

Ca^{2+} calcium
CAH congenital adrenal hyperplasia
CAIS complete androgen insensitivity syndrome
cAMP cyclic adenosine monophosphate
CaSR calcium-sensing receptor
CBG cortisol-binding globulin
CETP cholesteryl ester transfer protein
CHD coronary heart disease
CNS central nervous system
CoA coenzyme A
COMT catechol *O*-methyltransferase
CRH corticotropin-releasing hormone
CSII continuous subcutaneous insulin infusion
CT computed tomography
CTX c-telopeptide crosslink or cerebrotendinous xanthomatosis
CXR chest radiograph

DA dopamine
DBH dopamine β-hydroxylase
DD disc diameter
DHA docosahexaenoic acid
Dhal-1 dehalogenase 1 isoenzyme
DHEA dehydroepiandrosterone
DHEA-S dehydroepiandrosterone sulfate
DHT dihydrotestosterone
DI diabetes insipidus
DIDMOAD diabetes insipidus, diabetes mellitus, optic atrophy, and deafness
DIT diiodotyrosine
DKA diabetic ketoacidosis
DNA deoxyribonucleic acid
DOC deoxycorticosterone
DPP-IV dipeptidyl peptidase IV
DR diabetic retinopathy
DSD disorder of sex development
DSPN distal symmetric polyneuropathy
DST dexamethasone suppression test
DXA dual energy–x-ray absorptiometry

EPA eicosapentaenoic acid
ER endoplasmic reticulum
ESR erythrocyte sedimentation rate
ESRD end-stage renal disease

FAD flavin adenine dinucleotide
FGF23 fibroblast growth factor 23
FH familial hypercholesterolemia or familial hyperaldosteronism
FHH familial hypocalciuric hypercalcemia
FISH fluorescence in situ hybridization
FMTC familial medullary thyroid carcinoma
FNA fine-needle aspiration
FRAX fracture risk assessment tool
FSH follicle-stimulating hormone
FTC follicular thyroid carcinoma

GABA γ-aminobutyric acid
GAD glutamic acid decarboxylase
GAG glycosaminoglycan
Gb3 globotriaosylceramide
GCT glucose challenge test
GD Gaucher disease
GDM gestational diabetes mellitus
GEP gastroenteropancreatic
GFR glomerular filtration rate
GH growth hormone
GHRH growth hormone–releasing hormone
GI gastrointestinal
GIP gastric inhibitory polypeptide
GLP-1 glucagon-like peptide 1
GLUT glucose transporter
GnRH gonadotropin-releasing hormone
GRA glucocorticoid-remediable aldosteronism
GTP guanosine triphosphate

H&E hematoxylin-eosin
HbA_{1c} hemoglobin A_{1c}
HCC Hürthle cell carcinoma
HCO_3 bicarbonate
hCG human chorionic gonadotropin
hCS human chorionic somatomammotropin
HDL high-density lipoprotein
Hex A hexosaminidase A
HIF hypoxia-inducible factor
HLA human leukocyte antigen
HMG-CoA 3-hydroxy-3-methylglutaryl coenzyme A
HNF hepatocyte nuclear factor
HPT hyperparathyroidism
HVA homovanillic acid

I^- inorganic iodine
IF intrinsic factor
Ig immunoglobulin
IGF-1 insulinlike growth factor 1
IHA bilateral idiopathic hyperaldosteronism
IP3 inositol triphosphate
IPEX immunodysregulation polyendocrinopathy enteropathy X-linked syndrome
IPSS inferior petrosal sinus sampling
IRS insulin receptor substrate
IVC inferior vena cava

JNC7 Seventh Report of the Joint National Committee on Prevention, Detection, Evaluation, and Treatment of High Blood Pressure

K^+ potassium
$KClO_4^-$ potassium perchlorate

LCAT lecithin-cholesterol acyltransferase
LDL low-density lipoprotein
LH luteinizing hormone
Lp(a) lipoprotein(a)
LPL lipoprotein lipase

MAO monoamine oxidase
MAPK mitogen-activated protein kinase
MDI multiple daily injections
MEN 1 multiple endocrine neoplasia type 1
MEN 2 multiple endocrine neoplasia type 2
MI myocardial infarction
MIBG metaiodobenzylguanidine
MIT monoiodotyrosine
MLD metachromatic leukodystrophy
MODY maturity-onset diabetes of the young
MR mineralocorticoid receptor
MRI magnetic resonance imaging
MTC medullary thyroid carcinoma

NAD nicotinamide adenine dinucleotide
NADP nicotinamide adenine dinucleotide phosphate
NCEP National Cholesterol Education Program
NF1 neurofibromatosis type 1
NIPHS noninsulinoma pancreatogenous hypoglycemia syndrome
NIS sodium-iodide symporter
NPD Niemann-Pick disease
NPDR nonproliferative diabetic retinopathy
NPH neutral protamine Hagedorn
NTX N-telopeptide crosslinks
NVD neovascularization at the disc
NVE neovascularization elsewhere

OGTT oral glucose tolerance test
OI osteogenesis imperfecta

P450aro aromatase
P450c11AS aldosterone synthase
P450c11β 11β-hydroxylase
P450c17 17α-hydroxylase
P450c21 21-hydroxylase
P450scc cholesterol side-chain cleavage (desmolase)
PA primary aldosteronism
PAC plasma aldosterone concentration
PAIS partial androgen insensitivity syndrome
PAS periodic acid–Schiff

PCOS polycystic ovary syndrome
PDR proliferative diabetic retinopathy
PHP pseudohypoparathyroidism
PI3 kinase phophatidylinositol-3-kinase
PMDS persistent müllerian duct syndrome
PNMT phenylethanolamine *N*-methyltransferase
POEMS syndrome polyneuropathy, organomegaly, endocrinopathy, edema, M-protein, and skin abnormalities
PPAR α peroxisome proliferator–activated receptor α
PPNAD primary pigmented nodular adrenocortical disease
PRA plasma renin activity
PTC papillary thyroid carcinoma
PTH parathyroid hormone
PTHrP parathyroid hormone–related protein
POMC pro-opiomelanocortin
PPAR peroxisome proliferator-activated receptor
PVN paraventricular nucleus

RAAS renin–angiotensin–aldosterone system
RANK receptor activator of NF-κ B

RANKL NF-κB ligand
RBP retinol-binding proteins
rT$_3$ reverse triiodothyronine
RYGB Roux-en-Y gastric bypass

SD standard deviation
SDH succinate dehydrogenase
SHBG sex hormone–binding globulin
SMBG self-monitoring of blood glucose
SON supraoptic nucleus
SREBP sterol regulatory element–binding protein
StAR steroidogenic acute regulatory protein
SUR sulfonylurea receptor

T$_2$ diiodothyronine
T$_3$ triiodothyronine
T$_4$ thyroxine
TBG thyroxine-binding globulin
TC transcobalamins
TCA tricarboxylic acid
Tg thyroglobulin
TGRL triglyceride-rich lipoproteins
TH tyrosine hydroxylase

THOX2 thyroid oxidase 2
TPO thyroid peroxidase
TRH thyrotropin-releasing hormone
TSH thyrotropin
TZD thiazolidinedione

UAH unilateral adrenal hyperplasia
UFC urinary free cortisol
U:L ratio upper body to lower body segment ratio
UDP uridine diphosphate
UDPGlc uridine diphosphate glucose
UTI urinary tract infection
UTP uridine triphosphate

VHL von Hippel–Lindau
VLDL very low-density lipoprotein
VMA vanillylmandelic acid
VMAT vesicular monoamine transporter

ZF adrenal zona fasciculata
ZG adrenal zona glomerulosa
ZR adrenal zona reticularis

Gynecomastia, 125
  in Klinefelter syndrome, 116
  neonatal, 125
  pathologic conditions causing, 125
  pubertal, 107, 125

H

Hair
  in adrenal insufficiency, 91
  axillary, development of, 84, 106, 107
  facial, development of, 107
  growth phases of, 120
  in hypothyroidism, 49, 50
  male-pattern
    adrenal androgen effects on, 84
    in women. See Hirsutism.
  pubic, development of, 84, 105, 106, 107
  thinning of, in Cushing syndrome, 76
Hashimoto thyroiditis, 51, 56, 218
Head trauma, hypopituitarism from, 14
Heart, enlarged, in hypothyroidism, 49
Heart disease
  carcinoid, 219
  coronary. See also Atherosclerosis.
    diabetes mellitus and, 145
    hypercholesterolemia and, 188, 189, 194, 196
    risk factors for, 196
  valvular, in carcinoid tumors, 219
Heart failure, in Graves disease, 44
Height
  excessive, growth hormone–induced, 21
  loss of, in osteoporosis, 170
  velocity of, during puberty, 105
Hemangioblastoma, in von Hippel-Lindau syndrome, 216
Hemianopsia, from pituitary tumors, 13
Hemorrhage
  of adrenal glands, 90
  perifollicular, in scurvy, 203
  of pituitary gland, 20
  uterine, causes of, 124
Henle, loop of, in water homeostasis, 28
Hepatosplenomegaly, in hypertriglyceridemia, 192
Hermaphroditism
  pseudo-, 111–113
  true, 113, 114
Hirata disease, 218
Hirschsprung disease, 214, 215
Hirsutism, 85, 120–121
  causes of, 120–121
  in Cushing syndrome, 76
  definition of, 120
  evaluation of, 121
Histiocytosis, Langerhans cell, 29, 30, 31
HLA (human leukocyte antigen) phenotypes, in diabetes
    mellitus, 139
HMG-CoA reductase, 183
HMG-CoA reductase inhibitors. See Statins.
Homonymous hemianopsia, from pituitary tumors, 13
Homovanillic acid, 95
Human chorionic gonadotropin, reproductive cycle
    influence of, 122, 123
Human leukocyte antigen (HLA) phenotypes, in diabetes
    mellitus, 139
Hürthle cell thyroid carcinoma, 61
Hydrocephalus
  in craniopharyngioma, 12
  in neurofibromatosis type 1, 217
Hydrocortisone
  for adrenal crisis, 90
  for adrenal insufficiency, 93
  for corticotropin-secreting pituitary tumor, 24
3-Hydroxy-3-methylglutaryl coenzyme A (HMG-CoA),
    183
Hydroxyapatite, 155
5-Hydroxyindole acetic acid, in carcinoid tumors, 219
11ß-Hydroxylase, 74
  deficiency of, 81, 83
17α-Hydroxylase, 74
  deficiency of, 81, 82

α1-Hydroxylase deficiency, 172
21-Hydroxylase deficiency, 81, 83
3ß-Hydroxysteroid dehydrogenase, 74
  deficiency of, 81, 82
    late-onset, 85
11ß-Hydroxysteroid dehydrogenase, 74
  deficiency of, 83
    late-onset, 85
17ß-Hydroxysteroid dehydrogenase, 74
Hyoid bone, 36, 37
Hyperalgesia, in diabetes mellitus, 144
Hyperapobetalipoproteinemia, familial, 187
Hypercalcemia
  clinical manifestations of, 155
  differential diagnosis of, 159
  hyperparathyroidism and, 157, 158, 159
  hypocalciuric, familial, 159
  parathyroid hormone–mediated, 159
Hypercholesterolemia, 187
  coronary heart disease risk and, 188, 189, 194, 196
  etiology of, 187
  familial, 185, 187, 188–189, 191
  guidelines on, 187
  polygenic, 185
  xanthomatosis in, 188–189
Hypercortisolism
  in Cushing syndrome, 76, 78
  in primary pigmented nodular adrenocortical disease,
    80
Hyperglycemia
  in diabetes mellitus, 139, 140, 148
  maternal, 147
  treatment of, 148
Hyperinsulinism. See Insulin resistance
    (hyperinsulinemia).
Hyperkalemia, in adrenal insufficiency, 92
Hyperkeratinization, in vitamin A deficiency, 204
Hyperlipemia retinalis, 193
Hyperlipidemia
  coronary heart disease risk and, 194, 196
  familial combined, 187, 191
  monitoring in, 199
  prevention of, 199
  treatment of, 199
Hyperlipoproteinemia
  classification of, 191
  type I, 191
  type III, 185, 191
  type IV, 191
  type V, 191
Hypernatremia, in adrenal insufficiency, 92
Hyperparathyroidism
  histology in, 162
  hypercalcemia and, 157, 158, 159
  in multiple endocrine neoplasia, 213, 214
  in osteoporosis, 167
  in Paget disease of bone, 177
  primary
    clinical manifestations of, 158
    pathology of, 158
    pathophysiology of, 157
  in pseudohypoparathyroidism type 1, 166
  in renal osteodystrophy, 160, 161
Hyperphosphatemia
  in hypoparathyroidism, 163
  in renal osteodystrophy, 160
Hyperpigmentation
  in adrenal insufficiency, 91
  in carcinoid tumors, 219
  in Nelson syndrome, 25
Hyperprolactinemia, 23
  from clinically nonfunctioning pituitary tumor,
    26
  galactorrhea in, 126
Hyperreflexia, in hypocalcemia, 164
Hypertension
  in aldosteronism, 87, 89
  coronary heart disease risk and, 196
  in diabetic nephropathy, 143
  in hypothyroidism, 49

Hypertension (Continued)
  in neurofibromatosis type 1, 217
  renovascular, in renal artery stenosis, 89
Hyperthecosis, 121
Hyperthyroidism
  in Graves disease, 43
  gynecomastia in, 125
  hypercalcemia in, 159
  in toxic adenoma and toxic multinodular goiter, 47, 48
Hypertriglyceridemia, 191–193
  in apolipoprotein CII deficiency, 192, 193
  borderline, 191
  clinical manifestations of, 192
  familial, 191, 193
  in lipoprotein lipase deficiency, 192–193
  mixed, 191
  risk factors for, 191
  treatment of, 193, 199
Hypesthesia, in diabetes mellitus, 144
Hypocalcemia
  acute, clinical manifestations of, 164
  in autoimmune polyglandular syndrome type I, 218
  clinical manifestations of, 155
  in hypoparathyroidism, 163
  in pseudohypoparathyroidism type 1, 166
Hypoglycemia
  in adrenal insufficiency, 93
  differential diagnosis of, 151
  from insulinoma, 150
  from islet-cell hyperplasia, 151
  noninsulinoma pancreatogenous, 151
Hypogonadism
  gynecomastia in, 125
  hypogonadotropic, prolactin-dependent, 23
  from hypothalamic lesions, 11
  primary, in autoimmune polyglandular syndrome type I
    and II, 218
Hypokalemia, in aldosteronism, 87
Hyponatremia, in adrenal insufficiency, 93
Hypoparathyroidism
  in autoimmune polyglandular syndrome type I, 218
  congenital, 163
  pathophysiology of, 163
Hypophosphatasia, 175, 180
Hypophosphatemia
  in hypercalcemia, 159
  osteomalacia in, 175
Hypophosphatemic rickets, 173
Hypophyseal artery, 5, 9
Hypophyseal fossa, 8
Hypophyseal portal system, 5
Hypophyseal portal vein, 5
Hypophyseal vein, 5
Hypophysis. See Pituitary gland.
Hypophysitis
  granulomatous, 14
  lymphocytic, 14, 17
Hypopituitarism, 15, 16
  adrenal insufficiency with, 93
  from craniopharyngioma, 12
  from nontumorous lesions, 14
  selective and partial, 17
  severe, 18
  in Sheehan syndrome, 19
Hypotension
  in adrenal crisis, 90
  in adrenal insufficiency, 91
Hypothalamic artery, 9
Hypothalamic inhibitory regulatory factors, 9
Hypothalamic-pituitary-adrenal (HPA) axis, 72
Hypothalamic-releasing hormones, 9
Hypothalamic sulcus, 6
Hypothalamo-hypophysial tract, 4
Hypothalamus
  craniopharyngioma compressing, 12
  lesions of
    diabetes insipidus from, 29
    hypopituitarism from, 15, 16
    manifestations of, 11
  relationship of, to pituitary gland, 4, 6

Hypothyroidism
  in adults, 49–51
  in anorexia nervosa, 208
  central (hypothalamic or pituitary), 11, 51, 52
  congenital, 52
  etiology of, 50–51
  primary, 50–51
  in pseudohypoparathyroidism type 1, 166
  signs and symptoms of, 49–50
  treatment of, 51
Hypoxia-inducible factor (HIF), regulation of, 135

I
Iliac vein, 88
Immobilization, hypercalcemia from, 159
Immunoglobulin A deficiency, 205
Incretin effect, 132
Incretin-related agents, for diabetes mellitus, 148
Infarction
  myocardial, in diabetes mellitus, 145
  of pituitary gland, postpartum, 19
Inflammation, glucocorticoid effects on, 75
Infradian rhythms, 9
Infundibular artery, 5
  spasm of, postpartum, 19
Infundibular process, 3, 4, 5
Infundibular stem, 4
Insulin
  actions of, 133
  administration of
    for diabetes mellitus, 148, 149
    for diabetic ketoacidosis, 138
    for gestational diabetes, 147
  deficiency of, consequences of, 137
  in glycogenolysis, 136
  regulation of, 131
  secretion of, 132
  synthesis of, 131
Insulin-like growth factor-1, 9
  during puberty, 104
  secretion of, 9
Insulin receptor, 133
Insulin resistance (hyperinsulinemia)
  atherosclerosis and, 145
  congenital, islet-cell hyperplasia from, 151
  in diabetes mellitus, 140
  fetal, 147
  hyperthecosis and, 121
  in insulinoma, 150
  in metabolic syndrome, 197
  type B, 218
Insulin secretagogues, for diabetes mellitus, 148
Insulin sensitizers, for diabetes mellitus, 148
Insulinoma, 150
  in multiple endocrine neoplasia type 1, 213
Interpeduncular cistern, 6
Interventricular foramen, 6
Intralingual thyroid tissue, 40
Intratracheal thyroid tissue, 40
Iodine
  deficiency of, goiter from, 54, 55
  metabolism of, 42
  radioactive
    for follicular thyroid carcinoma, 59
    for papillary thyroid carcinoma, 58
    for toxic adenoma and toxic multinodular goiter, 47
  uptake of
    in Graves disease, 46
    in subacute thyroiditis, 57
    in toxic adenoma and toxic multinodular goiter, 47
IPEX syndrome, 218
Iris, Lisch nodules on, in neurofibromatosis type 1, 217
Iron overload, 14
Islets of Langerhans. See Pancreatic islets.

J
Jejunum, 129
Jugular vein
  anterior, 36
  external, 36
  internal, 36, 37

K
Kearns-Sayre syndrome, 218
Keratinization, in vitamin A deficiency, 204
Ketoacidosis, diabetic, 138
Ketoaciduria, from insulin deprivation, 137
α-Ketoglutarate, 135
17-Ketosteroid deficiency, in adrenal insufficiency, 92, 93
17ß-Ketosteroid reductase, 74
Kimmelstiel-Wilson nodules, in diabetic nephropathy, 143
Klinefelter syndrome, 115, 116
Knee, xanthoma of, 188
Krebs cycle, 135
Kyphosis
  in Paget disease of bone, 176
  thoracic, in osteoporosis, 168, 169, 170

L
Labia majora and minora, development of, 102
Labioscrotal swellings, 102
Labor induction, oxytocin in, 27
Lactation
  abnormal. See Galactorrhea.
  oxytocin in, 27
Lactic acid, 134
Lamina terminalis, 6
Langerhans, islets of. See Pancreatic islets.
Langerhans cell histiocytosis, 29, 30, 31
Laparoscopic adjustable gastric banding, 210
Laryngeal nerve
  recurrent, 36, 37
  superior, external branch of, 37
Laryngeal spasm, in hypocalcemia, 164
Larynx, 38
Laser photocoagulation, for diabetic retinopathy, 142
Lens opacities, in autoimmune polyglandular syndrome type I, 218
Leptin
  in anorexia nervosa, 208
  puberty and, 104
Lethargy, in hypothyroidism, 49
Leukodystrophy, metachromatic, 207
Levothyroxine
  for follicular thyroid carcinoma, 59
  for hypothyroidism, 51
  for papillary thyroid carcinoma, 58
  for thyroiditis, 56, 57
Leydig cells, 100, 107
  fetal, 112
  in Klinefelter syndrome, 116
  tumor of, 109
Ligament
  cricothyroid, 37
  round, 101
Limbs
  bowing of, in Paget disease of bone, 176
  deformities of, in osteogenesis imperfecta, 178, 179
Lingual thyroid, 40
Lipase, 130, 184, 192
Lipid(s). See also Dyslipidemia; Hyperlipidemia.
  dietary, 184
  fasting, monitoring of, 199
  metabolism of, 130, 134, 183, 184
    glucocorticoids in, 75
  transport of, 183, 184. See also Lipoprotein(s).
Lipid-lowering therapy
  coronary heart disease risk and, 196
  for familial hypercholesterolemia, 189
  mechanisms of action of, 198
Lipid screening tests, recommendations for, 196
Lipidosis, sphingomyelin-cholesterol, 206

Lipogenesis, insulin stimulation of, 133
Lipoid hyperplasia, congenital, 81, 82
Lipolysis, from insulin deprivation, 137
Lipoma, in multiple endocrine neoplasia type 1, 213
Lipoprotein(a), plasma, elevated, 185
Lipoprotein(s). See also Apolipoprotein.
  classification of, 183
  excess of. See Hyperlipoproteinemia.
  high-density, 183
    antiatherogenic properties of, 186
    deficiency of, in Tangier disease, 190
    metabolism of, 186
    raising, 199
    synthesis of, 186
  low-density, 183
    excess of. See Hypercholesterolemia.
    extracorporeal removal of, for familial hypercholesterolemia, 189
  structure of, 183
  very-low-density, 183
    overproduction of, in familial hypertriglyceridemia, 193
Lipoprotein lipase
  actions of, 191
  deficiency of, 192–193
  synthesis of, 192
Lipoprotein receptor, low-density, 183
  mutations of, hypercholesterolemia from, 187, 188–189
  regulation of, 185
Lisch nodules, in neurofibromatosis type 1, 217
Longus colli muscle, 36
Looser zones (pseudofractures)
  in osteomalacia, 175
  in renal osteodystrophy, 161
  in rickets, 174
Lordosis, in abetalipoproteinemia, 190
Lumbar splanchnic nerve, 70
Lung
  carcinoids of, 219
  Langerhans cell histiocytosis in, 30, 31
Lung bud, 38
Luteinizing hormone (LH), 9
  deficiency of, 18
    in boys, 15
  at puberty, 104, 107
  reproductive cycle influence of, 122, 123
Lymph node
  pretracheal, 37
  thyroid, 36, 37
Lymph vessels, thyroid, 37
Lymphatic drainage, of thyroid and parathyroid glands, 36, 37
Lymphocytic hypophysitis, 14, 17
Lymphocytic infiltration, in Graves disease, 46
Lymphocytic (Hashimoto) thyroiditis, 51, 56
Lymphoma, hypercalcemia in, 159
Lysosomal storage disorders, 206–207

M
Macroadenoma, pituitary, 13
Macroglossia, in hypothyroidism, 49, 50
Macrosomia, fetal, in gestational diabetes, 147
Macular edema, in diabetic retinopathy, 141, 142
Magnetic resonance imaging
  of clinically nonfunctioning pituitary tumor, 26
  of corticotropin-secreting pituitary tumor, 24
  of craniopharyngioma, 12
  in Cushing syndrome, 77
  of growth hormone–secreting pituitary tumor, 21, 22
  in Langerhans cell histiocytosis, 31
  in neurofibromatosis type 1, 217
  in pituitary apoplexy, 20
  of pituitary macroadenoma, 13
  posterior pituitary bright spot on, 10
  of prolactinoma, 23
Malabsorption
  in autoimmune polyglandular syndrome type I, 218
  in celiac disease, 205
Malnutrition, in abetalipoproteinemia, 190

Mammillary bodies, 6
Masculinization
    of external genitalia, 102, 111
    genital, 112, 113–114
    signs and symptoms of, 85
Maturity-onset diabetes of the young (MODY), 140
Maxillary nerve, 7
Maxillary process, 38
McCune-Albright syndrome, precocious puberty in, 109, 110
Median eminence, 3, 4
Medullary thyroid carcinoma, 60
    in multiple endocrine neoplasia type 2, 60, 214, 215
MEN1 mutations, 213
Menopause
    hormonal influences in, 123
    osteoporosis after, 168
Menorrhagia, in hypothyroidism, 49
Menstruation
    normal, 124
    onset of, 106
Mental retardation, in congenital hypothyroidism, 52
Mesenteric artery, superior, 69
Mesenteric ganglion, superior, 70
Mesenteric vessels, superior, 129
Mesentery, 129
Mesonephric body, 101
Mesonephric duct, 100, 101
Mesonephric remnants, 100
Mesonephric tubules, 100
Metabolic syndrome, 140, 197
Metacarpals, short, in pseudohypoparathyroidism type 1, 166
Metachromatic leukodystrophy, 207
Metanephrine, 94, 95
Metastatic disease
    to adrenal glands, 98
    to bone, hypercalcemia in, 159
    to pituitary gland, 32
    to thyroid gland, 63
Metformin, for diabetes mellitus, 148
Methimazole, for toxic adenoma and toxic multinodular goiter, 47
Miglitol, for diabetes mellitus, 148
Milk-alkali syndrome, hypercalcemia in, 159
Milk letdown, oxytocin in, 27
Milkman syndrome
    in osteomalacia, 175
    in renal osteodystrophy, 161
    in rickets, 174
Mineral loss, from insulin deprivation, 137
Mineralocorticoid receptors, 86
Mineralocorticoids. See also Aldosterone.
    for adrenal insufficiency, 92
    apparent excess of, 83
    for congenital adrenal hyperplasia, 82
Mitogen-activating protein kinase signaling pathway, 133
Mönckeberg arteriosclerosis, 145
Mononeuropathy, in diabetes mellitus, 144
Moon face, in Cushing syndrome, 76
Mosaicism
    45,X,/46,XX, 117, 118
    chromosomal, 100
Mucocutaneous neuroma, in multiple endocrine neoplasia type 2, 215
Müllerian duct, 100, 101
    persistent, 113
Multiple endocrine neoplasia type 1, 214
    carcinoid tumors in, 219
Multiple endocrine neoplasia type 2
    cutaneous lichen amyloidosis in, 214
    genetics of, 215
    Hirschsprung disease in, 214
    hyperparathyroidism in, 214
    medullary thyroid carcinoma in, 60, 214, 215
    pheochromocytoma in, 214

Muscles. See also named muscles.
    adrenal androgen effects on, 84
    androgenic (anabolic) steroid effects on, 84
    glucocorticoid effects on, 75
    wasting of, in Graves disease, 44
    weakness of
        in Cushing syndrome, 76
        in Graves disease, 44
Myeloma, multiple, hypercalcemia in, 159
Mylohyoid muscle, 36
Myocardial infarction, in diabetes mellitus, 145
Myocarditis, in pheochromocytoma, 97
Myopathy
    cardiac, in pheochromocytoma, 97
    thyroid, 44
Myxedema, in Graves disease, 43, 44
Myxedema madness, 49

N
Nasal septum, 6, 8
Nasopharynx, 6, 7
Neck surgery, hypoparathyroidism after, 163
Nelson syndrome, 25
Neonate, hormonal influences in, 123, 125
Nephrocalcinosis, in hyperparathyroidism, 157, 158
Nephrogenic cord, 100
Nephrolithiasis, in hyperparathyroidism, 158
Nephropathy, diabetic, 143
Nephrotic syndrome, in diabetic nephropathy, 143
Nerve supply. See also named nerves.
    of adrenal glands, 70
    of pancreas, 129
    of pituitary gland, 4, 7
    of thyroid and parathyroid glands, 36, 37
Nesidioblastosis, in islet-cell hyperplasia, 151
Neurocognitive dysfunction, in Turner syndrome, 118
Neurofibromatosis type 1, 217
Neuroglycopenia, in insulinoma, 150
Neurohypophysis. See Pituitary gland, posterior.
Neuroma, mucocutaneous, in multiple endocrine neoplasia type 2, 215
Neuropathy
    in abetalipoproteinemia, 190
    diabetic, 144, 146
    in pellagra, 202
Nevi, in Carney complex, 80
NF1 mutations, in neurofibromatosis type 1, 217
Niacin
    absorption of, 200
    deficiency of, 202
    recommended dietary allowance for, 202
Nicotinic acid
    for hypertriglyceridemia, 193
    mechanisms of action of, 198
Niemann-Pick disease, 206
Night blindness, in vitamin A deficiency, 204
Nitrogen loss, from insulin deprivation, 137
Nodules
    in goiter, 47, 53, 54
    Kimmelstiel-Wilson, in diabetic nephropathy, 143
    Lisch, in neurofibromatosis type 1, 217
    in papillary thyroid carcinoma, 58
    in primary pigmented nodular adrenocortical disease, 79, 80
    in pseudohypoparathyroidism type 1, 166
    in toxic multinodular goiter, 48
Nondisjunction, sex chromosome, 115
Noninsulinoma pancreatogenous hypoglycemia syndrome, 151
Nonsteroidal antiinflammatory drugs (NSAIDs), for subacute thyroiditis, 57
Norepinephrine
    biologic actions of, 94
    metabolism of, 95
    secretion of, 95, 97
    synthesis of, 95
    tumors secreting, 97
Normetanephrine, 94, 95
Nutritional-deficiency rickets, 171

O
Obesity, 209–210
    central (abdominal)
        in Cushing syndrome, 76
        in diabetes mellitus, 140
        measurement of, 209
        in metabolic syndrome, 197
    evaluation of, 209
    from hypothalamic lesions, 11
    surgical treatment options for, 210
    treatment of, 209
Occipital bone, 8
Oculomotor nerve, 6, 7
    compressed, in pituitary apoplexy, 20
    palsy of, in diabetes mellitus, 144
Omentum, lesser, 129
Omohyoid muscle, 36
Onycholysis, in Graves disease, 43
Oogonia, 100
Ophthalmic nerve, 7
Ophthalmopathy, in Graves disease, 45
Optic chiasm
    compressed
        in clinically nonfunctioning pituitary tumor, 26
        in pituitary apoplexy, 20
    pituitary gland and, 6, 7
    pituitary tumor compressing or invading, 13
Optic disk
    in hypocalcemia, 164
    neovascularization at, in diabetic retinopathy, 141
Optic foramen, 8
Optic glioma, in neurofibromatosis type 1, 217
Optic nerve, 6
Optic tract, right, 6
Orlistat, for hypertriglyceridemia, 193
Osmolality of body fluids, vasopressin and, 28
Osmoreceptors, 28
Osteitis deformans, 176–177
Osteitis fibrosa cystica, 161
Osteoblasts, 156
Osteoclasts, 156
Osteodystrophy
    Albright hereditary, 165, 166
    renal, 160–161
Osteogenesis imperfecta, 178–179
Osteomalacia
    calcipenic, 171
    clinical manifestations of, 175
    pseudovitamin D–deficiency, 172
    in renal osteodystrophy, 161
    tumor-induced, 173
    vitamin D–deficiency, 171
Osteon, 156
Osteoporosis
    clinical manifestations of, 168
    in men, 169
    pathogenesis of, 167
    in postmenopausal women, 168
    spinal deformity in, 169
Ovarian hormones. See also Estrogen; Progesterone.
    reproductive cycle influence of, 122, 123
Ovary, 101
    differentiation of, 100, 101
    follicular cyst of, precocious puberty from, 110
    granulosa cell tumor of, 110
Ovotestis, 113, 114
Ovulation
    failure of, causes of, 124
    onset of, 106
Ovum, 100
Oxytocin, 10, 27

P
Paget disease of bone, 176–177
Pain
    bone, in Paget disease of bone, 176
    in thyroiditis, 57
Palatine bone, 8
Palatine plate, 8

Pancreas
  abnormalities of, in von Hippel-Lindau syndrome, 216
  anatomy and physiology of, 129
  damage to, diabetes mellitus after, 140
  development of, 129
  exocrine functions of, 130
Pancreatic artery, 129
Pancreatic ducts, 129
Pancreatic islets
  histology of, 129, 131
  hyperplasia of, 151
  insulin production in, 132
  pathology of, in diabetes mellitus, 139
  tumors of, in multiple endocrine neoplasia type 1, 213
Pancreatic juice, 130
Pancreatic polypeptide, 131
Panhypopituitarism, 15, 16, 18, 93
Pantothenic acid, 200
Papillary cystadenoma, in von Hippel-Lindau syndrome, 216
Papillary thyroid carcinoma, 58
Papilledema, from pituitary tumors, 13
Paraganglioma
  catecholamine-secreting, 96–97
  in von Hippel-Lindau syndrome, 216
Parathyroid gland
  adenoma of, 157, 162
  anatomy of, 36–37
  in bone remodeling, 156
  carcinoma of, 157, 162
  development of, 39
  hyperplasia of, primary, 157, 162
  physiology of, 155
Parathyroid hormone
  abnormalities of. See Hyperparathyroidism; Hypoparathyroidism.
  end-organ resistance to, 163, 165, 166
  hypercalcemia mediated by, 159
  secretion of, 155
  serum, in rickets, 174
  supplementation of, for osteoporosis, 168, 169
Parathyroid hormone–related peptide, in hypercalcemia, 159
Paraurethral glands, 102
Paraventricular nucleus, 9, 27
Paresthesia, in diabetes mellitus, 144
Paroöphoron, 101
Parotid gland, 36
Pars distalis (pars glandularis), 3, 4
Pars intermedia, 3, 4
Pars nervosa, 3
Pars tuberalis, 3, 4
Pellagra, 202
Pendred syndrome, 55
Pendrin, 42
Penis, development of, 102, 106, 107
Pentose shunt, 134, 135, 136
Peptic ulcer disease, in multiple endocrine neoplasia type 1, 213
Periorbital edema
  in Graves disease, 45
  in hypothyroidism, 49
Peritoneum, 68
Petechial hemorrhage, in scurvy, 203
Petrosal sinus, superior, 7
Phalanges, resorption of, in renal osteodystrophy, 161
Pharyngeal cavity, 38
Pharyngeal constrictor muscle, 37
Pharyngeal pituitary, 3
Pharyngeal pouches, 38, 39
Pharynx, development of, 38, 39
Phenotypic sex, 111–112
Pheochromocytoma, 96–97
  in multiple endocrine neoplasia type 2, 214
  in neurofibromatosis type 1, 217
  in von Hippel-Lindau syndrome, 216
PHEX gene, in X-linked hypophosphatemic rickets, 173
Phophatidylinositol-3-kinase pathway, 133

Phosphate
  absorption and excretion of, 155
  disturbances of. See Hyperphosphatemia; Hypophosphatemia.
  glomerular filtration of, in renal osteodystrophy, 160
  serum, in hypercalcemia, 159
  supplementation of, for X-linked hypophosphatemic rickets, 173
Phospholipase A, 130
Phospholipids, dietary, 184
Photocoagulation, laser, for diabetic retinopathy, 142
Phrenic artery, 68, 69, 70
Phrenic nerve, 36, 70
Phrenic plexus, 70
Phrenic vein, 69, 88
Pigmentation disorders
  in adrenal insufficiency, 91
  in carcinoid tumors, 219
  in Nelson syndrome, 25
Pineal gland, 6
Pioglitazone, for diabetes mellitus, 148
Pituitary apoplexy, 20
Pituitary gland, 3–33. See also Hypopituitarism.
  acute hemorrhage of, 20
  adenoma of, 13, 24, 25, 26, 213
  anatomy of, 6
  anomalies of, 14
  anterior, 4
    deficiency of
      in adults, 16
      in boys, 15
    development of, 3
    divisions of, 4
    hormones and feedback control of, 9
  blood supply of, 5
  craniopharyngioma compressing, 12
  development of, 3
  divisions of, 4
  hormones of
    anterior, 9
    posterior, 10
    reproductive cycle influence of, 122, 123
  in hypothalamic-pituitary-adrenal (HPA) axis, 72
  infarction of, postpartum, 19
  nerve supply of, 4, 7
  nontumorous lesions of, 14
  posterior, 4, 10
    development of, 3
    divisions of, 4
    hormones of, 10
  relationship of
    to cavernous sinus, 7
    to hypothalamus, 4, 6
    to optic chiasm, 6
    to pineal gland, 6
  surgical approaches to, 33
  tumors of
    clinically nonfunctioning, 26
    corticotropin-secreting, 24, 25, 78
    growth hormone–secreting
      acromegaly from, 22
      gigantism from, 21
    metastatic, 32
    prolactin-secreting (prolactinoma), 23
    TSH-secreting, 41
    visual effects of, 13
Pituitary stalk, 4
  nontumorous lesions of, 14
Plaques
  fibrous, in atherosclerosis, 195
  subcutaneous osseous, in pseudohypoparathyroidism type 1, 166
Platysma, 36
Plexus
  basilar, 7
  celiac, 70
  of hypophyseal portal system, 5
  phrenic, 70
  renal, 70
Plummer's nails, in Graves disease, 43

POEMS syndrome, 218
Polycystic ovarian syndrome, androgen excess in, 120–121
Polyendocrine disorders, autoimmune, 91, 218
Polyglandular autoimmune syndrome, hypoparathyroidism after, 163
Polyneuropathy, distal symmetric, in diabetes mellitus, 144
Polypeptide-producing cells, 131
Polyradiculopathy, in diabetes mellitus, 144
Polyuria
  in diabetes insipidus, 29
  from insulin deprivation, 137
Pons, 6
Pontine cistern, 6
Portal vein, 129
Potassium
  deficiency of, in aldosteronism, 87
  excess of, in adrenal insufficiency, 92
  insulin secretion and, 132
  supplementation of, for diabetic ketoacidosis, 138
Pregnenolone, 73, 103
Pregnancy
  diabetes mellitus in, 147
  hyperandrogenism in, virilization in, 111, 113
  uterine bleeding abnormalities in, 124
Prelaryngeal thyroid tissue, 40
PRKAR1A gene mutations, in primary pigmented nodular adrenocortical disease, 80
Progesterone
  adrenal, 73
  at puberty, 107
  reproductive cycle influence of, 122, 123
  synthesis of, 103
Progestogens, 72
Prognathism, in acromegaly, 22
Proinsulin, 132
Prolactin, 9
  deficiency of, 16, 17, 18
  excess of, 23
    from clinically nonfunctioning pituitary tumor, 26
    galactorrhea in, 126
    hypogonadotropic hypogonadism associated with, 23
    reproductive cycle influence of, 122, 123
Prolactinoma, 23
PROP1 mutations, hypopituitarism from, 14
Proptosis, in Graves disease, 45, 46
Propylthiouracil, for toxic adenoma and toxic multinodular goiter, 47
Prostate gland, 101, 102
Prostatic utricle, 101, 102
Protein, metabolism of, 75, 130
Proteinuria, in diabetic nephropathy, 143
Proteolytic enzymes, 130
Proximal motor neuropathy, in diabetes mellitus, 144
Pseudofractures (Looser zones)
  in osteomalacia, 175
  in renal osteodystrophy, 161
  in rickets, 174
Pseudogynecomastia, 125
Pseudohermaphroditism, 111–113
Pseudohypercalcemia, 159
Pseudohypoparathyroidism, 163
  pathophysiology of, 165
  type 1, 165, 166
  type 2, 165
Pseudovitamin D–deficiency rickets and osteomalacia, 172
Psychosis, in hypothyroidism, 49
Psychosocial development, in disorders of sex development, 112
Pubarche, 84
Puberty
  delayed, 17, 18
  female, 104, 105–106, 107
  gynecomastia in, 125
  hormonal events in, 107, 123
  male, 104, 106–107
  normal, 104–107
  precocious, 108–110

Puberty (Continued)
    diagnosis and treatment of, 110
    gonadotropin-dependent, 108
    gonadotropin-independent, 108–109
    from hypothalamic lesions, 11
    incomplete, 109
    timing of, 104–105
Pubic hair, development of, 84, 105, 106, 107
Pulse, in hypothyroidism, 49
Purging, in anorexia nervosa, 208
Pyridoxine, 200
Pyruvate, 134

Q
QT interval, prolonged, in hypocalcemia, 164

R
Rachitic bone, in rickets, 174
Radiography
    in osteogenesis imperfecta, 178, 179
    in osteoporosis, 170
    in Paget disease of bone, 176
    in renal osteodystrophy, 161
    in rickets, 174
    in vertebral compression fracture, 170
Radioiodine
    for follicular thyroid carcinoma, 59
    for papillary thyroid carcinoma, 58
    for toxic adenoma and toxic multinodular goiter, 47
Radiotherapy
    for follicular thyroid carcinoma, 59
    for Hürthle cell thyroid carcinoma, 61
    for papillary thyroid carcinoma, 58
RANK ligand, 156
Rash, in Langerhans cell histiocytosis, 31
Rathke pouch, 3
Red striae, in Cushing syndrome, 76
Renal artery, 68, 69
    stenosis of, renovascular hypertension in, 89
Renal cell carcinoma, in von Hippel-Lindau syndrome, 216
Renal (Gerota) fascia, 68
Renal ganglion and plexus, 70
Renal osteodystrophy, 160–161
Renal stones, in hyperparathyroidism, 157
Renal vein, 68, 69
Renin-angiotensin-aldosterone system, 86, 89
Renovascular hypertension, in renal artery stenosis, 89
Reproductive cycle, gonadal hormonal influences on, 122, 123
Resiliency testing, in Graves disease, 45
RET mutations, 60, 213, 215
Rete ovarii, 100
Rete testis, 100
Retina
    angioma of, in von Hippel-Lindau syndrome, 216
    detachment of, in diabetic retinopathy, 142
    lesions of, in abetalipoproteinemia, 190
Retinohypothalamic tract, 9
Retinopathy, diabetic, 141
    macular edema in, 141
    nonproliferative, 141
    proliferative, 141, 142
Retroperitoneoscopic adrenalectomy, 69
Rhinorrhea, cerebrospinal fluid, in prolactinoma, 23
Rib
    first, 37
    fracture of, in osteoporosis, 168
Rickets
    calcipenic, 171
    clinical manifestations of, 174
    hereditary vitamin D–resistant, 172
    hypophosphatemic, 173
    nutritional-deficiency, 171
    pseudovitamin D–deficiency, 172
    from renal α1-hydroxylase deficiency, 172
    vitamin D–deficiency, 171

Riedel thyroiditis, 56
Rosiglitazone, for diabetes mellitus, 148
Round ligament, 101
Roux-en-Y gastric bypass surgery, 151, 210
Rubor, dependent, in diabetic foot ulcers, 146
Rumpel-Leede test, in scurvy, 203

S
Sagittal sinus, superior, 7
Saline, for diabetic ketoacidosis, 138
Salt wasting, 81, 83
Santorini, duct of, 129
Sarcoidosis, hypercalcemia in, 159
Satiety center, 11
Scalene muscle, 36
Scintigraphy, bone, in Paget disease of bone, 176
Sclerae, blue, in osteogenesis imperfecta, 178, 179
Sclerosis, in renal osteodystrophy, 161
Scorbutic rosary, 203
Scotoma, from pituitary tumors, 13
Scrotum, development of, 102, 106, 107
Scurvy, 203
Secretin, 130
Sella, empty, 14
Sella turcica, 8, 14
Seminal vesicle, 101
Seminiferous tubules, 100
Sertoli cell, 107
Sertoli-Leydig cell tumors, virilization in, 121
Sex
    chromosomal, 100, 111
        analysis of, 115
        errors in. See Sex chromosome disorder of sex development.
    gonadal, 111
    phenotypic, 111–112
Sex characteristics
    male, adrenal androgen effects on, 84
    secondary
        absence of, in Turner syndrome, 117
        development of, 104, 105, 106
Sex chromosome disorder of sex development, 112–113, 115
    45,X, 117
    45,X/46,XX, 118
    45,X/46,XY (mixed gonadal dysgenesis), 113, 118, 119
    46,XX/46,XY (chimerism), 113
    47,XXX (triple X syndrome), 115
    47,XXY, 116
    Klinefelter syndrome as, 115, 116
    Turner syndrome as, 115, 117–119
Sex cords
    primary, 100
    secondary, 100
Sex hormone–binding globulin, in Graves disease, 44
Sexual differentiation
    female, 112
    male, 111–112
        variations in, 113, 114
Sexual orientation, 112
Sheehan syndrome, 19
Shock, in adrenal crisis, 90
Short stature, 15
    in pseudohypoparathyroidism type 1, 166
    in Turner syndrome, 117
Sitosterolemia, 189
Skeleton deformities, in rickets, 174
Skene's duct, 101
Skin
    in adrenal crisis, 90
    in Carney complex, 80
    in Cushing syndrome, 76
    glucocorticoid effects on, 75
    in Graves disease, 43
    hyperkeratinization of, in vitamin A deficiency, 204
    hyperpigmentation of
        in adrenal insufficiency, 91
        in carcinoid tumors, 219
        in Nelson syndrome, 25

Skin (Continued)
    in hypothyroidism, 49, 50
    in Langerhans cell histiocytosis, 31
    in multiple endocrine neoplasia type 1, 213
    in neurofibromatosis type 1, 217
Skull lesions, in Langerhans cell histiocytosis, 30
Small intestine, carcinoids of, 219
Smoking, coronary heart disease risk and, 196
Sodium
    abnormalities of, in adrenal insufficiency, 92, 93
    aldosterone effects on, 86
Sodium-iodide symporter (NIS), block of, 55
Soft tissue overgrowth, in acromegaly, 22
Somatostatin, 131, 132
Somnolence, from hypothalamic lesions, 11
SOX9 gene, in gonadal differentiation, 100
Spermatogenesis, 107
Spermatogonia, 100
Sphenoid bone, 8
Sphenoid sinus, 3, 6, 7, 8
Sphenoparietal sinus, 7
Sphincter of Oddi, 129
Sphingolipidoses, 206–207
Sphingomyelin-cholesterol lipidosis, 206
Spinal deformity, in osteoporosis, 169
Splanchnic nerve, 70
Spleen
    enlargement of, in hypertriglyceridemia, 192
    topographic relationships of, 68, 129
Splenic artery, 129
Splenic vein, 129
Sprue
    celiac, 205
    nontropical, 205
SRY gene, in gonadal differentiation, 100, 101
Stare, in Graves disease, 44, 45
Statins
    coronary heart disease risk and, 196
    in diabetes mellitus, 145
    for familial hypercholesterolemia, 189
    for hyperlipidemia, 199
    for hypertriglyceridemia, 193
    mechanisms of action of, 198
Stature
    short, 15
        in pseudohypoparathyroidism type 1, 166
        in Turner syndrome, 117
    tall, 21
Steatorrhea, in celiac disease, 205
Sternocleidomastoid muscle, 36
Sternohyoid muscle, 36
Sternothyroid muscle, 36
Steroid withdrawal bleeding, 124
Steroidogenesis
    adrenal, major blocks in, 81
    regulation of, 103
Steroidogenic acute regulatory protein (StART), 73
    deficiency of, 81, 82
Steroidogenic enzymes, adrenal, 74
Steroids. See also Glucocorticoids.
    adrenal, biosynthesis and metabolism of, 72–74
    androgenic (anabolic), 84
Sterol regulatory element–binding protein (SREBP), 185
Stomach, 129
Stress, corticotropin secretion and, 72
Stridor, in hypocalcemia, 164
Subarachnoid cistern, 6
Subclavian artery, 37
Subclavian vein, 37
Sublingual thyroid tissue, 40
Submandibular gland, 36
Substernal thyroid tissue, 40
Sulfatidosis, 207
Sulfonylurea receptor agonists, for diabetes mellitus, 148
Supraclavicular nerve, 36
Supraoptic nucleus, 9
Supraopticohypophysial tract, 4
Suprarenal glands. See Adrenal glands.
Suprasellar disease, 11

Swyer syndrome, 114
Sympathetic trunk, 36, 70

T

Tall stature, 21
Tamoxifen, for Riedel thyroiditis, 56
Tangier disease, 190
Tanner stages
   of breast development, 104
   of female pubic hair development, 105
   of male pubic hair and genital development, 106
Tay-Sachs disease, 206
Temporal pole of brain, 6
Tendons, xanthoma of, 188, 189
Testis, 101
   adrenal rest tumor of, precocious puberty from, 109
   appendix, 101
   descent of, 112
   development of
      disorders of, 113
      during puberty, 106–107
   differentiation of, 100, 101
   dysgenesis of, 112, 114
Testosterone
   adrenal, 72, 73, 103, 104
      biologic actions of, 84
      excess of, 85
      neoplasms secreting, 85, 121
      in secondary adrenal insufficiency, 93
   deficiency of, 15, 114
   excess of
      in 46,XX disorders of sex development, 112, 113–114
      adult adrenogenital syndromes associated with, 85
      in hirsutism and virilization, 120–121
      in masculinization of external genitalia, 102, 111
      in precocious puberty, 109, 110
      virilization in, 111, 113
      in women, 120, 121
   gonadal, 104
   for Klinefelter syndrome, 116
   potency of, 73
   at puberty, 107
   synthesis of, 103
Tetany, 164
Tetracycline, bone biopsy with, in osteomalacia, 175
Thalamus, 6
Theca cells, 100
Thelarche, 104, 105
   premature, 109
   pubertal, 104, 105
Thiamine
   absorption of, 200
   deficiency of, 201
   recommended dietary allowance for, 201
Thiazolidinediones, for diabetes mellitus, 148
Thionamides, for toxic adenoma and toxic multinodular goiter, 47
Thirst, 28
   for cold liquids, in diabetes insipidus, 29
Thoracic kyphosis, in osteoporosis, 168, 169, 170
Thoracic splanchnic nerve, 70
Thrombosis, in atherosclerosis, 195
Thymus gland, 38
   development of, 39
   tumors of, 218
Thyrocervical trunk, 37
Thyroglobulin
   antibodies to, in Hashimoto thyroiditis, 56
   inhibition of, 55
   in subacute thyroiditis, 57
Thyroglossal cyst, 40
Thyroglossal duct, 38, 40
Thyrohyoid membrane, 37
Thyrohyoid muscle, 36
Thyroid artery, 36, 37
Thyroid-binding globulin (TBG), 42
Thyroid cartilage, 36, 37

Thyroid follicles, 38
Thyroid gland, 35–63
   anatomy of, 36–37
   anomalies of, 37, 40
   carcinoma of
      anaplastic, 62
      follicular, 59
      Hürthle cell, 61
      medullary, 60, 214, 215
      in multiple endocrine neoplasia type 2, 60, 214, 215
      papillary, 58
   development of, 38–39
   dysgenesis of, 52
   enlargement of. See Goiter.
   hyperplasia of, goiter after, 55
   metastatic disease to, 63
   pathology of, in Graves disease, 46
   pyramidal lobe of, 39
   thyrotropin effects on, 41
Thyroid hormones
   in anorexia nervosa, 208
   deficiency of, 16, 55
   disturbances of. See Hyperthyroidism; Hypothyroidism.
   physiology of, 42
   reduced sensitivity to, 55
Thyroid isthmus, 38
Thyroid peroxidase
   antibodies to, in Hashimoto thyroiditis, 56
   inhibition of, 42, 55
Thyroid-stimulating hormone (TSH). See Thyrotropin.
Thyroid tissue, aberrant, 40
Thyroid vein, 37
Thyroidectomy
   for follicular thyroid carcinoma, 59
   for Hürthle cell thyroid carcinoma, 61
   hypoparathyroidism after, 163
   for medullary thyroid carcinoma, 60
   for papillary thyroid carcinoma, 58
Thyroiditis
   acute nonsuppurative, 57
   chronic lymphocytic (Hashimoto), 51, 56
   fibrous (Riedel), 56
   subacute (de Quervain), 57
Thyrotropin, 9
   deficiency of, 15, 17, 18, 51
   effects of, on thyroid gland, 41
   in hypothyroidism, 50
   pituitary tumor secreting, 41
   in subacute thyroiditis, 57
Thyrotropin receptor, 41
   mutations of, goiter from, 47, 55
Thyrotropin-releasing hormone (TRH), 9, 41
Thyroxine, 41
   in hypothyroidism, 50
   physiology of, 42
   in subacute thyroiditis, 57
Tongue, 38
   in hypothyroidism, 49, 50
   in pellagra, 202
Tonsil
   in pellagra, 202
   in Tangier disease, 190
Tooth (teeth)
   in autoimmune polyglandular syndrome type I, 218
   loss of, in hypophosphatasia, 180
   malocclusion of, in acromegaly, 22
   opalescent, in osteogenesis imperfecta, 178, 179
Toxic adenoma, 47, 48
Toxic multinodular goiter, 47, 48
Trabecula, artery of, 5
Trachea, 36, 38
   compression of, by anaplastic thyroid carcinoma, 62
Transabdominal adrenalectomy, 69
Transnasal approach to pituitary, 33
Transseptal approach to pituitary, 33
Transsphenoidal approach to pituitary, 24, 33
Tremor, in Graves disease, 43

Tricarboxylic acid cycle, 135
Trigeminal nerve, 6, 7
Triglycerides. See also Hypertriglyceridemia.
   dietary, 184
   gastrointestinal absorption of, 184
   metabolism of, 191
   serum, 191
Triiodothyronine, 41
   in hypothyroidism, 50
   physiology of, 42
   in subacute thyroiditis, 57
Triple X syndrome, 115
Trochlear nerve, 6, 7
Trousseau sign, 164
TSH (thyroid-stimulating hormone). See Thyrotropin.
Tube, fallopian, 101
Tuber cinereum, 6
Tuberculosis, of adrenal glands, 91
Tuberculum sellae, 8
Tuberohypophysial tract, 4
Tuberous xanthoma, 188, 189
Tumors. See also Carcinoma.
   adrenal rest, testicular, 109
   adrenocortical, 85, 109, 121
   of brain
      diabetes insipidus and, 29
      in neurofibromatosis type 1, 217
      precocious puberty and, 108, 110
   carcinoid, 213, 219
   catecholamine-secreting, 96–97
   granulosa cell, of ovary, 110
   Leydig cell, 109
   metastatic. See Metastatic disease.
   osteomalacia associated with, 173
   pituitary. See Pituitary gland, tumors of.
   Sertoli-Leydig cell, virilization in, 121
   of thymus gland, 218
Tunica albuginea, 100
Tunica vaginalis, 100
Turner syndrome, 115, 117–119
   45,X, 117
   45,X,/46,XX mosaicism, 117, 118
Tyrosine, 95

U

Ulcer
   neuropathic, in diabetes mellitus, 144, 146
   peptic, in multiple endocrine neoplasia type 1, 213
Ultradian rhythms, 9
Uncinate process, 129
Upper body to lower body segment ratio (U:L ratio), 105
Urethra, 101
Urethral folds, 102
Urethral groove, 102
Urogenital sinus, 102
Urogenital slit, 102
Uterus
   bleeding from, causes of, 124
   contraction of, oxytocin in, 27
   development of, 101
Utricle, prostatic, 101, 102

V

Vagal trunk, 70
Vagina, 101
   development of, 102, 106
   remnant of, 102
Vagus nerve, 36, 37
Valvular heart disease, in carcinoid tumors, 219
Vanillylmandelic acid, 94, 95
Vas deferens, 100, 101
Vasa efferentia, 101
Vascular insufficiency, in diabetes mellitus, 146
Vasopressin
   deficiency of
      in diabetes insipidus, 29
      in Langerhans cell histiocytosis, 30

Vasopressin (*Continued*)
  overview of, 10
  secretion and action of, 28
Veins. *See* Blood supply; *named veins.*
Vena cava
  inferior, 68, 69, 88, 129
  superior, 37
Ventricle, third, 7
Vertebral body, 36
Vertebral compression fracture, in osteoporosis, 168, 169, 170
Vesiculosa, appendix, 101
VHL tumor suppressor gene, in von Hippel-Lindau syndrome, 216
Vibration sense, loss of, in diabetes mellitus, 144
Virchow nodes, 37
Virilization, 85, 120–121
  causes of, 112, 113–114, 120–121
  definition of, 85, 120
  simple, 83
  in Turner syndrome, 118
  under-, of male infants, 113, 114
Visual apparatus, pituitary tumor effects on, 13
Visual loss
  from craniopharyngioma, 12
  in diabetic retinopathy, 141
  from hypothalamic lesions, 11
  from pituitary tumors, 13
Vitamin(s)
  absorption of, 200
  fat-soluble, 200
  water-soluble, 200
Vitamin A
  absorption of, 200
  deficiency of, 204
  recommended dietary allowance for, 204
Vitamin B, in tricarboxylic acid cycle, 135

Vitamin B_1 (thiamine)
  absorption of, 200
  deficiency of, 201
  recommended dietary allowance for, 201
Vitamin B_2 (riboflavin), 200
Vitamin B_3 (niacin)
  absorption of, 200
  deficiency of, 202
  recommended dietary allowance for, 202
Vitamin B_5 (pantothenic acid), 200
Vitamin B_6 (pyridoxine), 200
Vitamin B_{12} (cobalamin), 200
Vitamin C (ascorbic acid)
  absorption of, 200
  deficiency of, 203
  recommended dietary allowance for, 203
Vitamin D
  absorption of, 200
  deficiency of, in hyperparathyroidism, 158
  intake of, in osteoporosis, 168
  intoxication with, hypercalcemia in, 159
  serum, in hypercalcemia, 159
Vitamin D receptor gene, mutations of, 172
Vitamin D–deficiency rickets and osteomalacia, 171
Vitamin E, 200
Vitamin K, 200
Vitiligo, in autoimmune polyglandular syndrome type I, 218
Vitreous hemorrhage, in diabetic retinopathy, 142
Voice changes
  adrenal androgens and, 84
  in hypothyroidism, 49
  during puberty, 107
Volume repletion
  for adrenal crisis, 90
  for diabetic ketoacidosis, 138
Von Hippel-Lindau syndrome, 216
Von Recklinghausen disease, 217

W
Waist circumference. *See* Abdominal obesity.
Water homeostasis, vasopressin and, 28
Waterhouse-Friderichsen syndrome, 90
Weight gain. *See* Obesity.
Weight loss
  in anorexia nervosa, 208
  in Graves disease, 44
  from insulin deprivation, 137
  for obesity, 209–210
Wernicke-Korsakoff syndrome, 201
Whipple procedure, for insulinoma, 150
Whipple triad, in insulinoma, 150
Wirsung, duct of, 129
Wolffian body, 101
Wolffian duct, 100, 101
Wolfram syndrome, 29, 218
Wound healing, in Cushing syndrome, 76
Wrist drop, in diabetes mellitus, 144

X
X-linked hypophosphatemic rickets, 173
Xanthoma
  hypercholesterolemic, 188–189
  in hypertriglyceridemia, 192, 193
Xanthomatosis, cerebrotendinous, 189

Z
Zollinger-Ellison syndrome, in multiple endocrine neoplasia type 1, 213
Zona fasciculata, 71
Zona glomerulosa, 71
Zona reticularis, 71
Zuckerkandl organ, 67